GODDESSES
NEVER AGE

ALSO BY CHRISTIANE NORTHRUP, M.D.

GODDESSES
NEVER AGE

The Secret Prescription for Radiance,
Vitality, and Well-Being

CHRISTIANE NORTHRUP, M.D.

HAY HOUSE, INC.
Carlsbad, California • New York City
London • Sydney • Johannesburg
Vancouver • New Delhi

Published and distributed in the United States by: Hay House, Inc.: www
.hayhouse.com® • *Published and distributed in Australia by:* Hay House Australia Pty. Ltd.: www.hayhouse.com.au • *Published and distributed in the
United Kingdom by:* Hay House UK, Ltd.: www.hayhouse.co.uk • *Published
and distributed in the Republic of South Africa by:* Hay House SA (Pty), Ltd.:
www.hayhouse.co.za • *Distributed in Canada by:* Raincoast Books: www
.raincoast.com • *Published in India by:* Hay House Publishers India: www
.hayhouse.co.in

Indexer: Jay Kreider
Cover design: Karla Baker • *Interior design:* Riann Bender
Interior illustrations: Scott Leighton, © Christiane Northrup Inc.

Lines from "We Have Not Come to Take Prisoners" from the Penguin
publication *The Gift: Poems by Hafiz,* by Daniel Ladinsky. Copyright © 1999
Daniel Ladinsky and used with his permission.

"The Kiss," from *Make Me Your Own: Poems to the Divine Beloved,*
copyright © 2013 by Tosha Silver. Reprinted by permission of Urban Kali
Productions.

Library of Congress Cataloging-in-Publication Data for the original edition

Tradepaper ISBN: 978-1-4019-4595-4

10 9 8 7 6 5 4 3 2 1
1st edition, February 2015
2nd edition, December 2016

Printed in the United States of America

SUSTAINABLE
FORESTRY
INITIATIVE
Certified Sourcing
www.sfiprogram.org
SFI-01268
SFI label applies to text stock only

To the ageless goddess that lives in every woman—
and to Gaia Sophia, the Earth herself

CONTENTS

INTRODUCTION

One of my 20-something pals told me, "Girl, you're a puzzle.
You're not young, you're not old. I don't know what the hell you
are. You're Somethin' Else. Just be somethin' else. That works!"

— TOSHA SILVER, AUTHOR OF *OUTRAGEOUS OPENNESS*

Recently, I went to a sporting goods store to get my ski boot
bindings adjusted, and the salesperson, who was clearly younger
than I am, asked me what age I was. Apparently, if you're over a
certain age, they assume you need your bindings to release quickly because your balance has deteriorated and you fall more easily.
I am physically active, more so than in my younger years, and
I regularly dance Argentine tango, so my balance is just fine. I
told the salesperson, who was looking at a formula to determine
my binding adjustment, "Just put in 40." I do that when I'm on
exercise equipment, too. I don't need the stair machine coddling
me as if I am a frail little old lady who might hurt herself if the
program pushes her a bit. If it doesn't feel right, I'll stop and adjust the machine. I don't let myself feel embarrassed or ashamed
about having to use a lower setting. And I don't let someone else's
idea about what "40," or "50," or "60," or any other number
means inform how I see myself.

When someone asks you what age you are, do you even remember? Or is it so unimportant to you that you forget unless a "milestone" birthday is coming up? Age is just a number, and agelessness means not buying into the idea that a number determines everything from your state of health to your attractiveness to your value. You can be younger at 60 than you were at 30 because you've changed your attitude and your lifestyle. To be ageless is to defy the rules of what it supposedly means to be this age or that age. It is, quite simply, to never grow "old"—to never feel as if the best days are behind you and it's all downhill from here.

Let me make one thing very clear: We begin to get *older* the moment we are born. But we don't use the term "aging" in this culture until we get to about 50, and what most of us associate with "aging" is "deterioration." The truth is that when it comes to aging, there are people in their 20s or even younger who already show signs of "aging": deteriorating muscle mass, unstable blood sugar, and loss of balance. Meanwhile, others who are in their 70s are the picture of health. According to Joan Vernikos, Ph.D., a research scientist and former director of NASA's Life Sciences Division, who prepared 77-year-old John Glenn to return to space, aging is nothing more than a slow form of weightlessness: it's what happens to your body when you don't get up off your chair, move around, live an active life, and experience the earth's gravitational pull. Getting older does *not* mean an inevitable decline in physical health or a slide into cultural irrelevance.

Goddesses Never Age is about agelessness, or ageless living, which is what you experience when you engage life without fear that you're going to fall—or fall apart. We are long overdue for a paradigm shift in what we believe about growing older. Centenarians are the fastest-growing segment of the U.S. population (increasing at the rate of 75,000 people per year).[1] There are currently about 53,000 centenarians in the U.S. and by 2050, there will be 600,000. You read that right: *ten times* as many Americans will be over 100 years old two generations from now. That's simply one piece of a global story about people living longer. If you want longevity, I'm sure you don't also want to spend the last years of your life in poor health, thinking about how "old" you are. You can change your future starting today by adopting a new, ageless attitude that will help you flourish physically, emotionally, mentally, and spiritually.

Growing older is an opportunity for you to increase your value and competence as the neural connections in your hippocampus and throughout your brain increase, weaving into your brain and body the wisdom of a life well lived, which allows you to stop living out of fear of disappointing others and being imperfect. Ageless living is courageous living. It means being undistracted by the petty dramas of life because you have enough experience to know what's not worth worrying about and what ought to be your priorities. It means establishing a new relationship to time, where you stop fearing it or trying to outrun it. When people over 100 were asked in a recent survey how they felt about reaching the triple digits, the top three answers were "blessed," "happy," and "surprised"—surprised because when you're living agelessly, you don't pay attention to your age, whatever it is.[2]

The soul is ageless, and it's an expression of the divine, feminine creative force of the universe. The sacred feminine has traditionally been associated with darkness, the body, mystery, fertility, receiving, and the primordial soup—the womb in which all life begins and is nurtured. Every woman is an ageless goddess, an expression of the sacred feminine physical form. Unfortunately, we often forget this in the onslaught of ageist cultural messages. We need to be more aware of our culture's negative messages about growing older and make a conscious effort to reject them.

Clinical neuroscientist Mario E. Martinez, Psy.D., the founder of the Biocognitive Science Institute, has written about cultural expectations, or what he calls "cultural portals," that we internalize—such as turning 30, or 50, or 65. Dr. Martinez says that you should always refuse the senior discount because it just reinforces the false belief that you're growing older and more frail, that you can't work and need to be taken care of by others.[3] My brother recently discovered the truth of this when he decided to take the discount on a flight to save $25. When he got to the airport, he had to stand in yet another line to prove that he was indeed a senior. He said he ended up feeling like a second-class citizen, which was certainly not worth saving $25.

My mother, who is nearly 90, got in trouble for not signing up for a Medicare drug prescription plan. She didn't see any reason to do so because she's not on any drugs and doesn't plan to be. Do you want to spend your 65th birthday thinking about what diseases and ailments you're likely to develop so you can choose which prescription drug plan will be right for you? Why is that the cultural portal you're expected to walk through? It's probably because back in the 19th century, 65 was chosen as the retirement age that qualified people for a state pension, as that was the average life expectancy. Since then, actuarial charts and statistics have solidified the age of retirement somewhere around 65, give or take 5 years, but now the life expectancy after age 65 is 24 years! So why continue to expect to wind down at age 65? Or 75, or 85, or any age?

If you aren't thinking about how old you are at the moment, then a milestone birthday, or a lifestyle-related illness of a same-age friend or relative, or a crisis in your life might make you reflect on how you could change your script and get older without deteriorating. Many women call my radio show to get my advice because they've suddenly developed an autoimmune disorder, a precancerous or cancerous condition, or allergies. If it's not a health crisis that's thrown them off course, it's the loss of a job or a relationship or an illusion. Sometimes they tell me they have just found out that their husband has been cheating on them or their college-age son or daughter has a mental illness or a substance abuse problem. Our souls design many potent wake-up calls to get our attention back on track.

And of course "the change," as menopause used to be called, is a natural transformation point in a woman's life. We are meant to begin life anew around the biological marker of our last menstrual period. Our bodies know it, even when our minds don't. When I was in active medical practice, brilliant professional women would come in for pregnancy tests, and when I told them the results were positive, they would declare, "I can't believe it. How did this happen?" Trust me, they understood contraception and the body's fertility cycle. They were just in denial of their unconscious need to undergo a dramatic change—a need that drove them to be lax about using birth control. How much easier it is when we can become conscious about the desire to give birth to something new and remember that there are many ways to do that without actually becoming a mother again.

As they enter perimenopause, the transition into menopause that typically lasts for 6 to 12 years, many women realize they're no longer willing to put their dreams on hold and live according to what everyone around them wants. Maybe you have a strong feeling you should switch careers, move to a new place, end a relationship, or explore your sexuality in a new way. Pay attention to that yearning. Your creative juices are flowing! Life force is coming through you. The new life you give birth to must include your own.

Or maybe you aren't yet aware of a desire to make changes. The natural shift in focus women experience can often come on unexpectedly—just as perimenopause does. One woman I talked to said her first hot flash was so unexpected and intense that she scolded her husband for giving her a cup of fully caffeinated coffee instead of decaf—she assumed that had caused the sensation. When he said, "Maybe you're having a hot flash. Aren't you around that age?" she was stunned into silence. Women often don't think about perimenopause until they are in it, or a girlfriend or sister around the same age enters it. *Am I that age already?* they wonder. *Really?* And then, *So what does this mean for me? What am I going to create in the next chapter of my life? What am I changing into?*

What you are changing into is the powerful, luscious, fertile, ageless goddess you were meant to be—an expression of the divine, feminine life force unencumbered by cultural expectations that keep you small, overly cautious, and afraid to upset anybody. You are in the process of discovering your ageless goddess self, and she has many ways to express her creativity and experience the pleasures in life, from feeling good in her body and rediscovering her sexuality to beginning a new relationship, project, or way of living.

Goddesses Never Age is a book for women of any age who are enjoying their lives today and are eager to experience how life can get even better. I didn't want to write a health book for women that would scare them about growing older and tell them how to prepare for every awful thing that could happen to them, from disease of the breast to the heart to the uterus. I didn't want to carve the female body into pieces and tell women to use these ten tips to make sure that this piece doesn't fall apart or to make sure that system doesn't go haywire. I am *so* over that approach to health. If you want specific advice on how to have healthy breasts, how to nourish your body with good, wholesome foods, and how to keep yourself looking fabulous year after year, you'll find all that in this book. However, you will also find ideas that will challenge you to let go of the myths about women and our relationships with each other, our bodies, and the earth—myths that women have internalized and that age them.

In fact, *Goddesses Never Age* is set up to help you move out of the old paradigm and into the new. It's about pointing out everything that can go *right* with your body and how to em-body balance and health regardless of your state of health and well-being now—even if you already have a chronic condition. No matter what your diagnosis might be, the approach in this book can support your healing. Chapter 1 busts the myths of aging and helps you understand what it means to be ageless and a goddess. The reality is that our bodies are not separate from our thoughts or emotions. They're not separate from the planet Earth, our great mother, or from the sky and the stars. Under-standing this will help you see why it's so important to let go of the toxic beliefs and feelings that keep you from experiencing op-timum health and well-being. And because the number-one thing you can do for your health is to live joyously, indulging in sus-tainable pleasure, Chapter 2 of this book is devoted to that topic.

In Chapters 3 and 4, I'll give you a very different perspec-tive on the usual concerns women have about their bodies and physical health as they reach menopause and postmenopause. In Chapter 5, you'll learn about how to release old emotions that can cause disease: grief, anger, and shame. Chapter 6 will help you reclaim your sexuality—your Aphrodite nature—so you stop thinking you're not sexy simply because you don't have the body of a slim 22-year-old. In Chapter 7, you'll continue releasing toxic emotions as you let go of the shame and perfectionism that are affecting your relationship with yourself and the important people in your life. Chapter 8 is about a new relationship with food and your body as you make peace with your belly, and Chapter 9 is about moving joyously instead of forcing yourself to "exercise." Chapter 10 is about seeing yourself as beautiful, and enhancing and adorning that beauty with confidence if you'd like to change the way you look. And in Chapter 11, you will receive guidance on listening to your goddess-like wisdom and the signals from your finely honed BS meter. You'll also learn how to forge a new relationship with the earth and her inhabitants as you step fully into your ageless goddess self. Finally, in Chapter 12, you'll receive a practical template for applying the ideas in this book through the 14-Day Ageless Goddess Program, and after that, you'll find a list of helpful resources for nourishing the goddess in you.

So here you are, at a crossroads, where you have to make a decision about what your life will be like in the years to come. The fact that you are reading this right now is absolute proof that the divine goddess within you would like you to let her take the lead now. I say this with great assurance because I've lived long enough to know that there are no coincidences that are simply random. If you weren't seriously thinking about changing your approach to your life, you wouldn't be here with me right now.

So are you going to grow older with gusto or deteriorate with age? Will you stick with the old paradigm of battling the body to get it to behave itself? Will you continue putting other people's needs ahead of your own and fueling yourself with processed foods, sugar, caffeine, anxiety, and sheer willpower? Or will you get off the road that leads to illness, frailty, and reduced quality of life and start living courageously, as if you really mean it?

Getting older is not something to fear. This is not an anti-aging book designed to arm you in the war against growing older—and anyway, a war metaphor isn't appropriate. Whenever you take an adversarial attitude toward something, you give it power. Instead of being fearful and resistant toward growing older, invoke the magical principle that knowing something's name gives you power—not *over* it but *with* it, as the author Starhawk says.

Then you can become a neutralizing force. You can make growing older a different experience. Then you won't be old and you won't be young. You'll be "something else": an ageless goddess.

CHAPTER ONE

GODDESSES ARE AGELESS

We are not proponents of long life. We are proponents of joyful life, and when you find yourself in joy, the longevity usually follows. We do not count the success of a life by its length; we count it by its joy.

— ABRAHAM

My mother is nearing 90, but she still likes to drive. At her home, she maneuvers her sitting lawn mower around her property at least once a week, steering clear of the landscaping on her three-quarters-of-an-acre lawn. Behind the wheel of her Pleasure-Way camper, she has made her way through the streets of Boston to meet me for dinner. Mom drove her camper on a trip across the U.S. a couple of summers ago with her friend Anne, who was a bit older (and who recently died at age 91). They wanted to see the redwoods. The two of them weren't afraid to pull up to a campground and park for the night. I prefer to leave lawn mowing and heavy city traffic to others, but I know that when I am my mother's age, I will be as active as she is. Mom and I are different in many ways, yet she is my role model for living fully and with a sense of joy and adventure. From her I learned the importance of exercise and taking care of my body so I can spend my later years doing what I like instead of reacting to one health crisis after another. To quote Esther Hicks and Abraham, my formula for my later years is "happy, healthy, dead."[1] You are not doomed to spend your last months with an oxygen cannula up your nose. You can rewrite that story!

As a physician and health educator, I know you can minimize the possibility of degenerative disease and premature aging if you make good lifestyle choices. You don't have to experience health as a temporary respite. It is your *birthright*. You can get out of the state of hypervigilance and stop worrying that your body is about to betray you any minute. Instead, you can reclaim your natural, harmonious relationship with your body and experience pleasure, joy, and vibrant wellness as a daily reality. Then you'll live agelessly, with the vitality of a goddess, and your body and spirit will reflect that.

CELLULAR AGING, CELLULAR REGENERATION

Although most people don't realize it, the body is constantly in a state of reinvention. Cells replenish themselves regularly. Old cells die and new ones are born. Of all your organs, your skin replaces itself the most quickly, but each one regenerates. You do not have the same physical body you had just a few years ago. Every cell has been replaced.

In a sense, we have a shelf life. Structures on the tips of our chromosomes called telomeres, which are like wicks on sticks of dynamite, grow shorter when cells divide. When the wick gets small enough, cells no longer receive the instruction to replicate and their death follows. However, telomeres do not have to shorten as quickly as they do. Research shows that an enzyme called telomerase repairs them and extends them slightly, which offers promise that we have the power to actually reverse aging by improving our ability to repair and lengthen our telomeres.[2] Mindfulness meditation, exercise, and thinking differently all show promise for slowing the aging process.[3] Studies by researchers such as Richard Davidson of the University of Wisconsin show that mindfulness practices rewire the brain, resulting in greater immunity[4] and improved ability to manage stress and emotions.[5] And a recent longitudinal study lasting eight years and following people over 50 showed that as little as an hour a week of moderate exercise can cut your risk of developing chronic disease sevenfold. "Moderate" exercising is as little as an hour a week of dancing around, washing your car, or walking. And even those who had been sedentary up until the beginning of the study had outcomes similar to those who had been exercising all along.[6] So if you want vibrant new cells in your body, nourish them by making positive lifestyle choices that include maintaining a positive attitude about yourself, your well-being, and your value.

It's cellular breakdown that produces the physical changes we associate with aging, from wrinkles to minor aches and ailments. The physical deterioration occurs in large part because of the accumulation of toxins, which results in cellular deterioration and damage along with tissue and organ breakdown. This toxic buildup's effect on the body is exacerbated by the development of dense fascia: that is, scarring of connective tissue caused by physical, emotional, and mental stress (more on this later). And as I mentioned in the Introduction, spending too much time sitting and lying down speeds up the aging process. That's why you need to move your body and experience the earth's gravitational pull through walking, pushing, pulling, and moving. One reason movement is vitally important is that your fluids can more easily move toxins to organs that process them if you aren't sitting all day long. In fact, urinary incontinence is exacerbated by prolonged sitting (as is erectile dysfunction, which is a reason why men need to move too). If the body's toxins aren't processed, cellular breakdown occurs.

There are toxins in our food and environment we should avoid as much as possible, but many of the toxins that contribute to the aging process are produced in our own bodies. Stress hormones such as cortisol and adrenaline are meant to be used by the body in the case of an immediate threat to physical safety. They give us quick energy to run for the hills or put up the fight of our lives. When these hormones are chronically elevated in the system due to unremitting emotional and physical stress, they cause cellular inflammation, and that is the primary cause of all chronic, degenerative diseases, including cancer.

A friend of mine had a medical emergency, and I took him to the ER and stayed with him for hours while the doctors and nurses treated him and ran tests. His blood tests were all normal and, after a few long, stressful hours in the ER, he was sent home with pain medications. The next morning, I had gained three pounds. My body was retaining water as part of an inflammatory process that was trying to reduce the amount of cortisol and adrenaline in my system left over from the stress of the day before. Over time, emotional and physical stressors such as poor-quality sleep can be powerful enough to cause us to gain and retain weight, slowing our metabolism. In a sense, many women are carrying the weight of the world on their bodies by empathically taking on the emotional stress of those around them, as Colette Baron-Reid pointed out in her book *Weight Loss for People Who Feel Too Much* (Harmony, 2013).

Oxidative stress is another process that wreaks havoc on our bodies over time. Free radicals, byproducts of metabolism within our cells, are molecules missing electrons that travel through the system to find cells from which they can scavenge electrons. They leave those cells damaged, and the damaged cells in turn go off in search of the electrons that would return them to stability. If your body doesn't have enough antioxidants to regularly counteract free radical damage, eventually it will not be able to repair itself.

You exacerbate inflammation and oxidative stress when you reach for sugary foods that offer temporary relief from anxiety, anger, sadness, pain, and displeasure. I'm not talking about fresh fruit, which contains fiber and lots of nutrients and antioxidants. You're probably not drowning your sorrows by indulging in a bowl full of freshly picked blueberries. The sugars we consume under stress tend to be highly refined. They're the sugars in foods that lack the protein or fiber that would slow the biochemical effect of the sugar on the body. The quick energy from sugar may make you feel good in the moment, but the candy bar, cup-cake, or glass of wine can spike your insulin, and that causes damage to LDL (low-density lipoprotein) cholesterol. The sticky, damaged LDL travels through your blood vessels and incites fur-ther inflammation until it ends up glued to the walls, forming plaques that create restrictions and, eventually, increased risk for Alzheimer's, diabetes, arthritis, heart attack, and stroke. In addi-tion, glycemic stress from even slightly high levels of blood sugar results in the release of inflammatory chemicals like cytokines from immune cells, which damage blood vessel walls.

Excess visceral fat (belly fat) also causes inflammation, which leads to the sorts of aches and pains that make you want to fore-go an evening walk and settle onto the couch with a bowl of ice cream. Ingesting refined sugars triggers a beta-endorphin re-sponse that dulls pain and feels good temporarily, but the sugar-and-sedentary-living habit creates vicious cycles of inflammation and oxidation. That rounded belly isn't due to age but to sugar consumption and inflammation catching up with you. It's a sign that you need to give birth to a new you: an ageless goddess who experiences so much pleasure that she doesn't succumb to the temptation of lesser, temporary pleasures from sugars and alcohols.

And while the aging effects of regular drinking start to become obvious to the eye, much of the damage is happening deeper within the body. The brain's pathways for processing do-pamine, a natural pain reliever and pleasure creator, stop func-tioning properly. Over time, you start to feel worse sober than you did before the drinking habit took hold. "Just a glass" of beer or wine improves mood and sense of well-being temporar-ily, but then the cycle begins all over again. Now, having a few sugary, sweet, or alcoholic indulgences isn't going to kill you. In fact, healthy rituals involving pleasure (like eating fine chocolate or enjoying a glass of good wine) are part of living well. But mindless overindulgence as a way to ease pain you don't want to feel is a whole different story. Do you really want sugar, or a sweeter life? Are you seeking spirits in a bottle of vodka, or do you want to find Spirit? Do you self-medicate and suppress your "inconvenient," difficult feelings? It's far better to detoxify from them and release them so that you can experience sustainable joy, like a happy two-year-old!

Detoxification is great. It fosters good health and reminds us of how good it feels to get the junk out of our system and return to our natural state of wellness. However, most of us do a detox as a sort of penance for being "bad," which is not an ageless attitude. The thought is: *I was "bad" and ate too many holiday treats so I have to punish myself with a grueling detox.* You don't have to do a four-day detox that brings on a migraine and flu-like symptoms. You can simply choose to begin the process of returning to clean eating and pleasurable living, knowing that you might feel a bit under the weather for a few days as all those toxins make their way out of your body. During that mild discomfort, you can look forward to the transition from feeling bloated, achy, and low on energy to feeling vibrant again. Let go of the concept of detoxification as punishment and focus on the pleasures of taking care of yourself, tuning in to your needs, and eating fresh, healthy foods. Notice how good it feels to tackle a cluttered drawer or closet—and then enjoy the "white" space that is left. The same thing happens in your body when you clear out the gunk.

All the junk you eat and all the health-eroding messages and behaviors you keep repeating will take their toll if you don't admit it's time to really care for and love yourself enough to put your adrenaline-fueled ways behind you. Then you will find that you have much more control over your health than you previously thought. Gerontologist Michael F. Roizen, M.D., has done research showing that you can extend your quality and quantity of life by adopting a positive attitude and even just flossing your teeth![7] Some of the changes may seem difficult as you try to develop new habits and fit new activities into your busy schedule, but the payoffs can be extraordinary.

NO MORE SENIOR MOMENTS

Everyone wants her healthspan to match her lifespan. Many women don't just fear losing their health, their stamina, or their looks. They also fear dementia, which is the physical degeneration of the brain. It seems every day there's another frightening report on how many older people who are otherwise in good physical health are in cognitive decline or have developed Alzheimer's. What isn't so apparent is that we can make many lifestyle changes to protect our brain health. There's quite a lot of ongoing research into dementia, but rather than wait for a treatment, why not live a lifestyle now that prevents it in the first place?

What we commonly refer to as stress—mental, physical, emotional, or spiritual—actually creates inflammatory chemicals in the brain and body that lead to memory deterioration. Whether that stress comes from too much sugar in the diet, chronic worry, or lack of sleep, stress leads to cellular degeneration. Fortunately, you have the ability to turn that around. You can read about how to "manage" stress, but reading about it and intending to manage your stress one of these days isn't going to do anything. You need daily health practices that boost immunity, lower cortisol levels and inflammation, support brain health, and cause you to embody wellness and joy. These practices can include regular movement, standing up from a sitting position regularly throughout the day, enjoying meals with good friends, dancing, breathing fully, stretching your fascia (connective tissue) through yoga or other practices, calming your emotions and calming the activity of your mind through meditation, taking antioxidant supplements, or something else. There are plenty of other ways to enhance brain health, too (more on that later).

If you find yourself standing in a room wondering where your cell phone is, please don't say, "I'm having a senior moment." Cognitive decline is not a normal part of getting older. What you're probably experiencing is mental overload from trying to juggle too many tasks and not getting enough quality sleep (more on that later as well). Words are powerful. Don't talk yourself into believing your brain is turning to mush just because you are over 40! Adopt an ageless and healthy mind-set so you can program your cells to be ageless and healthy too.

AN AGELESS MIND-SET

Mental habits play a huge role in our health and longevity. The famous Ohio Longitudinal Study of Aging and Retirement (OLSAR) by gerontologist and epidemiologist Becca Levy, Ph.D., found that people with positive perceptions about aging live, on average, seven and a half years longer than people who don't hold that belief. In fact, people's perceptions of aging had more of an effect, positive or negative, on healthy longevity than did having low cholesterol or blood pressure (which increase longevity by four years) or a low body mass index (BMI). Perceptions even had more of an effect than not smoking (which adds three years to your life).[8]

In other words, the belief in the positive aspects of aging strongly affects your biology and thus your survival. If this information were a drug, it would be unethical not to prescribe it! A different study was done with people 60 to 90 years old to determine their "swing time," that is, the time the foot is off the ground when a person is walking. Swing time measures balance and can indicate that someone is becoming frail. Both groups in the study were told to walk so that their swing time could be measured as a baseline. Then the subjects played a simple computer game, but unknown to them, the first group's game contained subliminal positive messages such as "wise," "astute," and "accomplished" and the second group's had subliminal negative messages such as "senile," "dependent," and "diseased." After playing the computer game, the second group lost swing time. They walked as if they were actually "senile," "dependent," and "diseased." However, the first group's swing time increased. The transformation seemed to be due solely to their unconscious thoughts and the immediate effect of these thoughts on their bodily functions.[9]

How powerful are our attitudes toward aging and growing older? Harvard professor Ellen Langer, Ph.D., in her classic book *Mindfulness* (Addison-Wesley, 1989), recounts how she conducted a famous study of men in their 70s and 80s. She had one group live as though it were the 1950s when they were in their prime: watching television shows from that era, looking at pictures of themselves in their prime on the walls, reading magazines from that time period, and so on. A control group lived away from their daily routine, but without any reminders of what life was like in their youth. Before the study began, the men underwent tests for hearing, blood pressure, eyesight, and pulmonary function. They also had their pictures taken. After two weeks, the tests were repeated. The men who had just lived as if in the era of their prime looked, on average, ten years younger. Their hearing, vision, lung function, and other functions and measures had also improved dramatically. They had a greater sense of well-being. And when they left the venue where they had been living, they all carried their own luggage—like the healthy vibrant men they remembered they could be. The control group showed no changes.

Here's another example of research that supports an ageless mind-set. The famous University of Minnesota longitudinal study of nuns, which began in 1986 and continues today, looked at women who entered the cloistered life in their early 20s to determine what distinguished the women who developed Alzheimer's in their 80s from those who maintained healthy brain function. Each nun had written an autobiographical essay upon entering the monastic life in her early 20s. Only 10 percent of those whose essays were rich with linguistic flourishes, energetic descriptions, and complex language structures went on to develop Alzheimer's disease, whereas 80 percent of those who wrote plain essays did develop it. This study suggests that being vivacious and fully engaged by our experiences and enjoying our creativity protects our brain health.[10] It's marvelous that we have so much control over our health and well-being! And now for some really unexpected news out of that study: autopsies showed that the nuns who relished life and showed no signs of dementia had just as many plaques in their brains as the less vivacious nuns whose dementia was apparent before they died. Please reread that last sentence. It is proof that a healthy mind and spirit can exist in a body that is less than perfect. *That* is the power of an ageless attitude.

BELIEFS AND BIOLOGY

The most important thing you need to know about your health is that the health of your body and its organs does not exist separate from your emotional well-being, your thoughts, your cultural programming, and your spiritual outlook. *Your thoughts and beliefs are the single most important indicator of your state of health.* That is amazingly good news because your thoughts and beliefs can be brought under your conscious control and, when necessary, surrendered to the healing power of Spirit (much more on that later). This is the part of health that Western medicine always leaves out, but trust me, it's where your real power resides, with no exceptions. Your beliefs and thoughts are wired into your biology. They become your cells, tissues, and organs. There's no supplement, no diet, no medicine, and no exercise regimen that can compare with the power of your thoughts and beliefs. That's the very first place you need to look when anything goes wrong with your body.

Let me be clear here. If something has shown up in your body as a health concern, you most likely aren't consciously aware of why it is there. If you had been conscious of the issue or emotion, it would not have had to show up physically because you would already have addressed it. Please try your best not to resist this truth. Have the courage to go deep within and ask yourself the following: "What is going on in my life, and my thoughts and beliefs, that I can learn from through this situation? What is the soul lesson for me here? How can I grow from this?"

Ayurvedic and Eastern medicine practitioners are well aware of the energetic connections between various systems in the body, but Western medical practitioners tend to look at one system in isolation. In fact, this mind/body split is built right into the fabric of our society. No podiatrist is likely to look at how you bear weight on your feet and ask you about whether you have any unprocessed emotions or stressful situations causing you sadness, anger, or grief. If he or she did, you'd probably recoil and feel defensive and blamed, thus blocking off access to that line of inquiry. Yet even if you're having hand problems that you can relate to not having an ergonomic workstation, or if you've injured your hand in an accident, getting in touch with unprocessed emotions that you may be holding in the tissues in your arm and hand might alleviate the pain and allow this part of your body to repair itself. And remember that you probably won't know what the lesson really is until *after* it has been resolved.

Over the years, my most profound soul lessons—the ones that really have brought in the light and, eventually, the joy—have come in several ways. I once had a huge breast abscess dissecting into my chest wall, which pretty much liquefied the lower half of my right breast, requiring emergency surgery. That taught me a lesson in self-care and self-nurture while trying to nurse a baby and work 80 hours a week. At one point, I developed a fibroid tumor in my uterus the size of a soccer ball, which had to be removed surgically. That woke me up to the fact that I had been shunting my creative energy into a dead-end job and a dead-end relationship. I also once had a rare infection in my left cornea that nearly blinded me. According to traditional Chinese medicine (TCM), the eye is in the liver meridian (a meridian is an energy channel through which the life force flows), and that's the meridian associated with anger. The condition developed while I was processing childhood anger regarding my mother. These memories arose when I was starting the writing process for *Mother-Daughter Wisdom* (Bantam, 2005), and medical treatment at a major eye hospital was unsuccessful. The infection went away only after I began taking high doses of vitamin C, or as I like to say, vitamin *See*. I was so angry at my mother for childhood things I had deep-sixed that I literally "couldn't see straight."

Because our bodies have interconnected systems that balance each other, it doesn't make sense to focus on this problem or that problem as if it exists in a vacuum, outside of your emotions, or to look for a miracle cure or intervention. We've been taught to worry about this disease or that one according to our genetics, but that's an outdated way of thinking about health that is based on outmoded science as well. It's crucial to know that our immunity and resilience are boosted by the exalted emotions of compassion, love, and honor, all of which render us far more capable of fighting germs and viruses. But righteous anger and standing up for yourself are also associated with health! When you build your overall health and wellness through appreciating your power to feel your emotions and to change your thoughts, beliefs, and, finally, your actions, you'll find you can enhance your health and immunity through experiencing emotions such as joy, elation, compassion, pleasure, and righteous anger. At the same time, you can decrease cellular inflammation, which, as I've said, is the root cause of all chronic degenerative diseases such as cancer, heart disease, arthritis, and diabetes. All wellness and vitality come first via your connection with your spirit. Let the program in this book serve as your template for vitality.

In the Introduction, I explained Dr. Mario Martinez's model of cultural portals, or expectations that we internalize about what different stages of life mean. Cultural portals can also work in positive ways. A patient of mine went to China and said her hip pain, which she associated with growing older, vanished while she was there. She believes that's because elders are so respected in China that while she was there, her perspective on herself changed and so did her biochemistry. And Dr. Martinez gives the example of menopausal hot flashes in Peru versus in Japan. In Peru, the term for hot flashes means "shame," whereas in Japan, hot flashes and menopause are considered signs of a second spring when a woman goes deeper into wisdom. The inflammation Peruvian women experience with hot flashes is higher than it is for Japanese women because of the negative association. Similarly, in the !Kung tribe in Africa, there's no word for hot flash. A woman's status in the tribe increases as she enters menopause. In the West, we need to recontextualize the experience of menopause so that we see it as positive instead of a portal into decline.[11]

ALPHA GODDESSES

We are in the era of the Alpha Goddess, the perimenopausal or postmenopausal woman who has come into her own. Advertisers are beginning to realize that women in their 50s and 60s are spending their money on themselves and the people they love, without apologies, embarrassment, or hesitation. Women over 50 were the first adopters of e-readers, changing the face of book publishing, and they continue to be the number-one group of book buyers. They know what they want, they're open to trying something new, and their buying power has a major effect on the economy.[12] In a recent editorial entitled "The Smart Money Is on the 50+ Crowd," Robert Love, editor-in-chief of *AARP: The Magazine,* wrote, "We the people over the age of 50 are 100 million strong. We will soon control more than 70 percent of the disposable income in this country. We buy two-thirds of all the new cars, half of all the computers and a third of all movie tickets. We spend $7 billion a year shopping online. Travel? More than 80 percent of all the premium-travel dollars flow from our credit cards. Add it all up . . . and U.S. adults who are over 50 ka-ching as the third largest economy in the world, trailing only the gross national product of the United States and China."[13]

Women who aren't as well off financially are not necessarily plunking down money for a tablet or a designer perfume, but they don't hesitate to nurture themselves, either. Self-care and self-development become priorities when a woman has entered her second spring. At wellness expos, crowds of women are exploring all the many ways they can increase their well-being. They are getting massages and acupuncture and becoming massage therapists and acupuncturists. They and their girlfriends are off to the meditation center on Sunday mornings or to a condominium in a resort area for a weekend of talking, hiking, and wine tasting. Alpha Goddesses are finding their tribes. They know that if they don't have anything in common with the other women they see each day at the local pool, they can simply enjoy having someone to chat with in the locker room, and they can expand their tribe of friends outward by meeting up with people in any number of ways. As the old summer camp song goes, Alpha Goddesses know how to "make new friends but keep the old"—but they only hang on to those longstanding friendships if they're vitalizing instead of draining. Alpha goddesses are *ageless* goddesses.

And Alpha Goddesses feel that "this is my time." They're realizing that they need to give to the world without squelching their own needs, and express themselves without being afraid of hurting someone's feelings. Their desires and passions are calling to them. They know their strength because they have experienced significant loss and come through it. The fear that they can't depend on themselves disappeared along with the first husband or the first job they were fired from. They know their weaknesses and have come to peace with them, having figured out ways to work around their ADHD, their impatience, their shyness, their disdain for small talk, or whatever it is that they were told in their teens would hold them back from being well-liked and accepted and catching a man. As one woman put it, "I found out that even cranky women get laid."

Some Alpha Goddesses are facing serious financial issues they will have to address, but they are feeling more encouraged than ever about their ability to take care of themselves. They may look around at women who have more financial security and realize that even though it would be nice to have the mortgage-free home, paid-off cars, and retirement fund, they feel more independent, smart, and capable than they ever have. Creating what they need and want doesn't feel like an impossible dream. They're coming into their own power, and realizing they don't need to achieve success according to someone else's definition in order to feel good about themselves and their lives. Often, they find that the opportunities that passed them by and the losses that seemed huge at the time prove not to have been quite so devastating in retrospect. The cheating lover moved on to a younger woman who is now reminding him to test his blood sugar and dealing with his irritability and demands for attention. Our second spring brings a reframing of the past—and the present and future.

Alpha Goddesses are able to put matters in perspective, whether it's a car that's been totaled or stolen, or another encounter with that one person in every workplace or family who has to stir up a conflict to draw attention her way. The things that used to make them pick up the phone and vent to their friends or write furiously in their journal no longer faze them. Their attitude is "Oh well, that's life" or "This too shall pass"—or my personal favorite, an old Polish proverb: "Not my circus. Not my monkeys." Many years ago, I lost my sister in an accident. Ever since, when someone calls with bad news, my attitude is "Hey, a family member didn't die. This isn't so bad." When we're over

50, we have enough life experience to instantly recognize what is small stuff and what isn't.

Over the years, we develop a finely calibrated BS detector. We recognize that some people are not being honest with themselves about what they are doing to create their own problems. If they pressure us to rescue them, or try to make us feel guilty for not changing our plans to accommodate their latest crisis, we find it's easier than ever before not to give into their emotional threats. Alpha Goddesses recognize that "No" is a complete sentence. How liberating!

I see this a lot in women with aging mothers or fathers who have placed far too many unreasonable demands on them. This is the time when you learn that being a good daughter doesn't mean letting yourself become depleted by your parents. They brought you into this world and took care of you, but making your life about their needs is not necessary or healthy for you *or them*. Very often, what older parents really want is to feel independent and useful. When you say no and you ask them to help you out in some way, however small, you restore balance in the relationship. It's a gift to realize you truly are on a journey separate from your parents'. Your paths intersect, but you can't be responsible for their lives. The same is true for your adult children.

Alpha Goddesses recognize their value in the "tribe." Although our culture is less ageist than it was a generation or two ago, there's still too much power in the old message that a woman's value decreases when she enters menopause because she's no longer physically fertile. That message has been drilled into us often over our lifetimes and is rooted in the belief that a woman is like an empty vessel, designed solely for the purpose of incubating and nurturing the next generation. Once we can no longer do that, what's our purpose? Most of us don't actually think we have no more value once our eggs dry up, but many of us do internalize the message that our value is in what we can produce for others. Consequently, we start feeling guilty that we aren't spending more time, energy, and money on our adult children who are struggling with their bills, or our teenagers who are having trouble navigating the choppy emotional waters of middle school. Other people's problems keep creeping up to the top of our To Do lists because we are trying to prove our worth to ourselves and others. Without the balance that comes from rest and receiving help from others, we burn ourselves out. There's no better way to suck up your vital energy than to try to prove to everyone that you are a good mother, good neighbor, good daughter, and so on. As Tosha Silver, the author of *Outrageous Openness: Letting the Divine Take the Lead,* says, "Accept yourself absolutely and unconditionally. It's one of the most radical acts you can do in an insane culture that actually profits from your self-loathing."[14]

As we enter our ageless years, we can also finally free ourselves from the need to prove ourselves. We look back and see that we didn't do so badly after all. Maybe we have some regrets, and maybe we disappointed some people, but that's part of being human. Now is our time to focus on ourselves more instead of always worrying about everyone else. According to Chinese and ancient Ayurvedic medicine, at age 60, women end their householder life and begin to develop their souls. Our fertility stops being about having children and starts being about what we create for ourselves that benefits us and the people around us.

CREATIVE GODDESSES

This new form of creating means seeing new possibilities all the time. Ageless goddesses aren't jaded. They recognize that there are always new things to learn and discover, and new relationships to begin. They're exuberant about life and they let loose their curiosity and playfulness. A friend of mine went on a cruise to a tropical island with a turquoise lagoon and was practically "drunk with joy," as she described it. She eagerly climbed into a boat that would take the group out to snorkel in a coral reef. But two women near her, both 20 years or so younger than she was, could only talk about how they wished the boat taking them out snorkeling had a quieter motor, and how the wind was too strong, and how the waves were going to be hard to navigate once they jumped into the water. Hello—you're in a sparkling tropical lagoon communing with the fish! If you can't enjoy that, you need to reconnect with your spirit and earthly pleasures so you can participate in the creative process of the earth herself.

Agelessness is all about vitality, the creative force that gives birth to new life—the divine feminine that makes it all happen. Blades of grass will push up through a brick patio even if there is a foot of gravel underneath the brick because nature is determined to push outward, upward, and forward in the act of creation if it has to. Vitality is our natural state. Taking all the right supplements and pills, or getting the right procedure done, isn't the prescription for anti-aging. It's ageless living that brings back a sense of vibrancy and youthfulness.

I'm all for exercise and healthy eating, but forcing yourself to go to a badly lit basement gym and work up a sweat on an elliptical machine while staring at a concrete wall or a depressing 24-hour news channel, and avoiding all of the foods you really love, is not going to make you ageless. Don't "battle" aging when you can dance with life, moving your body joyously. The perfect combination of weight training, low-impact aerobics, and interval training isn't going to do it either. If you have a passion for tweaking your workout routine, by all means go ahead and do that, but don't think you have found the magic formula. The real fountain of youth is the fountain of happiness, well-being, and connection with what Tosha Silver calls "the Divine Beloved" (or God—and you get to call it whatever you want, whether it's God, Goddess, Source, your Higher Power, the Universe, All That Is, or any other name that speaks to your heart and spirit). The anti-aging prescription is to love life, try new things, and savor your experiences. Joy comes from feeling connected to the life force.

While your skin may not glow as it did when you were 20, you can glow with vitality if you see yourself as an expression of the Divine and a being through which the Divine Beloved operates. For you, agelessness may mean you finally find the courage to stop dyeing your hair to hide the gray, or it may mean you finally start dyeing it because it makes you feel better and you don't care what anyone thinks of your decision. *You* get to decide what makes you feel ageless and how you want to express yourself. If your daughter says, "Oh, Mom, you're too old to wear that," tell her, "No, I'm not!" Learn the skill of standing up to and defying the cultural editors of our joy and freedom—especially in your own family. We have to teach our daughters to become ageless too. They need to reject the notion that at a certain age, their value begins to decline. Those lessons start with you.

You can turn back the hands on the clock when it comes to physical health and vitality by being open to what's new but not afraid to hold on to what's old if it still works for you. If you're an analog woman in a digital age and you despise figuring out how to operate a new piece of technology, enjoy the fact that, having been around for a few years, you can you trust your judgment about whether you need to learn this skill. If you feel like trying something new, try it simply because you want to, not because you're afraid of being left behind. On one hand, listening to new bands and musical performers will help you to remain ageless, just like spending time around people 20, 30, and even 40 years younger than you are will help you stay connected to what is happening now. What you will also discover is that interests in things like art and music are completely ageless. I know 20-year-olds who adore the music of Jimi Hendrix and Bruce Springsteen and are into vinyl records. My tango community encompasses people from 25 to 75. Age couldn't matter less. Agelessness means you make your decisions based not on a fear of looking foolish but on feeling comfortable in your body and being keenly interested in the world around you.

SACRED FEMININE ENERGY

The energy of receiving and accepting balances the energy of doing and acting that we get pulled into much too easily. A crisis or intense call to change can make us realize that we can't go on using up all our vital energy and not replenishing it, always doing and rarely receiving. I call this "donating bone marrow." Energetically, it really is that!

It's not just women who are in transition. Around the globe, people are aware that life is changing. Astrologically, we are experiencing what's known as "the turning of the ages," when the planet Earth moves back into the eleventh house of the zodiac.

This is a point at which the feminine rises in partnership with the masculine—both within us and between men and women. Even if you don't follow astrology, you can see that human beings are undergoing a massive change and turning away from old perceptions and ideas. Technologies, especially communication technologies, have had a huge effect on how we perceive each other and have helped us see ourselves as part of a larger whole. Our hearts break over an online video of something happening halfway around the globe, or we're moved to tears at some child's triumph that was recorded on his father's smartphone and appears on the screen of our own as we're sitting at the airport. We all sense the truth so beautifully documented in my friend Dr. Larry Dossey's book *One Mind: How Our Individual Mind Is Part of a Greater Consciousness and Why It Matters*. We really are connected to everyone and everything, and unless we get serious about how to collaborate more effectively, the problems that seem to be "over there" will appear "over here" if they haven't already. The world needs a lot of creativity right now if we're going to solve our problems, and it yearns for the wisdom of seasoned women who own their goddess nature.

We're entering a new age of experience and bringing back the sacred feminine energy, also known as yin or the female principle, that was central to the lives and beliefs of humanity for the vast majority of prehistory. The sacred feminine influenced the rituals, ceremonies, religions, myths, legends, and artwork of ancient civilizations all around the world for thousands and thousands of years—far longer than the relatively new era of "written" history, which is a mere blip on the screen. And according to many anthropologists, the sacred feminine was worshipped as a Great Goddess or Earth Mother.[15] Well, it's time to bring Mama back!

If the lost feminine principle sounds far removed from your life, think about the buzzwords you have been hearing lately. Business leaders are saying we need workers who are creative and who have good people skills (read: they're intuitive and can collaborate and communicate easily). Political leaders are talking about how we have to stop the partisan bickering and work together. Both men and women are questioning the endless quest for financial rewards at all costs and the sacrifice of time that could be spent building community or developing relationships with others, including our kids. Feminine energy involves heeding the messages of our emotions and taking the time to care for our physical bodies and the earth herself. It means listening to and receiving new ideas and taking in what other people feel, and then putting it all together to better understand how to interact with someone else in a way that benefits both people. That's just what all good mothers do automatically. *This* is how the lost sacred female energy can work in the modern world, and each of us is part of it. We've tried war and conflict and being alienated from our bodies, our emotions, our pain, and our needs. How about trying something else?

Although the divine feminine is often associated with women and how we perceive, think, or behave differently from men, it's absolutely part of men's lives too. The hearts of men feel very deeply, and most men are hardwired to serve and protect those they love. If you look at the symbol for the Tao, which represents the balance between the male and female principles, you find that there's some feminine energy in the masculine and vice versa. You can see this balance reflected in our bodies' hormones: both men and women have the male hormone testosterone and the female hormones estrogen and progesterone. Now we need that balance in our communities. Women have to work with men to bring forth new life—and together, we have to invent new ways of relating to each other and working together.

The values of patriarchy—or what scholar Riane Eisler, author of *The Chalice and the Blade* (HarperCollins, 1987), calls a "dominator culture"—have to be balanced by feminine values that support life and collaboration. We need to learn to reconnect with the divine feminine and be like the moon, which waxes and wanes. Our bodies are connected to this mysterious, beautiful orb that was worshipped by the ancients. But we think that if we are to be good people and valuable to society, the sun can never set on our generosity and hard work. We have to be on call constantly. For thousands of years, we've been expected to produce more and more whatever the cost, driving ourselves relentlessly. Instead of collaborating, cooperating, and creating, humans have been competing. Now that the human population has topped 7 billion, we're going to have to come up with some plans for sharing the planet's resources and living together healthfully and harmoniously into the future.

Today, it's relentless progress without reflection and competition without collaboration that are "old school." Fueling ourselves with adrenaline, sugar, and caffeine is no longer sustainable for anyone. Fueling ourselves with thoughts of "I'd better get mine before someone else grabs it" or "I'd better try to reverse aging or some younger person will beat me to the job or take all the good romantic and sexual partners" isn't working either. We have to know when to rest, recharge, and begin envisioning what we want to create next—together.

Whether your life force is draining because you are constantly trying to please others, or gobbling down fast food, or not nurturing your soul, it's time to get off that stressful course that leads to exhaustion and degenerative disease. Exercise your goddess-like power to renew and rejuvenate yourself through joyful, pleasurable everyday practices that are crucial to mental, emotional, and physical wellness. Get rid of the idea of health as the absence of illness—as a temporary respite from the discomfort of the body's decline—and instead see it as the natural expression of your innate divinity. The divine force is loving and joyous. It has the power to repair, restore, and fortify your body. However, we can access it only if we allow ourselves to experience what has been denied women for millennia: guilt-free pleasure, self-love, and joy.

CHAPTER TWO

GODDESSES KNOW THE POWER OF PLEASURE

Nothing can cure the soul but the senses, just as nothing can cure the senses but the soul.

— OSCAR WILDE, *THE PICTURE OF DORIAN GRAY*

The connection with my tango partner was delicious. We were in close embrace, and my eyes were closed as he held me firmly against his chest and we moved to the music together. Argentine tango is an earthy dance that blends male and female energy in a moving meditation in which both partners move as one. This dance, which is completely improvisational, allows a man and woman the opportunity to both give and receive exquisite pleasure.

Although I wasn't consciously thinking about it, I knew my brain and body were awash in naturally produced chemicals that were creating a feeling of euphoria. I was in a completely safe environment, enjoying the bond between me and the men who served as my partners during that night at the dance studio. With an open heart, I consciously experienced a powerful high that I would be able to re-create again and again. I was mindful of how wonderful it felt to be in my body.

When the evening ended, I glanced out the window onto Congress Street in Portland, Maine, and saw the misty cloud around the streetlamps as I heard the quiet swish of car tires on the rain-slicked street. I felt a kind of buzz that didn't lift for hours, a lightness and radiance that would leave me with no negative aftereffects. I wouldn't gain weight, develop high blood pressure, feel guilty, or get bored as a result of my enjoyable indulgence. In fact, just the opposite was true: Argentine tango has many documented health benefits. I had discovered a sustainable pleasure I could sink into with delight over and over again for the rest of my life—a pleasure that would actually contribute to my health and well-being!

I was first drawn to Argentine tango because I had always wanted to do partner dancing—and when I first saw this dance form while peering through the window of a dance studio on a snowy January night, every cell in my body said *yes!* It was deeply sensual and sexy. Little did I know then that this passionate dance form would also be a way of connecting my soul and my body in a highly focused and pleasurable way. Over several years, I taught myself to relax into the sensation of being supported by a man while feeling completely present in my own pleasure. Learning this dance form, which is more like a mindful martial art than anything else, was one of the most difficult, but ultimately most rewarding, endeavors I had ever attempted. Years later, my daughter Annie, who had recently moved home for a sabbatical, said to me, "Mom, I don't want to horn in on your 'thing,' but after hearing you talk about how incredible tango feels, and having experienced it myself, do you mind if I go to tango with you?" That's right: my sophisticated adult daughter from New York City wanted a piece of my over-50 lifestyle.

Normally, when we hear the word "pleasure," we think about sex, but sexual pleasure is a whole-body experience of all the senses. All pleasure is sensual in nature as we allow our bodies to dance with the creative energy of the universe. Life itself is sexually transmitted. Immersing ourselves in a state of vitality, whether through a discipline like Argentine tango or any other activity that takes us out of our heads and back into our bodies, allows us to feel the miracle of our physical being. It also allows us to participate in the birthing of a new world even as we rejuvenate our cells and our spirits.

I don't want to knock ministering to others and contributing to the health of the world, or the joy we receive when we give of ourselves. I have experienced the intoxicating feeling of satisfaction that comes from assisting someone in the emergency room or during a difficult labor. What I want to encourage is the reclamation of the power of pleasure, which comes from the divine force of the universe. Pleasure is a divine gift to us. It should be a discipline practiced regularly to establish happiness and joy in your body and your life. Sustainable pleasure is the ultimate prescription for good health.

All the goddesses of pleasure are associated with sensuality, with being present in our physical experience and not cut off from our bodies or our environments. Embody the goddess energies and enjoy pleasure, sensation, and the joys of self-replenishment. Embrace your joyous, sensual, earthy nature and stop giving away all your energy to other people. This isn't frivolous. It can save your life. The late poet laureate of New York State, Audre Lorde, was diagnosed with metastatic breast cancer that had spread to her liver and was given six months to live. She continued to thrive for another eight years. She wrote, "I had to examine, in my dreams as well as in my immune function tests, the devastating effects of overextension. Overextension is not stretching myself. Caring for myself is not self-indulgence, it is self-preservation, and that is an act of political warfare."[1] Several years ago, I took Audre Lorde's teaching about the health-promoting value of self-care to yet another level. I was invited to teach at Mama Gena's School of Womanly Arts Mastery Program in New York City. I intuitively felt that what these women were learning and practicing, the deliberate pursuit of pleasure, was most likely having a very positive effect on their health. To test my hypothesis, I asked those who had experienced health improvements to please line up at the microphone to share. I was astounded as, one after another, they spoke of resolutions or remissions of diseases and conditions ranging from arthritis and ovarian cysts to abnormal Pap smears and even bowel cancer—all of which happened after these women chose to fully experience pleasure, with no apologies. Pleasure is powerful medicine indeed. We know this to be true because our bodies are actually wired to repair and renew themselves optimally when we are happy. To be ageless is to know the incredible power of pleasure to better our lives and the lives of people around us. As the saying goes, "When Mama ain't happy, ain't nobody happy." And when women choose pleasure, pleasure becomes abundant for everyone.

RECLAIMING PLEASURE

Most of us have learned well how to make our bodies conform to the needs of our minds. Our entire educational system is set up this way. In our school days, we taught ourselves to sit still in our chairs, use the bathroom only during designated breaks, and devote all our attention to the teacher. Discipline, or training ourselves through practice to develop a habit, keeps us focused on doing what we think we're supposed to do. However, we're not designed simply to think about and take actions that support everyday survival, or that please others. Nor are we designed to sit still in chairs for hours, staring at screens. Our brains are wired to allow us to connect with the life force and experience rejuvenating pleasure for ourselves. We have forgotten the importance of pleasure and we need to remember how to experience it regularly—as a daily part of life.

Not long ago, neuroanatomist Jill Bolte Taylor, Ph.D., gave a presentation that turned into a viral video and then a book in which she talked about the disorienting but delightful experience of having a "stroke of insight" that shut down her rational, thinking brain and allowed her to feel the wonder, mystery, and euphoria of an activated right hemisphere. We've learned to quiet the activity on the right side of our brains. That has reduced our ability to relax into pleasure and the sheer joy of being alive and participate in the ongoing creation of beauty that is our true nature.

In her book *Dying to Be Me* (Hay House, 2012), author Anita Moorjani explains that after her near-death experience—in which she literally was pronounced dead of terminal cancer—her insight was that we are here to enjoy life. Asceticism, frugality, self-denial, and ignoring the desires of the body should not be our goals. Siddhartha, a wealthy prince who became the Buddha, discovered this as well after trying asceticism and living on as little as a grain of rice a day. Renouncing his riches didn't lead to enlightenment—sitting on the earth under a tree did. Think of that as a metaphor for getting back in touch with Mother Earth and her nourishing energy.

As long as we're living beings on this planet, we should relish the simple pleasures of feeling present in our bodies and connected to each other and the earth. Our bodies are actually designed to thrive and repair themselves through the earthly pleasure of being in a body.

THE BIOCHEMISTRY OF PLEASURE

Cells in our brains, blood, blood vessels, and lungs produce a signaling molecule, or gas, called nitric oxide or NO (not to be confused with the nitrous oxide used in dentistry, better known as laughing gas). The production of nitric oxide is triggered by laughter, orgasm, and other experiences of pleasure, as well as by eating fruits and vegetables high in antioxidants, meditating, and exercising (nitric oxide is at work in the sensation of "runner's high"). Nitric oxide relaxes blood vessel walls, which allows the vessels to widen and encourages more blood to flow through them. In fact, Viagra works by using this natural process in the body: it triggers release of nitric oxide, and the extra blood flow to the penis results in an erection. Similarly, nitroglycerin can stop a heart attack because it, too, releases nitric oxide that widens blood vessels and eases constrictions.

The sensation of nitric oxide being released lasts only a few seconds, but it is a *marvelous* few seconds! It sets off a chain reaction of other feel-good chemicals in the body. You feel a shift in your energy and an exquisite sense of relaxation. After its release into the system, nitric oxide works with anticoagulants to prevent strokes, signals white blood cells to fight infections and destroy tumors, balances levels of neurotransmitters, and reduces cellular inflammation. The more often your body creates and releases nitric oxide, the softer, more flexible, and wider your blood vessels become because you've trained them to relax. Your circulation improves. Saying yes to NO actually helps your body function better and avoid serious illness and disease.

I find it helpful to think of nitric oxide as the physical manifestation of the vital life force (also called *chi* or *prana*) that animates our bodies. Stanford University research on sea urchins shows that nitric oxide is released when the egg and sperm meet in a peak moment of creativity. On the other end of the life spectrum, the brilliant white light that people who have had near-death experiences report seeing upon the moment of death may be the result of a burst of nitric oxide. And nitric oxide given to premature babies gets their lungs working, since lung tissue is erectile in nature. Nitric oxide is like the very breath of life. It's even what lights up a firefly.

Researcher Herbert Benson, M.D., describes nitric oxide as a crucial element in what's known as a "peak experience" of ecstatic flow, and explains that it allows new neural connections to be made in the brain. Neural connections are the pathways along which information travels. It's possible that these brain changes lead to new habits of mind. As Benson says, NO is "a biological mechanism that somehow encompasses the dynamics of human belief, the creative process, the essence of physical and mental performance, and even spiritual experience."[2]

Anger, fear, and grief deplete nitric oxide. If the endothelial lining of your blood vessels has been damaged by free radical molecules created by stress and physical toxins, your body can't release enough nitric oxide to actually reduce free radical activity and tissue damage. The nitric oxide mechanism is a positive feedback loop: Create more and you make it easier for your body to create more. Pleasure leads to more pleasure. Life renews itself, while anger, fear, and grief suck the life out of you.

To be an ageless, healthy goddess, you must learn to cultivate your ability to experience emotions such as joy and compassion, release grief and resentment, and allow yourself to feel righteous anger when appropriate. For example, if you see someone harming an animal or a child and you stand up for the innocent being, you are contributing to your health and well-being (as long as you're physically safe confronting them). The worst thing you can do for yourself is hold on to destructive emotions.

The biochemistry of pleasure can counteract the biochemistry of aging. Nitric oxide is the über-neurotransmitter that increases and balances levels of all the others: endorphins, dopamine, serotonin, oxytocin (a bonding neurotransmitter released while breast-feeding, experiencing an orgasm, or even enjoying the company of others), and DMT, which is generated in the pineal gland in the brain and probably plays a role in dreaming.[3] Although we tend to think that neurotransmitters are generated and used only in the brain, we actually have cells throughout the body that can both produce and receive them. The gut produces more serotonin than the brain does—generated largely as a result of the huge number of healthy bacteria that live in what's known as your microbiome. When you have a visceral negative reaction to something—you can't "stomach" it—that's your neurotransmitters sending you the message "this doesn't feel right for me." Conversely, you can get a warm, happy feeling in your belly when neurotransmitters that affect mood are released as a result of a positive experience, thought, or feeling. The idea is to create that warm feeling through the emotional experience of genuine pleasure that supports your well-being, health, and agelessness.

YOU DESERVE PLEASURE!

We've been taught that anything pleasurable is suspect. We say "it's a guilty pleasure," "it's sinfully delicious," or "we're having too much fun." Someone is "drop-dead gorgeous," or we're going to "die laughing." These sayings are based in the idea that we can't handle the fullness of someone's beauty or our own laughter. The thought of simply enjoying ourselves, savoring sensual experiences, makes us look over our shoulders for the pleasure police.

I remember sitting in church when I was about 11 years old and saying the "general confession" from the Book of Common

Prayer, which read, "We have erred and strayed from thy ways like lost sheep. We have followed too much the devices and desires of our own heart. And there is no health in us. But God Almighty have mercy upon us, miserable sinners." I remember thinking, *I'm only eleven years old. I'm not that bad!* I wanted to feel a sense of the Sacred and the Divine in church. I didn't want to feel like a miserable worm asking for forgiveness for things that I couldn't possibly have done or even thought about. I wanted to feel good in my body and feel loved by the God who made the moon and the stars and the tides—*and* my own body.

Feeling bad and undeserving of pleasure is part of our dominator-culture heritage. We start to enjoy what we're doing and that little voice starts whispering, "Careful. Beware the pleasures of sin." If we allow ourselves physical pleasures, what's to stop us from becoming sinful, selfish hedonists who deserve to be punished for our wickedness? Denying and demonizing pleasure has caused too many women (and men) to doubt our natural instincts that tell us that when we feel good in our bodies and hearts, we overflow with joy and abundance that spills out onto other people. Our cup runneth over, and it keeps getting refilled with pleasure, when we reconnect to Spirit. We enjoy having optimism and a sense of possibility because we know that we're connected to the Divine. We're refilling the cup from the ultimate Source of all rescue, protection, and abundance—a Source that we ourselves are part of. What a delight to realize that God comes through us *as* us!

I remember when I was married, I used to avoid telling my husband if I was going to get a massage. It felt so decadent and self-indulgent—as if self-indulgence is a bad thing. I thought he wouldn't agree with my spending money on something "frivolous" like a massage. He never actually criticized me for doing this, but I had internalized the cultural message that women shouldn't "waste" money on their own pleasure. Many women would instantly hand over the same amount of money to their teenager to enjoy himself on a class trip, or would spend it on a present for a family member or donate it to charity. But spend it on themselves and their bodily pleasures?

It's important not just to get the massage but to get it without feeling guilt. If you hesitate to spend the money, find a discounted way to get a massage. One woman's husband signed up for text messages from the local beauty school so he could be alerted to discounted same-day massages and set them up for her. It's a smart man who knows the value of making his woman feel deliciously relaxed.

If you still find it hard to justify the time and expense required to give yourself the pleasurable experiences you crave, think about how easy it is for so many men to let themselves go off with their friends to have fun and indulge in nine holes of golf or a pricey concert. They haven't received a constant cultural message that taking care of their needs is selfish, so they don't worry and ask themselves, *What will people think?* or *Should I really be spending money on this?*

Deprivation is a puritanical value that is not conducive to alleviating stress and inflammation or to experiencing bursts of nitric oxide. Frugality and morality have become inextricably linked in our minds. It's an obsolete mind-set. Women's bodies, like Mother Earth, are designed to be a source of abundant pleasure. They are a reflection of that earth, the mother that brings forth life by working with the energy of the sun and all the elements. The sun feeds the plants, the plants feed the animals and us, and we flourish in abundance. The creatures lay plenty of eggs to hatch into new life or to serve as food that nourishes other animals. The trees drop more seeds than will ever grow into seedlings, and the birds eat them up. We get to enjoy the harvest of the earth, from the fresh fruits and vegetables she brings forth to the earthy smell of the rain-soaked soil that has been fertilized by earthworms. *That* is heaven on earth!

Don't hold back from pleasure. Be direct rather than apologetic or coy. Know and ask for what you enjoy, want, and deserve. Don't settle for what you think should be "enough" to satisfy you. If you want to spend the entire evening watching junk TV and giving yourself a pedicure instead of going to a community meeting you said you'd attend purely out of a sense of obligation, go for it.

Such simple pleasures may seem obvious, but they actually do reduce stress and, by extension, inflammation. You may even experience a burst of nitric oxide.

My prescription for general health is to experience more pleasure every day. Take a minute to put this book down and make a list of as many joyful activities and experiences as you can. Think of big ones as well as small ones: Heating the seat in your car on a cold day. Opening the door on a particularly clear morning and smelling the air. Relishing the first moment when you step into a warm bath. Acknowledging that you've hit a new level of fitness and feel completely in tune with your body. How can you have these experiences more often? How can you make boring, everyday activities you do mindlessly into succulent pleasures? How about putting on a great rock-and-roll playlist or Pandora station when you have some cleaning to do? It will change your mood entirely. And you'll enjoy the cleaning process far more!

RITUALISTIC PLEASURES

You don't have to swear off chocolate, rich foods, or alcohol completely to be a goddess of pleasure. In fact, studies of healthy centenarians show that these individuals enjoy things like alcohol, cigars, and chocolate as rituals of pleasure. The key is *ritual*. If you slow down and mindfully indulge in the ritual, even if you do it daily, your body will experience that food, drink, or cigar differently than it would if you consumed it while on the run—or if you used it as a means of distracting yourself from your anger or sadness. In a ritual, you consume consciously. Think of a Japanese tea ceremony—you don't rush the experience. You enjoy it fully as you take your time.

If you're going to have some chocolate cake, don't purchase some highly processed or cheap version. Buy or make the best possible quality treat, sit down in a comfortable place of beauty and grace, and pay attention as you slowly savor it. Again, make it a ritual. Remember the scene in *When Harry Met Sally . . .* when Meg Ryan fakes an orgasm during lunch? Have what she's having! And I don't mean fake an orgasm, either. Let yourself feel the desire to moan or sigh in delight over how wonderful it is to pamper yourself. Otherwise, the sugary treat just isn't worth it, and you're better off enjoying some pleasures that are truly guilt-free for you.

What I'm describing is very different from drinking, smoking, or eating as an addiction. I've found that people can be divided into two groups: the moderators and the abstainers. Moderators are able to enjoy a small bowl of ice cream and leave it at that. Abstainers find that one bowl of ice cream inevitably leads to finishing off the carton, and one cookie is never enough. Abstainers tend to do best when they abstain from all sugar for five or six days per week, leaving a day or two for eating whatever they want. Are you a moderator or an abstainer? If you "can't eat just one," like the TV commercial says, it's especially important to make use of all your other options for pleasure seeking.

You have so many options! Sit in your backyard with some friends on a hot summer night and stick your feet in a kiddie pool filled with cool water. Find yourself a porch swing and sit there gently rocking back and forth as you watch the colors of the sunset. Walk barefoot on the grass or a sandy beach. Go out into the forest for a hike. Let the earth renew you. Open yourself to receiving the prana and energy of nature that is all around you.

Find pleasure in your body, not just sexually but sensually. Truly delight in tastes, smells, sights, sounds, and tactile sensations such as the deep touch of a massage or the light touch of soft fabric or a feather against your skin. When you feel good inside your clothes, it shows in your attitude and mood. If you can't have pleasure, go for comfort. Ditch the stiff clothing and wear something that flows. Put on perfume when you're not expecting to go anywhere special, if you enjoy the scent. Spritz the room with it. There are companies that charge a lot of money for a "scent design," which gives a store an inviting ambience. Use scent to make your car or home a more pleasurable environment. And play music or recordings of natural, soothing sounds when you're working or doing chores. These activities can become rituals of pleasure too.

WINGWOMEN

I strongly believe in having "wingwomen" who support you in making time for pleasure. Get a friend or two to commit to going with you to the group meditation, organic food tasting, or folk dancing night at the community center so you'll encourage each other not to break the date. And if your girlfriends or your partner aren't interested in an activity, there's no reason to deny yourself the enjoyment. To me, one of the greatest things about social media is that it can be a means for finding others who share your interests. If you use it right, you can start a conversation with someone in the virtual world and carry it over to a real-life meeting at a coffee shop, event, or class. Just be sure you arrange to have experiences offline that are pleasurable and social. Most of our communication is nonverbal, so when you physically get together with people, you can communicate more richly.

Take pleasure in your friends' experiences too. People often get depressed and jealous reading the social media posts of others when those posts are about vacations, accomplishments, and so on. Yet people who post positive statements or share positive stories and videos on social media report greater happiness as a result. If you want to be happy, you have to let go of the belief that life is a zero-sum model—that if you're happy, somehow you're taking happiness away from someone else. Discard the old idea that there's only so much money, pleasure, joy, or rest to go around: it's simply not true. When it comes to pleasure and happiness, you can actually train your body to feel more and more of these emotions by being mindful and fully present. Your triumph isn't someone else's loss. When someone's doing really well, a part of you is uplifted—unless you give in to jealousy and resentment. When you pass a gorgeous young woman on the street, don't think, *I wish I had her body and her skin.* Think, *She's a part of me.* Smile and enjoy her beauty. Enfold it into your own experience. You're a part of her too, and she is able to experience your wisdom because you put that out into the world. She can experience the joy of experiencing your pleasure as you smile at her.

Exercise: Brag, Be Grateful, and Let Yourself Desire Something

I first read about this exercise in *Mama Gena's School of Womanly Arts: Using the Power of Pleasure to Have Your Way with the World* (Simon & Schuster, 2002) by Regena Thomashauer. I think it's fantastic for bringing perspective to your daily experiences and remembering how challenges set us up to more deeply appreciate blessings. Doing this exercise will help you remember how important it is to enjoy life instead of just getting through your To Do list. Mama Gena calls this exercise a "trinity": a Brag, a Grateful, a Desire.

First, identify something to brag about. What can you be proud of right now?

Second, identify something you appreciate or are grateful for. What blessing in your life would you like to acknowledge?

Third, identify something you desire. If money, time, and the laws of physics were no object, what would you desire right now?

Try doing this exercise daily, answering the questions in your journal and reflecting on them. And share this experience with others in conversation. I love asking these three questions at lunch or dinner with my daughters or my friends. Invite your wingwomen, or wingmen, to share their lists for the day too. It never fails to uplift everyone and probably generates nitric oxide as well.

OPTIMISM AND PLEASURE

Pessimism can be a bad habit. So can negative thinking or self-talk. And trust me, that's all they are—habits of thought that can be broken. You may have grown up in a family that had a propensity toward depression and chose to identify with it, saying, "That's just how we are in this family." I don't care what your family's culture is or whether your brain is currently wired for negativity. You have the power to change that. The research of Dr. Joe Dispenza, documented in his book *You Are the Placebo: Making Your Mind Matter* (Hay House, 2014), demonstrates that "neurons that fire together wire together" really is true. First, you have to set an intention to change your habits of mind, and then you have to take action. You have to generate new feeling states associated with the more exalted emotions of happiness and joy. You have to see and feel yourself behaving in new, uplifting ways and reinforce the new behaviors through affirmations and self-reflection, such as journaling. Research shows that adopting habits of gratitude leads to greater optimism. You can make a conscious choice to establish habits that support optimism and pleasure and enhance your mood through healthy foods, therapy, exercise, humor, Al-Anon or other 12-step programs, or even the simple awareness and expression of gratitude.

Use positive language when describing your life. If you feel you have a "heavy" schedule or are "crazy busy," that's going to weigh you down, mentally stress you, and make it harder for you to slow down, relax, and feel the lightness of pleasure. Use your language to reinforce the joy of being busy. Say, "My schedule this week is absolutely rich!"

Have you received awards in the past? Do you have objects that remind you of your accomplishments, your brilliance, or your beauty? Display them in your home or office rather than putting them in a drawer because someone might think you're "full of yourself." Be "full of yourself" and enjoy it.

Abe Lincoln is said to have declared, "Most people are about as happy as they make up their minds to be." Make up your mind to be happier and you will be—*if* you follow through by practicing pleasure. You must take action! Choosing to be positive and optimistic is a discipline, and it takes courage. It's much easier to be negative than joyful. Don't allow yourself the negative self-indulgence of seeing the glass as perpetually half empty.

When you commit to the discipline of optimism, you'll also be less likely to slip back into the Western medical model's focus on "What's going to fall apart next?" Our medical system is centered on finding and identifying problems, and it works on the self-fulfilling prophecy of "Your body is going to break down,

A Word about Depression

Depression involves brain chemistry and neurotransmitters, which can be affected in many ways, such as through regular exercise. While you may decide you want to take an antidepressant to affect your brain chemistry and depression, keep in mind that pharmaceutical drugs used to treat depression and anxiety should be an adjunct to, not a replacement for, working through your emotions and developing new habits of mind and body as part of a healing process. Even if being positive and optimistic is difficult for you, make an effort to develop habits that support a positive mood—and push yourself to make the changes you know you need to make.

Depression can be a symptom of blood sugar instability, a sign of feeling disconnected from the Divine, or even an indication that your vitamin D levels are low, or all three, so make sure you get your vitamin D levels up. It can also be a sign that you're avoiding a difficult decision, such as leaving a bad marriage or work situation. Staying in that situation will only make it harder to keep your mood positive and to live agelessly.

That said, if your symptoms of depression and lethargy are severe, you need to get very serious about addressing the issue. Don't delay in getting help from a medical professional. Please know that medication for psychiatric problems can be a lifesaver. If you need it, do not hesitate to take it. Bless it and stay on it.

And most importantly, do something—anything—to begin the process of recovery. Clean a drawer, sweep your front step, volunteer at an animal shelter. My colleague Bob Cooley says that creativity is the cure for depression. I completely agree. Sadness is meant to alert you to the need to grieve a loss and also take better care of yourself—it is not supposed to be a chronic condition. Your natural state of being is joyfulness! Recovery from depression is possible if you're simply willing to get moving in some way.

so be vigilant." Choose to think differently. Your body isn't a flawed creation just waiting for a chance to betray you or punish you. Health setbacks and bad test results are messages from your body that you're not taking the best care of it. Listen to the message and change your habits to help your body heal itself. Remember, your body is constantly regenerating at a cellular level. You have a new stomach lining every three days! Forget waiting for a bad diagnosis. Enjoy your body in its current state of health even as you're happily working toward greater pleasure, greater wellness, and greater fun. The body regenerates in an environment created by your thoughts, emotions, and expectations, so make sure they're positive.

TRUE SELF-CARE

I've already touched on the notion of what we "deserve." Be forewarned that the guilt and shame of millennia will hit you between the eyes once you open to pleasure. You may start to wonder if you're selfish or self-centered for wanting to have more joy in your life and indulge your desires. Fear of being selfish is embedded in our language: "Don't break your arm patting yourself on the back." "Don't toot your own horn." "Don't get too big for your britches." "You'll get a swelled head." Are you afraid people will think you're "full of yourself"? One in five people is genuinely narcissistic. These people take up all the oxygen in the room, satisfy their own desires at the expense of others, and blame problems on everyone else. They have an abyss inside that no amount of love or caring from others can fill, and they tend to be surrounded by those who over-give. If you have one of these individuals in your life, please know that it's neither possible nor even desirable to try to fill that abyss for him or her.

You have to overcome the habit of chronic over-giving in order to bring balance into your life and the lives of those around you. If you're always worried about others' feelings, you may be overly empathetic, excessively self-sacrificing, and badly in need of more self-nurturing. As Amanda Owen, author of *The Power of Receiving* (Tarcher, 2010), writes, "Those who have trouble giving attract those who have trouble receiving." And if you're concerned that *you* may be turning into a narcissist, that means you're not one. Believe me, narcissists do not reflect on how other people perceive them, or on their own failings.

Self-sacrifice is the shadow of self-centeredness. The desire to draw attention to yourself by becoming a martyr is supported by a dominator culture that benefits from women who are constantly giving to others in order to gain social approval. And we all know how difficult it is to be around martyrs who try to make us feel guilty and who get angry if we don't constantly notice how much they are doing for the benefit of others. When you give too much, you enter a state of imbalance. Then the pleasure gets sucked out of your life and you experience chronic resentment that too often leads to disease. To be an ageless goddess, figure out what makes you feel joy and then let go of the guilt.

Consider a discipline of pleasure to be an investment in your health. A joyful heart and a body that experiences pleasure and nurturing are your most reliable health insurance. The late Peter Calhoun, a former Episcopal priest turned shaman, pointed out that all native cultures have known that healing happens through regular primal experiences of pleasure and ecstasy in the body— not through the intellect. Five minutes spent dancing in your kitchen to a song you love, or petting your dog or cat who offers you unconditional love, can make a difference if you do it often enough.

Any pleasure can be yours if you own it. I like to tour those charity showcase houses, where they have designers redecorate every room of some gorgeous mansion, and appreciate the aesthetics. I used to find it hard to imagine myself being comfortable in such a house. They seemed too grand for me. Even just walking through them made me feel a bit like an intruder. I could never afford to live there—who was I kidding? Now I walk in as if I own the place. I'll take the card of the cabinetry guy. Why not imagine ways in which I could achieve pleasure, whether it's redesigning my kitchen or enjoying someone else's designer bedroom on display? Kids make believe all the time, but as adults, we've been taught to feel self-conscious about exercising one of our biggest sources of pleasure—imagination! The pleasure centers in your brain don't know that you don't actually own the hot tub at the hotel when you lower yourself into it. They don't know that the painting on the wall at an art museum isn't yours to keep. They only know that in that moment, you're in heaven enjoying the experience.

In Italy, public art is treasured by people of all social classes. Even those who are struggling financially "own" the art that's the legacy of their people. The Italians are on to something. Think about all those movies where some pleasure-deprived American or English woman goes to Italy and loses herself in the luxury of aesthetic and sensual pleasure—which then attracts a man she chooses to enjoy or not, depending on her mood. *Eat, Pray, Love; Enchanted April; Under the Tuscan Sun; Summertime; A Room with a View*—all these movies demonstrate the importance of slowing down to take time for pleasure. The Greeks understand this too—check out the movie *Shirley Valentine,* about a British woman in a stultifying marriage who finds pleasure again by vacationing in Greece alone and reconnecting to herself. She makes a brave move in devoting herself to her own pleasure—which also ends up saving her marriage.

We all need to remember the quiet, relaxing joy of being with others, taking in a beautiful view, and sharing good food, laughter, and conversation. If someone in the group is a curmudgeon, mentally cast her as a character in your story of pleasure. Maybe she's the Maggie Smith character whose dry wit you can enjoy without taking her comments too seriously. Smile at the predictability of that person's complaints, but don't take in any depressive energy.

And dance! Goddesses move their bodies. Every indigenous culture has used dance to celebrate life. We heal through dance, movement, sound, and tears. Eve Ensler, author of *The Vagina Monologues,* ushered in Valentine's Day in 2013 with a global movement called One Billion Rising (www.onebillionrising.org)—a call for people around the world to celebrate the resilience and life force of women who have been sexually abused (approximately one billion women) by getting up from their chairs and spending a few minutes in joyous dance. There's a time for grief, but then we have to dance. Many women love to dance but don't. Why do we deny ourselves?

I dance in my living room, which is in the exact feng shui center of my home. (Feng shui is the Chinese art of placement to enhance the flow of life force in a space.) For more than 30 years, the space was used only during the holidays, so most of the time, it was essentially empty of life. Then I removed all the furniture so I could use the room, which has a hardwood floor, as a dance or yoga studio. Now I use it regularly. One year, I threw a tango party on the anniversary of 9/11 to celebrate the people who survived and helped each other as well as those who were lost. One of the men who attended told me afterward, his voice cracking, that his brother had died in the September 11, 2001, attacks— which I'd not known about. He said softly, "I really needed this," and gave me a big hug. What better way to celebrate the memory of those who have died than to join in close embrace, dancing to beautiful music with another human being?

You can do this too. Open your home, your heart, and your front room. Life isn't meant to be lived with plastic covers on the couch or a veil of grief dampening your spirits.

Commit this to memory: *experiencing pleasure is crucial for vibrant health.* It is not selfish. It's a gift to yourself and the people around you. Your joy gives them permission to experience joy too. It creates an ever-broadening circle of celebration and joy that spreads out from you in waves, lifting up everyone.

Exercise: Peak Pleasure

Think back to two or three moments in your life when you experienced peak pleasure. Take some time to recall those moments in exquisite detail. Re-create the smells, sounds, sensory details, and emotional experiences you had. Regenerate the feelings and relive every tasty moment. The body makes no distinction between the actual event and what you're imagining, so in re-creating these moments, you alter your biochemistry and release nitric oxide, endorphins, and serotonin that stimulate circulation and cellular repair.

Often, we forget how to take pleasure in the simple things and are reminded of enjoyment only in contrast to an unpleasant experience. As a teen, I went on a canoe trip in the spring and accidentally overturned the canoe. I had to spend the rest of the trip soaking wet and freezing. We finally got to a hotel where I could take a hot bath, and to this day, I remember the comfort of that bath in sharp contrast to the bone-marrow-deep cold I had experienced leading up to that moment of warmth. If everything were pleasurable, you'd get bored and stop enjoying the simple delights of life, such as being dry, warm, and comfortable. Think back to a time when the contrast between displeasure and the pleasure created afterward was powerful for you. Relive that moment. In this way, you can train yourself to not be jaded—and learn to truly draw pleasure from small moments.

LAUGH AND LIGHTEN UP!

Laughter has many proven benefits, including reduced inflammation, lower blood pressure, greater immunity, improved memory and circulation, and better blood oxygenation. Laughter also reduces pain by increasing your beta-endorphins, which are feel-good neurotransmitters.

My motto is that anything worth taking seriously is worth making fun of. One evening many years back, when I was studying the harp, I was helping a fellow harpist in our harp ensemble at the Cleveland Institute of Music move her instrument out of a retirement home where our ensemble had played for the residents. As we carried the ungainly harp down a hallway, I overheard an older woman say to another, "It was a good day. Nobody fell." I burst into laughter and had to put my end of the harp on the ground. I managed to catch my breath long enough to say to my friend, "When my definition of a good day is when nobody falls, it's probably a good time for you to help me check out." My friend was horrified by my dark humor, but I really believe that when you lose your sense of humor, you lose your vitality. At that point, you're just waiting for the end to come.

Deep laughter from the belly floods you with nitric oxide. Buddhism has the laughing Buddha to remind us of the healing, life-affirming nature of laughter. I wish more spiritual traditions would help us lighten up. Just because something is meaningful doesn't mean it can't be screamingly funny.

Laugh and have fun. When you open up to receiving pleasure, it comes to you. Don't be afraid to lighten your To Do list and put "pleasure" at the top of it.

MEN'S ROLE IN WOMEN'S PLEASURE

Many men are having a hard time of it these days. Historically, men have always had a higher suicide rate than women, in no small part because women are far more likely to consult a therapist. In the U.S., the suicide rate of men in midlife is at an all-time high because men are feeling cut off from the life force.

Keep this in mind: Too many little boys have heard "Be a man" or "Don't be a sissy" over and over again since they were very young. They have to shut down their feelings of sadness or fear at an early age to survive in our culture. The result is that far too many have repressed anger and sadness that can easily turn into violence or depression. Men require support to access their feelings—rather than being told repeatedly to "suck it up."

Being cut off from their feelings makes it hard for men to connect with ours—which in turn makes it hard for them to support women's pleasure. A man's deepest desire is to serve the Goddess—that is, to serve life. That truth is written into the King Arthur legends and the stories of brave warriors who protected their people. Look at the comic books and science fiction movies that serve as our new myths. The man is always trying to serve and protect women, or the feminine.

The problem is that when it comes to serving women in real life, many men go about it ineptly much of the time because they're not listening to what women actually want and need. If we help them serve our goddess energy, and praise them for what they do for us, including the small things that make life more pleasant, men will want to work even harder for us.

To receive assistance and pleasure from men, you have to start with making requests, not demands, so that their egos don't get the better of them. Otherwise, they tend to shut down. Set the expectation that the men in your life can give you pleasure and acknowledge them for doing so. This can be as easy as thanking them for opening a door. And yes—I know you are fully capable of doing it yourself. But remember, receiving is a skill that has to be cultivated.

When you put pleasure and fun at the top of your list, the man wants to get in on it. Men find you attractive whatever your age because you are living agelessly and joyfully. Who wouldn't be attracted to someone like that? To use a dance metaphor, I waited my whole life for a man who would be willing to go out dancing with me. When I finally went on my own, I discovered there was an entire community of men and women looking to dance. I always find male partners willing to participate in the dance. (Of course, I also had to keep up my end of the bargain by getting good enough to be a pleasure to dance with!) I don't have to date a man who will dance with me because I own the dance in my body. I can go to any city on earth and dance the tango with strangers who don't even speak English. Men rise to the occasion when they're appreciated by the feminine energy.

For you, receiving pleasure might take a different form than having a partner dance with you and honor your goddess-like self. Your supportive partner may not be a man at all—it may be a woman who is attracted to you and unapologetic about desiring and receiving pleasure. Even so, open yourself up to having the men in your life and your community serve and assist you and other women.

It's not as if men have to lose out as women own their pleasure, and women become the "winners" who beat out men in some competition. Everyone benefits when we're balanced by embodying the feminine principles of receptivity, pleasure, and connection to the earth. A woman who owns her pleasure makes a man's life more fulfilling. It's not having a woman pay the bills and run the household that will unburden him, but having a woman who is overflowing with enthusiasm and passion for her life.

For too long, women have been trying to do it all. Getting angry or resentful toward men, or rejecting them, won't lead to a fulfilling and enjoyable life. Inviting men to step up and support women in receiving pleasure will.

RADIATE PLEASURE!

Your nature is joyous radiance. You don't have to ask permission to seek or receive pleasure. Your happiness serves the world and yourself, keeping your vibrational energy high.

Here's how it works: Your heart's electromagnetic field reaches out from your body and interacts with the field of energy we all share—you're actually wired to reach out and connect to pleasure. This energy field radiates throughout the universe via the electromagnetic field. Scientists know about these fields, but don't necessarily think of them metaphysically. They've discovered the Higgs boson particle, which is the evidence theoretical physicists have been searching for because it explains how energy coalesces into matter. Unity Minister Catherine Ponder's term for the Higgs boson is "divine substance." Others have called it "the God particle." When you have fun, your energy changes and so does the field around you, and that shapes physical reality—creating nitric oxide and endorphins in your own body. How that energy of pleasure manifests in the physical world outside your body is a marvelous mystery.

So adopt this motto: *Fun is important.* Fun is what keeps you ageless. Dream up a pleasurable adventure, get out there and do it, and chances are someone else will do it with you. Drive into the city to take a tango lesson. Book the cabin for a girlfriends' weekend in the woods during the dark months of winter. Pull out the card game or board game, get some people together, and laugh yourself silly over a trivia question.

The time for pleasure is now. I remember when I finished my medical residency at age 30. I'd been a nonstop student since I was in kindergarten and now my peers were choosing postdoctoral specialties. I wondered when I would get a chance to stop following the carrot on the stick and finally have some fun in the present instead of someday. I'd had enough. I said no to doing an ob/gyn subspecialty fellowship. It was time to live my life. How about you?

Learning tango or singing in public may not be giving food to the homeless or helping as a hospice volunteer, but these pleasurable pursuits are important. We're taught that good women spend their free time endlessly giving, selflessly serving, never caring about themselves. Tango is all about me, being in my body and feeling pleasure, but my dancing the tango gives others permission to indulge in their own gratification. Joy starts in our bodies, as nitric oxide and neurotransmitters, and then its positive energy heals our cells and then radiates outward to heal others and the planet. Dancing is a form of healing—in fact, any ecstatic experience can be healing not just for you but for others. Therapy is good to help you think differently and break patterns of pessimistic thinking or negative self-talk. But we have to be joyful, dance, and bring pleasure into our lives deliberately.

Life's too short to settle for the lousy theater seats, so buy the best or figure out how to become a volunteer usher so you can sit in the orchestra section. Get in touch with what really makes you feel good. Become an ageless Alpha Goddess of pleasure. In fact, make pleasure a sacrament. That will be a gift to yourself and the world.

CHAPTER THREE

GODDESSES
USE THE HEALING
POWER WITHIN

Women, delve deep into your primal power, beyond the
appearances, customs, and religions of this day. Delve into the
knowing that you have always had and always will—a knowing
that no religion can ever encompass and that no culture can
ever define. Delve deep into your belly and the brain that lies
there: the primal brain, your original voice, the voice that will
never betray you and will always lead you to the truth of love in
action, the being of joy, and peace: The Voice of Life itself.

— Padma and Anaiya Aon Prakasha, *Womb Wisdom: Awakening*
the Creative and Forgotten Powers of the Feminine

Toni had a recurrence of her Hodgkin's disease, a type of cancer that affects the blood and lymph nodes. Hodgkin's tends to lower your hemoglobin, or red blood cells, and

Toni was in the hospital with a fever and anemia. Her hemoglobin was dangerously low. A transfusion was ordered. No stranger to the power of the mind to influence the body, she asked her physician if she could hold off for a couple of hours and take the test again. Then she called a couple of natural healers who work over the phone and, with their guidance, envisioned rich, healthy blood cells traveling throughout her circulatory system. Sure enough, when the test was repeated, it showed her hemoglobin levels had jumped upward. In fact, she had as many red blood cells as if she had received the recommended transfusion of a unit of blood.

When Toni shared this story with me, I wasn't surprised. I thought about how when I went to medical school, we were trained to see health mechanistically, without regard to the power of the mind to affect our health. The influence of emotions and thoughts on our physical bodies is known as the placebo effect. This powerful effect is considered at best a medical curiosity and at worst a phenomenon that makes it difficult to test the efficacy of new pharmaceutical drugs. I have learned through decades of experience with patients, as well as countless scientific studies, that the placebo effect is powerful physical medicine. It can be harnessed consciously to create better health. Why wouldn't we take advantage of that?

"BODY, HEAL THYSELF"

As children, we're fascinated by our bodies' ability to heal a scraped knee or broken bone. But as adults, we often forget about the body's remarkable capacity for self-repair. The key to this repair is understanding there is a balance between immunity and pathogens. None of us is completely free of threats to our health. Every body has cancerous cells in it along with microorganisms that could cause illness if not kept in check. Everyone's body has manmade toxins in the bloodstream and organs. There's no way to live a perfectly clean life, free of all pathogens. In fact, the fear of pathogens making you sick will depress your immune system, making it more likely that you *will* get sick.

The very origins of Western medicine are rooted in the study of pathology: the paradigm of war and fighting invaders. Health and those things that contribute to it are almost never studied or taught. So starting in utero we are programmed to think of our bodies and our environments as war zones requiring an armamentarium of pills and surgery to wage war on germs and on the body itself. We have largely overlooked the power of our immune systems and our innate ability to boost our immunity. The medical mind-set—and the fear that drives it—has to go. It's time to reclaim the wisdom and power of the healer within.

There's no doubt that Western medicine can be very useful in addressing certain conditions that are acute. When you fall off a ladder and break your arm or get a concussion, of course you want to go to an emergency room for assistance. I'm a huge fan of Western medicine and its remarkable ability to replace a worn-out hip or address acute trauma. When an illness is life threatening, you want to be able to access the best medical tests and treatments available. However, most medical problems are not acute: they develop over time after a long process that we can intervene with at any point. As Myron Wentz, Ph.D., a world-renowned microbiologist, puts it, "We die too long and live too short." Most ailments aren't simply caused by a virus or single physical agent. They always have mental, emotional, and spiritual or energetic aspects to them. The best approach to health conditions is to acknowledge and address them through a holistic mind-body-spirit approach to wellness, not just a physical intervention.

Diseases and disorders are part of nature's way. Illness can give us that all-important nudge to look inward and deal with the emotions we've been avoiding for a lifetime. Years ago, Bernie Siegel, M.D., with whom I served as co-president of the American Holistic Medical Association, said, "The fundamental problem that most patients face is the inability to love themselves." This is so true—and not just for patients but for all of us. Our challenge is to learn to love ourselves just as Spirit does: unconditionally. We should love ourselves not because of some achievement or service we provide to others, but simply because we are precious beings. This is the primary message that those who have passed over in death and then returned have to share. We are loved and appreciated more than we can ever know. And we can learn to care for ourselves from a loving standpoint—physically, emotionally, mentally, and spiritually—as we would a precious child. Then our vitality is automatically boosted.

Women have been taught to be perfectionists, constantly on the go, doing for others without stopping to rest until it's absolutely necessary. Too often, we treat food as something to grab on the run. And we spend many hours sitting as we drive, work on computers, and so on. Exercise can seem like just another item to fit onto an overcrowded To Do list. We exhaust our bodies and our spirits trying to pack in all that we think we're supposed to do.

But our bodies were never meant to sit for prolonged periods. Nor were we designed for nutrient-poor fast food purchased at a drive-through window and eaten in quick bites at red lights. Sleep and rest are essential, as Arianna Huffington so powerfully demonstrates in her book *Thrive* (Harmony, 2014). A life devoid of movement, sleep, and nourishing food is draining and will age you quickly as it overtaxes your immune, endocrine, and central nervous systems. I consider sleep my number-one medicine. Having a good night's sleep solves most of my problems within a night or two because it boosts vitality, as does releasing any emotions and beliefs that restrict you from expressing your divine, goddess nature. And continual daily movement—as simple as standing up and then sitting down at your computer or while watching TV—about 32 times per day—will boost your immunity and put the health-giving effects of gravity to work for you!

Your immune system will naturally have highs and lows. The lymphocytes, or white blood cells, can be observed in whorls in the walls of the uterus waxing and waning with the menstrual cycle, just as the moon does. Consequently, your immunity is low just before your period, which is why you might notice that you're more prone to colds, migraines, and other ailments during those days just before and at the beginning of your period—if you're still menstruating, that is. This monthly dip in immunity tends to disappear after menopause. To boost immunity, you have to do extra self-nourishing—which is why the menstrual cycle is such a powerful natural tool for learning the art of self-care. Anything less than loving, nurturing care for yourself will often result in cramps and PMS.

The incredible inner healer in each of us is empowered by the ultimate healer: Divine Love (God). Working with this force, allowing it to fuel our lives, is the key to healing our unhealed wounds. Asking Divine Love to take away our anger, sadness, and resentment over unhealed traumas of the past is the answer. It's only when we're awakened to our exquisite sensitivity and empathetic nature that we can acknowledge the need to heal. Pain in all its many forms—whether emotional or physical—is actually a most powerful path to Divine Love. Only a direct connection with the Divine will heal us permanently.

The ultimate healer, Divine Love, is an inner gardener of sorts. She tends to the plants without worrying that weeds will overtake her seedlings and block their sunlight. She prepares for new growth. She's not a warrior out to battle a disease or virus and stomp it out with the help of a well-oiled medical army of procedures and pills. She's a healer who knows the power of the body's ability to generate and regenerate healthy cells, tissues, organs, and biological systems, and we can turn to her for help instead of just expecting a physician to heal us. Doctors can aid us in healing, but it's the body and the Divine who do the work.

Speaking of the body, a goddess has to let go of the ingrained belief that her body is unclean, ugly, or flawed. We've been taught that the experience of the Divine is transcendent and the body is unclean and impure: it poops, pees, and bleeds. But while we've been taught to see our bodies as ugly, it's through the body that we discover our divine nature. We should marvel at how beautifully designed our bodies and their systems are, and enjoy the gift of having an inner healer—the ability to boost our immunity, cleanse toxins, and repair our cells. We reflect Mother Earth's ability to recycle and regenerate, reabsorbing the hormones we don't need after they have served their purpose, pruning away what's no longer needed, and creating new cells and neural networks in the brain.

The body is not uncivilized and in need of taming, but the vessel for our creative life force and the temple in which we're designed to live heaven on earth. When we recognize that we came here to live heaven on earth, we start to realize that our bodies are the only place in which we can do this. We stop denying our needs, start releasing the old emotional and physical toxins that have clogged up our energy centers, reclaim our energy and vitality, and awaken our inner healer. That's when the real magic happens, from reinventing our lives to rebooting our health.

MORE THAN JUST A PRESCRIPTION

My understanding of our ability to access the healer within evolved over the course of several years. In medical school, I had learned to take a case history, diagnose, identify an appropriate intervention, give advice and perhaps a prescription, and send the patient on her way with the expectation that she would do the right thing for her health. I came to realize that helping women to get healthy involved much more than some educating and a prescription.

In the 1980s, women would flock to my clinic because I had a reputation for taking their PMS symptoms seriously, which wasn't the case with many ob/gyns back then. I would prescribe a regimen of reducing stress; avoiding caffeine, sugar, alcohol, and tobacco; and taking B vitamins, natural progesterone, and other supplements. Soon after following my advice, my patients would report that their symptoms had disappeared. But three months later, many were back where they had started. They had let the substances they were supposed to avoid creep back into their lives while their daily stresses remained the same. Needless to say, their symptoms also returned.

Why didn't my patients just continue to follow the doctor's orders? I didn't know how to motivate my patients to make the lifestyle changes permanent. I thought bloating, headaches, irritability, and mood swings would be enough motivation to make them stick to the program.

As I talked to my patients, however, I began to see common patterns of childhood traumas, sexual abuse, memories of abuse, unaddressed marital problems, and all sorts of hidden emotional issues that rose to the surface during those days before their menstrual periods. I began to make the correlation between unresolved trauma and PMS symptoms. That's when I realized that the menstrual cycle actually provided a powerful monthly opportunity for deep healing.

At that point, I began to question why it was that so many women suffered as part of a perfectly natural biological cycle that followed the 28-day cycle of the moon. Why would the Creator make women this way? Over time, I realized that I, too, was emotionally sensitive and deeply in touch with my spirit premenstrually and during the first couple of days of my period. I started to see that not only was my experience common, it was a gift, an opportunity to reboot my life on all levels. Think of it this way: Just before and during your period, the tide is out. And everything on the bottom that you don't want to see will be revealed. Your true needs—for rest, for nourishing food, for pleasure, for nurturance, and more—are signaled by the depth of your emotions. This isn't a bad thing. Experiencing anger, sadness, fear, or jealousy is a biologically supported opportunity to transform yourself. Use your emotions as a guidance system that directs you to your true needs. Learn the lessons your feelings have to teach you.

As I was educating myself about how women have experienced menstruation in various places in the world throughout history, I read that certain Native American tribes relied on the intuitive knowledge of menstruating women to guide the tribe. It occurred to me that a woman who is not struggling with unhealed abuse or trauma could spend that sensitive time just before and during her period in a state of restoration and replenishment—just like the womb itself. She could become deeply in touch with the voice of her soul. As I wrote in *Women's Bodies, Women's Wisdom,* "The ebb and flow of dreams, creativity, and hormones associated with different parts of the cycle offer us a profound opportunity to deepen our connection with our inner knowing. This is a gradual process for most women, one that involves unearthing our personal history and then, day by day, thinking differently about our cycles and living with them in a mindful way."[1]

Latham Thomas, the author of *Mama Glow: A Hip Guide to Your Fabulous Abundant Pregnancy* (Hay House, 2012), is a modern yoga teacher and life coach who lives this wisdom in the hustle and bustle of New York City. Every month, she books time off during her periods and chooses to use those days to rejuvenate. Like indigenous women who moved into a separate tent for the days when they were menstruating, she is recognizing the sacred nature of this time. In addition, she realizes that this consciously applied self-care ritual provides her with more than enough energy and stamina to make up for any perceived loss of time. Her impressive monthly self-care is all the more stunning given how difficult it is for most of us to unplug at any time—especially in this age of information overload!

According to Eric Schmidt, executive chairman of Google, we human beings create as much information in two days as we did from the dawn of civilization up through 2003.[2] Despite the revolution in information technology, our cyclic nature has remained the same for millennia. We are still strongly connected with the tides and the moon. Our deep emotional needs don't disappear just because our To Do lists have grown much longer.

To achieve transformation, a woman has to get in touch with the emotions that lie hidden below the surface of her awareness. She needs to understand that each and every emotion signals a genuine need. She needs to rest and receive support and listen to her wise inner healer that is urging her to make changes in her life.

When we find the courage to do this, we experience the health and well-being that are our birthrights as goddesses.

YOUR EMOTIONAL GUIDANCE SYSTEM

The inner healer knows that emotions are a potent guidance system to what healer Mercedes Kirkel calls our "divine attributes." The heavier, darker emotions such as grief and anger have to be expressed and transformed so we can flourish. We experience this healing release through tears, movement, and sound. The matriarchal cultures of old understood the power of dance and song to heal the tribe and reconnect the community to the life force itself. As they danced, sang, or chanted, people experienced the full range of emotions from joy to sorrow. As the tears flowed, anger and grief left the body and returned to the sacred Source. Author Rita Schiano wrote, "Tears are God's gift to us. Our holy water. They heal us as they flow."

These so-called "negative" emotions are powerful indicators of unmet needs, and those needs are part of our humanity. For most of us, this is a revelation. We all have needs for connection, intimacy, validation, safety, love, belonging, and rest, to name just a few. (There's a marvelous list of human needs you can find on the website of The Center for Nonviolent Communication at www.cnvc.org, where you'll also find an emotions inventory.) But most of us have been led to believe that we should somehow sublimate our needs to the needs of others. When we do this, our emotions have to shout louder and louder—often through physical symptoms—in order to get our attention.

The next time you feel anger or resentment, just sit with the feeling—do *not* blame yourself or anyone else for it. Don't kill the "messenger." Just stay with what you are feeling so you can discover its message for you. Then ask yourself, "What is it that I need right now that I don't have?" Then name the need. Here's an example: You're in a hurry and someone pulls ahead of you into a parking spot you were waiting for. In that moment, you feel anger or frustration. You take a moment and simply allow the feeling of that to wash over you. You feel the emotion fully, without trying to change it. Then you say to yourself, "What do I need?" The answer might be one of the following: *More leisure time so I'm not always in a hurry. Respect from the other driver. More sleep—so I don't feel so frazzled all the time.* Simply acknowledging the need is the first step toward getting that need met.

Dr. Mario Martinez also points out the value of righteous anger—the kind that flares up when the innocence of someone around us, or our own innocence, is threatened. If someone is nasty to a waitress who is serving you, for example, it's perfectly healthy to express how you feel about this rather than remaining silent. We must allow ourselves to feel our righteous anger when appropriate and take some kind of healthy action that is suitable to the situation. Sometimes that might mean waiting till we get home to blow off some steam.

Affirm that you have the power to get that need met—either through another person or through your connection with the Divine. By listening to the messages your emotions bring you, and honoring them, you can experience ageless living rather than be weighed down by old resentments and grief that will affect you at a cellular level. You can bring in joy, generate nitric oxide, and tap the wisdom of your inner healer to repair your body, mind, and spirit.

HOW THE INNER HEALER WORKS

Diseases don't just appear out of nowhere. They're the final result of a process that takes time to develop. They are, quite literally, an imbalance in the system that is usually the result of years and years of neglecting to engage in the causes of health, which include pleasure, exalted emotions, and righteous anger—most of which our culture has never taught us! If you listen to your body's messages and heed them, you can very often prevent disease and reverse it long before it becomes established.

Most of us share a culturally supported belief that disease and infirmity are inevitable. They are normal in our culture, yes. But if you look at the so-called Blue Zones around the globe, such as Okinawa, Japan, and Ikaria, Greece—places with unusually high concentrations of healthy older people, first identified by explorer and traveler Dan Buettner—you find that ill health doesn't need to be the norm.

The most common chronic degenerative diseases today—heart disease, arthritis, cancer, dementia, and diabetes—start with chronically high levels of the stress hormone cortisol. High cortisol levels, combined with a diet high in sugar that causes uneven blood sugar levels, create insulin resistance, chronic inflammation, and oxidation, which are the root causes of all chronic degenerative disease. If inflammation isn't checked, it causes tissue damage in the lining of the blood vessels. Those damaged blood vessels then attract platelets that stick together and adhere to the walls of the vessels as plaques. The result is hardening of the arteries—and this happens in the brain too. Oxidation causes cellular damage, particularly to the mitochondria, which are the power centers of the cells.

The vast majority of cancers also develop over time and in stages. In a healthy body, cells replicate and then die so that they can be replaced by newer, younger cells that are less prone to mutations. One of the important effects of cell death, or apoptosis, is to cause mutated cells to die before they can replicate and begin to form tumors. Cell death is triggered by the mitochondria. If a cell's DNA has been damaged by a mutation (in most cases, more than one mutation), that cell's mitochondria may not do their job properly. The damaged cell continues to live and reproduce, fed by promoters such as excess estrogen, trans fats, and excess blood sugar. The cluster of mutated cells that results has long been referred to as a carcinoma in situ, meaning cancer (carcinoma) in a specific limited location (in situ). It also means that the microscopic cancer has not invaded the surrounding tissue. Carcinoma in situ is commonly called stage 0 cancer—an unfortunate name that has led thousands of people to have treatments they didn't need. That's because up until recently, we did not understand the biology of this type of cell. Researcher H. Gilbert Welch, M.D., an expert on cancer screening, calls these kinds of clusters things we will die *with* but not *from*.[3] In the vast majority of cases, the immune system simply prevents abnormal cells from growing any further. Unfortunately, it is this indolent, benign kind of change that is most often picked up on medical screening tests.

And it is also true that when abnormal cells are not destroyed by the immune system, if a network of blood vessels forms to supply them with nutrients, they can become a cancer that is invasive. Cells may then break off and travel through the bloodstream to other areas of the body, which is known as metastasis. Cancers are staged according to how far they have metastasized in the body, with stage 4 being the most invasive and widespread. Nearly all cancer deaths occur at this stage.

Now let's put things into perspective. The conventional approach to cancer is "early diagnosis" because of the belief that removing a cancer through surgery, radiation, or drugs when it is at its earliest stages is the best way to cure it. Unfortunately, this approach is far from benign. Consider that each of us makes cancer cells every day, but we never know it because our bodies heal themselves. A study published in the November 2008 edition of the *Archives of Internal Medicine* followed more than 200,000 Norwegian women between the ages of 50 and 64 for two consecutive years. Half received regular mammograms and breast exams while the other half had no regular screening. The women who underwent screening had 22 percent more breast cancer than the unscreened group. The researchers concluded that the women who weren't screened probably had the same number of cancers, but their bodies had corrected the abnormalities on their own.[4]

What happens when we become too aggressive in trying to "fix" conditions that our bodies might heal naturally? Since mass mammography screening was started in 1980, 1.3 million women have been diagnosed with so-called breast cancer that was really just ductal carcinoma in situ, which would never have become clinically evident. Far too many women have been diagnosed and then overtreated with bilateral mastectomies, radiation, or pharmaceutical drugs to eradicate cancer. Seventy thousand women were overdiagnosed with breast cancer in 2008 alone. Though some women obviously benefitted from earlier diagnosis, the vast majority did not.[5] (I'll go into more detail about breast health in Chapter 4.)

We all know women who have died of breast cancer, so it feels like a very real threat to our health. Even so, most women overestimate their risk of dying from the disease. Sixty to 80 percent of breast cancer cases occur in postmenopause, are not aggressive, and do not metastasize. So while breast cancer can occur in younger women or be aggressive, neither of these scenarios is the most common. It's easy to forget this when you walk by the local park during breast cancer awareness month and see a field of pink cutouts of women representing deaths from breast cancer, a display designed to scare you into getting a mammogram. Education and awareness about any disease can distort our perceptions of risk and generate a lot of unnecessary fear.

(For more information on postmenopausal breast cancer, see www.breasthealthcancerprevention.com.)

If we're going to advocate awareness, here's what to be aware of at all times: The body is a marvelous creation designed by the Creator to be in a continual state of regeneration and repair to keep all its systems humming. Cells are constantly replacing themselves with healthy ones. Your body is designed to intervene with the disease process at every point and to prevent, slow down, and reverse this process to restore you to your natural state of health. Your immune system is designed to kick into gear and fight any pathogens or germs that enter the system. As you make choices that strengthen your immune system—such as finding things to feel joyful about—it becomes better able to surround, weaken, and kill pathogens.

The tools of Western medicine should be used when appropriate, but not as the first and only way of maintaining health and fostering agelessness. A physician can help you monitor symptoms of imbalances and pay attention to signs that you need to do more to enhance your health, but it's the Creator working within you that heals. Real health comes from Divine Love and infuses your body with vitality.

PRESCRIPTION MEDICATIONS

Seventy-five percent of people over 65 are on medications, and on average, they're taking five different drugs.[6] Most of these medications aren't necessary. The "tribe" I hang with vibrates in another reality entirely. I've heard my friend and colleague Gladys McGarey, M.D., say, "Ninety-three and prescription-free." She's still actively involved in changing the culture of medicine by lobbying in Washington and traveling around the world improving maternal and fetal health. Our unthinking acceptance of concepts like "prescription drugs for seniors" points to a mentality that drives people to see aging as an inevitable process of deterioration and decline.

If you do have chronic health issues that need to be addressed, you may benefit from medications that control symptoms and, in some cases, halt processes such as inflammation or control conditions like high blood pressure. But do yourself a favor. When you take your medication each day, affirm your ability to be whole and healthy and well. It's entirely possible that your need for the pill will just go away on its own. In the meantime, be grateful for the availability of a medication that is helpful!

Although Western medicine is too focused on medications and surgery, there is some good news on the medical front. Improvements include team treatment, such as ob/gyns now assembling obstetrics teams that include different types of medical professionals. Kaiser encourages group appointments for diabetics and other groups who can swap recipes and form wellness circles, whether in person or online. Medical schools are teaching new doctors about inflammation and the disease process. And ob/gyns are finally questioning the high rate of C-sections and labor inductions, which have doubled the rate of maternal death over the past 30 years. Labor inductions have also contributed to the birth of far too many premature babies—simply because we're so intervention driven! Pregnancy serves as a good metaphor: the body has its own timing and we have to stop aggressively intervening to try to control it. As more patients and healers recognize this truth, we'll see more changes in our health care systems—but don't hold your breath waiting. Access your own healing power now. It's right there waiting for you.

DON'T FEAR YOUR GENES!

Genes are a blueprint, not a destiny. It concerns me that so many women have been influenced to have unnecessary drastic surgery because of fears of their genes betraying them. We now have women undergoing a voluntary double mastectomy not only after breast cancer but also, sometimes, just out of fear that they might get breast cancer because they carry a gene mutation that might put them at high risk. Every woman should be respected for making her own health choices, but the story that so often plays out in the media goes something like this: "Brave mother sacrifices breasts so her children won't suffer." In any given case, we don't know how the risk of developing breast cancer was calculated, and putting a number on an individual's risk is very difficult given the research we have. What the media tends to ignore outright is the role of epigenetics, or gene expression, in disease. Scientists now know that our DNA contains not only coding in the form of genes, but also some of the triggers that turn on certain genes at certain times to specific degrees. We have more control over epigenetics than most believe.

When the Human Genome Project began in the 1990s, researchers believed they would identify more than 120,000 genes. To their surprise, they found we have only 25,000—fewer than can be found in an ear of corn or a fruit fly. It's not the genes, but the *expression* of the genes that determines the vast majority of our experiences. The science of epigenetics is still in its infancy, but we know that gene expression is strongly influenced by beliefs and emotions as well as by lifestyle choices. The so-called "junk" DNA, which scientists first believed was unnecessary duplicate coding, may be the key to understanding gene expression—and learning how to influence it. The fact that we initially assumed that this important part of our DNA must be "junk," just because we didn't see a purpose to it, says a lot about how closed-minded we can be about the incredible systems in the human body.[7]

Scientists know your DNA reflects the genetic legacy of your parents, their parents, and your ancestors. It's possible that it also reflects their emotional experiences. As researchers learn more about our DNA, maybe we'll find that our cells have encoded the traumas of our ancestors. Experiments in mice have shown that aversion to certain smells is passed down to the offspring after the parental mice were trained to avoid a certain smell by being shocked every time they smelled it.[8] While we know that a family history of heart disease may mean close relatives share genes and genetic markers, if we look back, we can often see in family stories hearts that are broken, conflicted, and prevented from loving fully. In my family, people tend to die of heart disease prematurely. My maternal grandmother died of a heart attack at 68. But my mother, who is nearly 90, says, "That has nothing to do with me." She is not living under the emotional constrictions that her mother did, and she's living a healthy, active life. If she has a "bad gene" for heart disease, she hasn't expressed it yet and may never do so.

Energies outside of our bodies affect our health as well. None of us is an island, and we are affected by the beliefs of our families, friends, and cultures. You may also find yourself taking on the emotions of others empathically, which will affect your stress levels. Have you ever walked away from a conversation or even a phone call feeling as though you could lie down and fall asleep? That's because that person was, literally, draining your life force. Dr. Mario Martinez points out that our experience of our health is also very much dependent upon the beliefs held within our culture. Migraines are one example; they're perceived and treated differently in different countries. In France, they are seen as related to the liver. In England, they are considered digestive. And in the U.S., they're thought to be neurovascular. Consequently, the treatments differ from country to country.

Radiation and pollution are just two external forces that influence what happens in our bodies and which genes are expressed. Radiation causes DNA damage that can lead to cancer unless the process of cellular damage is quelled. Thankfully, sunlight—which produces radiation—also helps your body generate vitamin D, a vital nutrient for good health. In fact, experts estimate that having optimal levels of vitamin D in the body cuts your risk of cancer in half!

It's counterproductive to worry about your genetics and whether you'll inherit the diseases and medical conditions that run in your family. It's not the genetics per se that are a problem so much as worrying about what terrible disease may befall you, along with the long-term stress caused by a fearful, pessimistic belief system. The fact that you have a gene for a particular disease doesn't mean the gene will express. It's estimated that 80 percent of all illnesses begin in the mind. Metaphysical healer Edgar Cayce said, "The spirit is the life, the mind is the builder, the physical is the result." In other words, work with Spirit to design the house (your health) and let your thoughts, beliefs, and emotions serve to build it. If you like a garden metaphor, you can think of Spirit as the wind, rain, and sun. The mind plants the seeds. The body is the garden. Are you going to plant fear or are you going to plant faith and water it with a positive mind-set and good health habits?

When you choose to take care of yourself not just by focusing on the physical health of a particular organ or system but by relaxing into your oneness with the Creator—physically, emotionally, and spiritually—you are influencing your genes' expression. Love and live with a fullness of heart, free of any fear of what might be encoded in your DNA. You can't change your genes, but you can change your inherited emotional patterns. Here's a prayer to inspire you: "Divine Beloved, please change me into someone who completely trusts my body and my genes."

LET YOUR INNER HEALER GUIDE YOUR CHOICES

Should you test for genes that, if expressed, would cause a serious illness or disease? My feeling is that you should make your decision based on what you plan to do with the information— and ask yourself if it's really information you need. Are you going to make positive lifestyle changes to reduce your chances of developing the disease? If so, why not do that anyway? If you're going to use the negative results as an excuse for not taking the best care of your body, why would you do that? Fewer than 5 percent of cancers are associated with genetics. Finding out you have, say, the BRCA1 gene mutation associated with breast cancer doesn't mean you will get breast cancer. Finding out you don't have it doesn't mean you won't get it, either. What's more, genetic tests can be very unreliable because they usually sequence only a small sample of your complete genome, so making a decision based on a genetic test is like trying to figure out someone's personality from looking at one snapshot.

A woman named Naomi has a family history of a fatal, untreatable autoimmune disorder that affects the lungs. You can't slow its development, nor can you cure it—the only hope is a lung transplant. Naomi has lost several close relatives to the disease, including her mother, and knows she can do tests to track her lung health to determine her risk if she chooses to. There is also a genetic test that will show whether she inherited a gene mutation that may be associated with the disease. However, she's decided not to do genetic tests or baseline lung function tests. Instead, she's choosing to live as healthfully as possible and to stay apprised of the research that is showing promise for people who develop the disease. She breathes freely, figuratively speaking—free of fear that she might hurt someone's feelings or disappoint them. Perfectionism and people pleasing, she says, are a family trait she's refusing to carry on or pass down to her own children.

Naomi says that growing up, she saw that whenever her mother or her mother's sister got angry with the other, they avoided a confrontation and complained to their mother, who conveyed the message to the other sister. Because the women never directly confronted each other, anxiety ran high among the three women. How can you relax when you never know whether someone you love is angry at you? Naomi grew up following her mother's pattern of trying to read people's minds, walking on eggshells, and worrying endlessly about whether anyone was upset with her. At one point, Naomi realized her anxious behavior patterns were too painful to live with anymore. She began exercising regularly and underwent cognitive behavioral therapy to learn how to break her anxious thought processes. After her mother developed the disease and had to use oxygen tanks to breathe, Naomi began a mindfulness meditation practice. "When I saw how terrified my mother was not being able to breathe easily, and heard her tell me her worst fear was to die not being able to draw breath, I knew that learning to breathe in every sense of the word was key to my own well-being. I knew I had to slow down and focus on my life and stop running around worrying about everyone else and what they might think of me."

Naomi feels she is using her inner healer as inspiration—to see all aspects of herself so that she doesn't need to manifest an autoimmune disorder. Autoimmune disorders, 80 percent of which occur in women, result when the immune system attacks the body's own tissues—essentially, the self attacking the self. It's interesting that many women develop autoimmune diseases after the chronic stress of spending years caretaking for their ailing parents. That's a route Naomi had no interest in taking. The anger and cellular inflammation that were present in her body and spirit weren't working for her, and she decided she would rather be healthy and happy than hold on to all that old resentment, even if she did believe she was entitled to it. "It really stunk that I had to lose so much time to caretaking, and that my decision to put my parents' needs so high on my list meant neglecting the needs of my family and myself, but it was my decision and I decided to accept that I'd made it, even though I wasn't happy with all the consequences," she explained.

The worst thing you can do for your health is hold on to anger, fear, and sadness rather than release them. You want your vital life force to be strong so it can support cellular repair and regeneration, lower inflammation and cortisol levels, more stable blood sugar levels, and reduced oxidative stress (the activity of free radicals in the body, which you'll learn more about later). Naomi is listening to her inner healer and making inspired choices for herself—choices that are divinely guided, not fear based. She knows the importance of boosting her immunity by learning to accept herself, letting go of her anxiety about how other people see her, and getting in touch with her natural healer.

Alleviating emotional stressors and avoiding environmental toxins can assist your inner healer to both tend the garden of your health and choose not to express genes for disease. And it's also important to relax and realize that it's not possible to avoid all toxins all the time!

DON'T FEAR YOUR TEST SCORES!

Numbers on a diagnostic test can be helpful indicators of a condition that needs to be addressed, but don't give them too much weight and let them worry you. According to Gerd Gigerenzer, director of the Harding Center for Risk Literacy in Berlin and the author of the book *Risk Savvy* (Viking, 2014), both doctors and patients tend to overestimate risk for disease of all kinds—which leads to far too many unnecessary procedures in general. Here's the truth: your thoughts and beliefs have a far bigger impact on your health than your medical test scores do (just as they also have a bigger impact on your health than your genes do). I once witnessed a man who was intubated and in the intensive care unit, with an oxygen level so low he should have been unconscious, sit up and write his last will and testament on a yellow legal pad. This should have been impossible, but his mind compelled his body to follow its dictates. I've also seen more than my share of vibrantly healthy people in their 80s with cholesterol levels above 300. It's a good thing no one ever put them on statins to lower their levels, which clearly weren't causing them health problems.

Medical tests are far less reliable than most people think. How often has someone said, "I went to the doctor and I got a clean bill of health" and been reassured by a test score, only to have a heart attack the next day? Conversely, how often has someone felt just fine and then been given a diagnosis of some dread disease—and died within months? When a patient is told bad news, it's often the news itself and the stress hormone reaction to it that hastens the progress of the disease. In fact, research has shown that stress hormones actually produce substances that speed up the growth of certain types of cancers.[9]

Sometimes test results show a problem, but when you repeat the test, the numbers are in the normal range. I've had several patients go to the operating room only to find that the original abnormality was gone by the time they got there. This happens more than we're led to believe. Also, doctors are human—and fallible. Five different pathologists can read your biopsy report and give you five different interpretations. Which lab you use, who is on duty reading lab results, and the time of day can all affect the accuracy of any test.

The problem with all medical testing is that once you find an abnormality, you're obligated to keep looking for more things—doctors don't want to "miss" something. That's all part of the training and the system. It's hard for doctors and patients to adopt an attitude of "wait and see" and emphasize making better lifestyle choices. One example is a bimanual pelvic exam. If you aren't experiencing any symptoms of a disease or disorder, there is no reason why your ob/gyn has to put on gloves, insert two fingers into your vagina, and push down on your belly to feel your uterus and ovaries. I was trained to do this on every woman. And more times than I'd like to admit, I'd feel something that I wasn't sure about, so I'd have to send the woman for an ultrasound.

Then, if that wasn't definitive, I'd have to schedule her for a laparoscopy—a surgery that requires general anesthesia. Most of the time, everything was normal. On the other hand, I sometimes found things I wasn't expecting—like endometriosis—in a completely healthy and symptom-free woman! I have learned that just having a diagnosis doesn't actually mean you are sick.

Increasingly, we're realizing we've been far too aggressive in treating conditions that indicate a problem *may* develop in the future. I've already mentioned the drawbacks of screening mammograms, which, because of the new high-resolution machines, are picking up an increasing number of lesions that would never have caused any problems. The Pap smear is another test that requires rethinking. There is almost no reason for a woman to have a yearly Pap smear if she's healthy. In the U.S., we're spending $5.4 billion annually administering Pap smears and $1.2 million in follow-up examinations to find the 1 percent of women tested whose scrapings of cervical cells indicate there could be a problem. Cervical cancer is on the decline, and the 2002 rate was 8.2 per 100,000 women. The American Society for Colposcopy and Cervical Pathology now recommends that women be screened for cervical cancer every five years, not every year, if they test negative for cervical cytology (which is what the Pap test is screening for) and also for HPV.[10] And happily, the vast majority of women with healthy immune systems clear HPV from their systems on their own. In other words, it usually does *not* present a problem in the vast majority of women.

Of course, if you're having pain, discharge, bloating, or spotting, you should look into what's going on in your body and your emotions. But if you make the mistake of thinking that disease screening is actually health care, you won't tap into your most vibrant, healthy self. You'll be in neutral waiting for something bad to happen instead of in a state of flourishing and vibrancy. Go ahead and get medical tests, but if you don't like the results of a test, address the issue with the power of the mind and emotions—and then take the test again. Don't be surprised if you see a very different result.

There are certain tests that truly can assist you in creating better health. Fasting blood sugar is one of them. Your fasting blood sugar should be no higher than 85 mg/dl, and an hour after a meal, your blood sugar should go no higher than 120 mg/dl. It's useful to get a glucometer (you can pick one up at a drugstore for about $10) and test your blood sugar regularly to know exactly what foods and activities spike it too high. It's also useful to measure your fasting insulin level. Testing for vitamin D levels is a very good idea too. For vitamin D, get a 25(OH)D blood test, not a 1,25(OH)2D test. It's the 25(OH)D that will tell you how much vitamin D is in your blood. This can be done through your doctor or an online lab (see Resources for online labs I recommend). Your level should be 40–80 ng/ml—and it will usually take at least 5,000 IU of vitamin D a day to get it there and keep it there. You'll want to be sure that your blood pressure is around 120/70, give or take a few points either way. Note that the values I'm citing here for blood sugar are lower than standard medicine allows and the levels of vitamin D are higher. These reflect the difference between optimal levels and minimal levels. Ageless goddesses shoot for what's optimal.

So while modern medicine and medical tests have their place, never underestimate the power of your beliefs to affect your health for the better—or the worse. Alternative health practitioner and author Andrew Weil, M.D., told me years ago that one of the primary sins of modern medicine is its ability to undermine people's experience of how they feel. If your sense of how well you're doing conflicts with the numbers shown on your medical test, question that. Former New York City mayor Ed Koch, known for his casual folksiness, used to stand at subway entrances, shaking the hands of commuters and asking, "How'm I doin'?" Medical tests are for asking, "How'm I doin'?" and checking in with how well you're engaging in self-care. They are not meant to provoke anxiety about any potential signs of disaster.

And remember this: no matter what your diagnosis may be, there's always hope. In the last 20 years, we've come a long way with our understanding of the mind/body connection and its impact on the body. For example, in *You Are the Placebo*, Dr. Joe Dispenza documents his extensive research (done using modern brain scanning techniques) that proves it's entirely possible to learn how to change the biology of our brains and bodies by harnessing the power of the placebo—meaning that when you expect something to work, it often does. And in her studies of those whose advanced cancer has inexplicably reversed, Kelly Turner, Ph.D., author of *Radical Remission: Surviving Cancer Against All Odds* (HarperOne, 2014), has identified a number of factors that favor survival even when modern medicine has nothing further to offer. Many of these factors are identical to those recommended in the Ageless Goddess Program, such as releasing suppressed emotions, embracing social support, deepening spiritual connection, changing your diet, and so on.

The earlier you respond to any condition you have, the greater your chances of resolving it for good—and that includes pesky things like allergies! Trust Divine Love and make use of the placebo effect by generating positive beliefs about your health and ability to return to a state of well-being. Recognize the power of the mind to create illness or health. And avoid chronic negative self-talk, which too many women habitually engage in. It's incredible how many times an hour we can beat ourselves up with self-criticism. Writer Anne Lamott says the mind is too often a bad neighborhood and you shouldn't go there alone!

I don't mean to imply that if you have a health condition, somehow you are to "blame" for it—far from it. The mind is powerful, but so are the collective mind and the mind of the Divine. We can't always know why everything happens, what the larger plan is, or why we develop a medical condition despite our best efforts to stay positive. What we do know is that by looking at every situation in life as an opportunity for deeper healing, deeper love, and deeper compassion for ourselves and others, we optimize our health and the health of our communities.

LISTEN TO YOUR INSTINCTS

To awaken your inner healer, you have to listen to your intuition and instincts about your own body. If a medical practitioner gives you advice that doesn't ring true for you in your unique situation, listen to your resistance and explore it. Sometimes you just know something isn't right for you, even if you can't explain why. Other times, when you do a little research, you realize that research and logic back up your instincts. We've had it drilled into us that we shouldn't trust ourselves, only our doctors, but our bodies and our spirits don't lie to us. You might find yourself having a symbolic dream that gives you insight into your situation, or you might feel a heaviness or emotional resistance that isn't coming from fear but from an inner knowing. When that happens, don't ignore it. I used to say to all of my patients who were facing surgery that they could call me anytime beforehand and cancel. I told them I'd happily wheel them out of the operating room before their procedure if, on the day of their surgery, they changed their minds! Believe me, this permission to listen to yourself really reduces fear and clears the path for your inner healer to speak!

Not all medical advice fits every person, but I need to call out the media on its constant fearmongering that scares people into herd mentality. Flu shots are an example. Vaccines for shingles are another. I can't help but notice that the number of people getting shingles has skyrocketed ever since the chicken pox vaccine became standard. They are the same virus, for heaven's sakes! You have to ask yourself, "What is going on here?" And the evidence to support widespread use of the flu vaccine, which is formulated based on the best guess of which flu viruses will affect people in flu season, is much less robust than the public has been led to believe. What is really being sold here is a sense of safety and security. If *not* getting a flu shot makes you feel really vulnerable, then the shot might be fine for you. After all, it's our sense of safety and security that directly and powerfully affects our immunity. But given that vaccines are not 100 percent safe, I recommend shoring up your sense of safety in other ways that don't involve needless risks. The flu vaccine—which, by the way, almost always contains mercury, a known neurotoxin, as a preservative—has also been known to set off autoimmune disorders in some people. And the flu vaccine isn't 100 percent effective. We all know people who got the shot and then had the worst flu of their lives. The herd mentality that drives people to automatically get a vaccine or take a pill because they're afraid of not getting one is not creating herd immunity. If you get a flu vaccine every year, ask yourself whether you're doing it to avoid taking care of yourself in other ways. Just as with doing medical tests, the question is, why aren't you taking care of yourself anyway?

The alternative to giving in to your fear and automatically getting a flu shot (or taking a statin drug, or getting a hysterectomy, or making any choice simply because you've been told it's "the best thing to do" in your situation) is to follow the basic formula of health:

~ Increase your body's ability to fend off germs and viruses.

~ Reduce inflammation and free radical activity that damages cells and tissues.

~ Allow your body the time, space, and environment to repair and heal itself when necessary, which includes taking good antioxidant supplements.

~ Use whatever you are drawn to—surgery, pharmaceutical drugs, whatever feels and seems right to you—to control deterioration, damage, and symptoms when necessary.

When it comes to any vaccine, medication, or operation, read about its pros and cons—and get more than one medical opinion if you're considering an operation. Then check in with your inner healer. If it feels right and makes sense for *you* to have this treatment, let go of any fear. Say a prayer of blessing as you receive it, imbue it with Divine Love, and ask Spirit to use it to protect you and help you to be your healthiest self. If you receive a medical diagnosis or test results that frighten you, take a few relaxing breaths, and connect with the Creator and that still, small voice within. Turn over your diagnosis and your body to the Creator—as an offering. The Divine made you. The Divine knows what to do. Now wait for guidance.

Here's a prayer I use all the time: "With my spirit and the angels' help, I focus Divine Love throughout my system and bring Divine Love into my (area of the body you are concerned about). I ask that this problem now be resolved with Divine Love according to the Creator's will." After saying this, draw in your breath, hold it for about four seconds, and then exhale in bursts through your nose, as though clearing it of mucus. Gently focus on that area of your body and imagine Divine Love filling it with light and healing.

Keep in mind that what I'm describing is a spiritual process, not a mind/body process. When you sincerely ask for Divine Help, it always comes. Divine Love does the rest of the work. After asking for Divine Love to help, pay attention to any guidance you receive. While taking a friend through this recently, I asked her to do the petition and then tell me what she "heard" or "saw" afterward. She said, "Sadness." Then she simply asked that the sadness be released with Divine Love.

Now that you know about your inner healer, which works with the guidance and assistance of Divine Love, let's look at some common health conditions and the tests used to diagnose them from the perspective of knowing that your inner healer is on the job. Whatever your health concerns, you can transmute any fear or anxiety into actions that nourish the garden of your health. And remember that the inner healer works only in an environment of faith and trust. You can always use the following to calm your mind while you're waiting for clarity: "Divine Beloved, change me into someone who trusts my divine guidance and knows that I will be shown the next step."

CHAPTER FOUR

GODDESSES UNDERSTAND THE CAUSES OF HEALTH

I have come to believe that cancer is the physical metaphor for the extreme need to grow.

— LEWIS THOMAS, M.D., FORMER DIRECTOR OF
MEMORIAL SLOAN-KETTERING HOSPITAL

R ecently, I was asked to provide ten health tips for a well-known women's publication. It's a common request I receive, because everyone wants simple keys to good health. The editor wanted me to come up with a list of things like cutting back on sugar, drinking more water, and having good friends—and all that's good stuff. But I also mentioned that it was important to have a relationship with the Divine. The editor said, "We're a traditional magazine. And talking about God is a little far out for our readers. Can you please replace that tip with something like 'get regular checkups'?" Now, keep in mind that regular checkups have not been found to improve health! And 90 percent of Americans say they believe in God. But a magazine editor doesn't want to "go there" because we've been taught to put spirituality in one box and health in another.

When you reconnect with Spirit and your own spirit, seeing yourself as a goddess, you have a completely different perspective on health. You realize you have more power than you thought to create wellness because you're not doing it alone—you're doing it with the help of the divine feminine force that knows how to cleanse the toxins in her waters, prune away the old growth, and bring forth new life. Of course, you want your healthspan and lifespan to match up—and they can, allowing you to relish great health. However, you also have to acknowledge your need to access your inner healer, whose wisdom and power are informed by Spirit. Good health starts upstream, with emotions and thoughts—not supplements and medical tests (although those can help).

If you have a chronic disease or ailment, you probably already know the basics of managing your medical condition—and you know that stress will worsen the symptoms, while tending to your body's needs will improve them, sometimes dramatically. But whether you have a medical condition or not, let's dispel the idea that health is determined by your genes or by the march of time.

Too often, discussions of women's health after 40 focus on fluctuations in the sex hormones (estrogen, progesterone, and testosterone), diseases, and decline. It's easy to forget that our bodies are designed to repair and replenish our cells and balance our biochemistry. But you're on your way to adopting a completely new way of looking at health—and at how to balance your systems to optimize your body's functioning.

Yes, your hormonal system is involved in your state of health, but the hormones you most need to start paying attention to are your stress hormones. You also have to look at the amount of sleep or rest you're getting, because you need to give your body time to recharge and generate new, healthier cells. And instead of worrying about the diseases of the heart, breast, uterus, ovaries, and brain, you have to support all your organs with good nutrients, pleasurable thoughts and emotions, and activities that are vitally important for your physical health—and I'm not simply talking about moving your body. I'm talking about listening to your ageless soul and expressing love, creativity, and joy. When you look at typical women's health issues, even as you give your body the physical support it needs, I want you to think beyond the literal and start seeing your state of physical being as reflective of your state of emotional, mental, and spiritual well-being. Your heart isn't just a muscle and your pelvis isn't just the place where your body nurtures a baby. You are so much more than the sum of your parts!

Dr. Mario Martinez describes disease as an imbalance of our bodies' systems over time that eventually leads to measurable pathology. Modern medicine is nothing more than the study of that pathology. When we engage in what Dr. Martinez calls the "causes of health," we stay way ahead of the pathology curve. He identifies the causes of health as: exalted emotions such as compassion, joy, and love; elevated cognition (focusing on what's positive); and righteous anger, allowing yourself to feel angry when your innocence has been violated. It doesn't matter if the violation took place years earlier; feeling your righteous anger and getting it out of your system can improve your health. No matter what your diagnosis or state of health, know that you can improve it by indulging in behaviors and thoughts that actually improve your health—not just treat disease.

THE SECRETS OF HORMONES

Hormones have received a lot of press, but the truth is that in perimenopause or menopause, the number-one hormone to be concerned about is not estrogen or progesterone, or even testosterone, but cortisol. A stress hormone, cortisol is designed to be used by the body in situations of acute stress to help you deal with physical danger quickly. Imagine yourself as a cavewoman throwing a big rock at a hissing poisonous snake that's about to strike, or running away at top speed. Cortisol also temporarily activates the immune system in case the danger isn't a snake but a bacteria or virus that has entered your system. It sets off an inflammatory response in which white blood cells gather around the pathogen to isolate it before attacking it. This sympathetic nervous system reaction happens very quickly. The problem is that if the cortisol and its partner, epinephrine (adrenaline), are not cleared from your system quickly and instead linger for days or even weeks or months, they have the opposite effect of lowering your immunity and energy. Chronic fear, anger, sadness, and resentment keep stress hormones in your system for too long, breaking down your immunity, thinning your skin and bones, causing weight gain, and setting the stage for poor health—including depression, cancer, and heart disease. If you've ever seen someone blow up like a balloon on high-dose steroids such as prednisone, you've seen the effect of excess stress hormones.

Estrogen, progesterone, and testosterone get much more press than cortisol and adrenaline do even though they're far less likely to adversely affect your health. It's true that the amounts of these hormones in the body change during the transitional period of perimenopause, and sometimes that shift causes uncomfortable symptoms. But there's nothing about menopause per se that will plummet you into hormonal hell, rage-aholic behavior, and a feeling of being lost in a sexual desert. It's a myth that in a healthy, happy woman, menopause will shut down her ovaries for good and make her shrivel into an asexual crone. After perimenopause has ended, hormones return to the level of pre-adolescence, and there's nothing wrong with those levels. Fatigue, insomnia, low libido, mental sluggishness, irritability, and hot flashes—particularly when they interfere with sleep—do not have to be a part of the perimenopausal or menopausal experience. You can reduce these symptoms naturally with a minimal amount of outside hormonal help when necessary.

Let's look at how things can get out of balance. With your ovaries now decreasing their hormonal output, your adrenal glands take over some of the work of generating progesterone, estrogen, and testosterone—as well as DHEA, which serves as a building block for the other hormones. But if your adrenal glands, which are walnut-sized organs that sit on top of your kidneys, are overproducing cortisol and adrenaline, they will start to become tired out and overwhelmed by their task of generating the stress hormones. Your multitasking adrenals have to set priorities. They will favor your need for stress hormones, which can then throw off the production and metabolism of your other hormones.

When your hormones are out of balance due to overproduction of cortisol, you feel the effects. You get cravings for sugar—particularly around 4:00 P.M. when cortisol naturally peaks. If you reach for a cupcake rather than taking a short walk to help your body break down the cortisol, you'll stimulate the adrenal glands further, causing them to release even more cortisol, which will spike your blood sugar levels. Four o'clock is like the PMS stage of the daily cycle; you're meant to go for a walk, take a nap, or get in touch with your feelings and inner wisdom, not reach for sugar. When you're aware of and in control of the relationship between your blood sugar, your emotions, your diet, and your exercise patterns, you'll be far less likely to respond to your cortisol spikes by consuming sugar or alcohol—a move that only worsens your hormonal state.

If you've had your uterus and/or ovaries removed—or if you're too stressed out by hormonal shifts to put the effort into exercising, changing your eating habits, or experiencing pleasure through sex or other means—you may need to check your hormone levels and take steps to adjust them, specifically with either bioidentical hormones or phytoestrogens such as *Pueraria mirifica* (see Resources). There are three ways to test hormones: saliva tests, blood tests, and urine tests. After working with all three of these for many years, my favorite—and the one I consider the most reliable at the moment—is serial urine testing, which tests for not only estrogen, progesterone, and testosterone but also patterns of stress hormone release. (You can learn more at www.precisionhormones.com and in Resources.)

If test results and symptoms confirm that you're low in estrogen, I suggest that you try taking a phytoestrogen, derived from plant sources (you'll find specifics on that and other recommended supplements and products in the Resources section). There's been a lot of confusion on this issue and many women worry unnecessarily that taking a supplement such as black cohosh, maca, flaxseed, or *Pueraria mirifica* could lead to cancer. Let me be very clear: there is no solid evidence that links phytohormones with cancer. If you were to look at the molecules for plant sterols such as phytoestrogens under a microscope, you would see that their chemical structure is completely different from mammalian estrogen. They can't stimulate the growth of estrogen-sensitive tissues in the same way a prescription hormone would. For the record, broccoli, peanuts, almonds, apples, and many other common foods also contain phytoestrogens.

Keep in mind, too, that there's often no correlation between how a woman feels and what her hormone levels are. I've seen women with very low estrogen and testosterone whose sexual appetite is just fine, and others who have perfectly healthy amounts of testosterone and estrogen but no sex drive at all. If you rely entirely on a test instead of how you feel to determine what's going on with you, you can scare yourself into taking medications or supplements you don't need.

SLEEP AND CELLULAR REPAIR

One of the most common complaints shared by many women is insomnia. Sleep is, hands down, the most effective way to metabolize excess stress hormones, which are the real culprits when it comes to hormone imbalance. Good quality sleep is absolutely essential to hormone health, and reducing stress improves sleep.

Fortunately, simple lifestyle changes can make a difference in your ability to fall asleep and stay asleep through the night. Try the following: Remove all electronic devices, including clocks with lighted displays, from your bedroom. At the very least, cover them at night. Don't work on a computer or mobile device such as a tablet when you're winding down for bed.[1] And create a sleep routine of going to bed around the same time every night and sleeping for at least eight hours. Don't watch the news or an intense movie before turning in for the night, and don't do any strenuous exercise either. If you feel a hot flash coming on, close your eyes and envision something cool, like sitting inside an igloo. Or take off a layer of clothing and stand in front of a fan. I'm a big supporter of the Chillow pillow, which you fill with water and insert into your pillowcase, where it stays cool throughout the night. Research has also shown that meditation, such as the "relaxation response" in which you close your eyes and repeat a mantra to yourself (such as "peace" or "inhale" and "exhale") for 20 minutes, reduces hot flashes significantly by reducing the stress hormones that contribute to them. In fact, anything you can do to decrease stress hormones decreases hot flashes. (You can find more ideas for managing menopausal symptoms naturally in *The Wisdom of Menopause*.)

When sleep disruption and hot flashes due to perimenopause are too disruptive, I recommend the herbal supplement *Pueraria mirifica*. Other helpful tools are valerian, melatonin, and Epsom salts, and you might want to try gels, oils, or bath crystals that promote relaxation.

Pueraria mirifica: A-ma-ta

Having been on the front lines of women's health for many years, I've long been interested in natural approaches to perimenopausal and menopausal symptoms, and also substances that help promote women's health on all levels. Several years ago, I received a call out of the blue from a Dr. Sandford Schwartz in Thailand, a researcher (originally from New York City) who has vast experience with the herb *Pueraria mirifica* (PM). Dr. Sandy, as he is called, convinced me to investigate the properties of this substance and try it using the patented form known as Puresterol. There are many different subspecies of PM, and to be effective, the right type of plant must be harvested at the right time by skilled foragers. Then the active ingredients must be standardized. This is what Puresterol is—a patented standardized extract of the right type of PM from Thailand, where it is sustainably harvested. Impressed with the research—and with the results that women were reporting—I eventually started my own company as a way to get the word out about this substance. The company is called A-ma-ta, a name derived from the Thai word for "ageless." I wanted women everywhere to have the opportunity to find relief for their perimenopausal and menopausal symptoms through using this herb, and to experience its "youthifying" effects. I never thought I'd start my own company—but in doing so, I have the quality control to make sure that women are getting the right amounts and the right formulation. *Pueraria mirifica* has also been shown to build bone mass, tone the breasts, and relieve vaginal dryness[2] as well as thicken vaginal walls, which tend to become thinner over time and can cause discomfort during intercourse.[3]

Women are reporting wonderful results with A-ma-ta products. And this is thrilling to me. "I didn't know what to expect, if anything," one user posted on the A-ma-ta website. "But within 2 weeks of starting the drops, well, let's just say I was shocked by the dramatic 'youthing' going on down there. Surprised, delighted, impressed." Another woman wrote, "I've been taking A-ma-ta 12 days and ladies . . . it truly is working. I have more energy, feel calmer, more rested, and the hot flashes are infrequent with much less intensity." Still another reported that after day three of taking A-ma-ta, "I actually fell asleep at a decent hour and woke up rested and without burning eyes. After a couple of weeks . . . I am more functional, calm, balanced, and joyful. . . . I can't wait to see and feel the positive changes in the future."

If you've tried these simple approaches to insomnia and are still having a problem, chances are good that your body is trying to get you to address some deeper issues. When Sue was going through a midlife divorce, she found herself waking up at 3:00 A.M. every night, and no matter what she did, this pattern continued. She finally stopped fighting it and instead decided to keep pen and paper nearby to record her dreams and inspirations that came pouring in at that time of night. Within a month, Sue realized that there were stories that wanted to come through her. She began to look forward to her late-night inspirations, and she eventually collected enough material to write a book.

My friend Wayne Dyer, Ph.D., writes all of his books in the wee hours of the night. He believes this is when God comes to us most clearly. And though I am not an early-morning writer— my best dreams are always around 7:30 to 8:30 A.M.—I'm well aware that 4:00 A.M. is considered the most yin (dark) time of night, when creative flow is likely to be especially powerful. In fact, this is when both animals and humans are most likely to give birth. And maybe it's when our souls want to come through to us to help us give birth to our highest selves. So rather than fight insomnia, you may want to consider whether it is a gift connecting you to your creative flow.

A HEALTHY HEART

Breast cancer has been branded with a pink ribbon, and now heart disease in women has also been branded—with a red dress—because heart disease is the number-one killer of women, surpassing breast cancer. Most people have been brainwashed into thinking that we have to have a disease in order to die. This belief, which robs us of vitality, is reinforced by all our "run for the cure" campaigns—none of which has ever done any good in actually decreasing the risk of getting a disease. It may even be the other way around, since what we resist persists. It's the Law of Attraction: we become what we think about and worry about the most. So as a first step in dealing with heart disease, breast cancer, or anything else, let's start fertilizing the idea that it's completely possible to die disease-free in our sleep when it's our time! Remember the goal: "Happy, healthy, dead!"

Heart disease comes on very slowly in most women. In fact, in Tulane University's Bogalusa heart study, which took place over a 44-year span, doctors found arteriosclerosis—the beginning of clogged arteries, which eventually leads to heart disease—in five-year-olds.[4] So you have years to address and reverse it if you monitor your health.

There are also some hormonal factors all women should know about. In his research on rhesus monkeys (and, later, on humans), researcher Kent Hermsmeyer, Ph.D., showed that natural progesterone, in contrast to synthetic progesterone such as Provera, causes coronary arteries to relax.[5] Many women with angina (heart pain) would do well to use natural progesterone, but they need to avoid the synthetic versions. The famous Women's Health Initiative study that was stopped abruptly in 2002 used Prempro as the hormone combination of choice for addressing women's menopause symptoms. The researchers found that using this artificial hormone combo correlated with an increased rate of death from heart disease. In fact, the study showed that the women taking this manmade hormone had a higher risk of heart disease *and* breast cancer. Since then, the medical profession has changed its tune and is now recommending the lowest dose of hormone for the shortest period of time necessary to relieve symptoms.

Here's more good news: the heart is very forgiving. Forgiving is a big part of its job, after all. It wants and needs to feel free, and carrying around resentment is just too much of a burden. Many people who have suffered heart attacks have healed by living in a wholehearted way that supports the wisdom of their hearts—wisdom that is all about passion, compassion, and loving deeply and freely. Getting things "off your chest" through forgiveness is more important than the effect of hormones on your heart. And the most important person to forgive is yourself. Letting go of your disappointments and harsh self-judgments is crucial for heart health and agelessness.

MENDING A BROKEN HEART

In the year following my divorce, I had my first bout of chest pain. I had picked up my then 16-year-old daughter at camp and had fantasized our reunion and joyful trip home together. My oldest had already gone off to college, so I had both an empty nest and an empty bed after 24 years of marriage. My sun and several other planets are in Libra, the sign of partnership, so my natural state is one of partnering. But my soul had decided that I was ready for an upgrade in this department. I needed to learn to be alone and not panic. The universe had ensured that I would start to lose people close to me so I could learn to loosen my attachments to others.

When I picked up my daughter at camp, she promptly fell asleep in the car, leaving me to drive for three hours without any conversation. I was very aware of being alone with my thoughts. When we got home, she bounded into the house and started calling her friends. So much for a cherished reunion! I felt like a fifth wheel, just someone who paid the bills and drove the car.

As I stood in the driveway, I had my first bout of chest pain. It radiated into my neck, and I knew that the pain was connected to my heart—but I also knew that it wasn't a heart attack. Still, I had an EKG and blood pressure taken to be sure. Everything was okay. My heart pain's purpose that day was to awaken me to my need to grow and to let go so that my daughter didn't have to stifle her own growth to meet my need for partnership.

Over the ensuing years, I developed this same heart pain about twice a year. And each time, the chest pain served as a kind of warning about a difficult emotional lesson that I still needed to learn. The pain never lasted more than 15 minutes. Heart disease runs in my family, but so does something else: a pattern of "smoothing things over," "keeping the peace," and "keeping things close to the chest." Getting things "off my chest" and being 100 percent honest about my true feelings, no matter how uncomfortable, was hard for me. All of those painful feelings were rooted in heartbreak about not having the love relationship I longed for.

The truth is that I had a big load of healing to do. I knew intellectually that I had to complete myself—to figure out how to be "whole, and complete, and lacking in nothing" (a description Unity minister Jill Rogers uses in her workshop The Seven Sacred Steps). But it's one thing to know a concept intellectually and quite another to embody it—to really, truly *feel* whole, and complete, and lacking in nothing whether or not you're in a relationship. This is especially true for a single woman in her ageless years who loves romance novels!

I had no lack of male attention, especially once I learned how to surrender to a man's lead in tango. It's just that almost none of the men who were attracted to me held any appeal for me other than as friends, and the two who did were not available. It was a heartbreaking pattern for me. I would think, *Oh, thank God. I've finally met a man who really turns me on, isn't jealous of my success, is fit and healthy, and is attracted to me. But once again, he's emotionally unavailable because of issues in his own life. Really? Are you kidding me?* Oh, the drama of my heartbreak! "Am I destined to be alone forever?" she says as she falls to the earth emitting heart-wrenching sobs.

The first step toward truly healing my heart was simply acknowledging the truth of what I was feeling: no judgment, no covering up, no shaming. And I am absolutely convinced that if I had not done serious emotional work to heal my past and my relationship patterns (which you'll learn more about in the next chapter), I would indeed have had a heart attack sooner or later. Or maybe I would have developed breast cancer. Instead, I transformed years of heartbreak into a wise, healed heart full of compassion for myself and others. Then I was able to let go of my need to cling to the people I loved with a death grip!

While many people are addicted to tobacco, alcohol, and food, my addiction of choice was relationships (an addiction often called codependence). By unflinchingly identifying this for what it truly was, and turning it over to God (about a million times!), I was able to nourish my heart's health. My heart is now free, happy, and whole. What a revelation! What a relief! This is true heart disease prevention. I want the same for you!

How to Love Your Heart

- *Appreciate that your heart is the energetic center of your body.* Like the Sun that is at the center of our solar system, your heart is the central "sun" that fuels every system in your body.

- *Recognize that your heart always wins.* When there's conflict between what you think and what you feel, what you feel wins—every time. If you don't listen to your heart trying to express its feelings, it may take an illness to get you to pay attention. That phrase "her heart just wasn't in it" when a relationship, job, or life dies is the truth. If your heart's not in it, why are you in it?

- *Forgive yourself and others.* Forgiveness is powerful physical medicine. Research has shown that resentment and hostility are very substantial risk factors for heart attacks. On the other hand, that old phrase "a merry heart doeth good like a medicine" is also true. Holding on to resentments and anger will age you. Forgiveness is not about the other person. It is about calling back your own worthiness from whoever or whatever hurt you and freeing yourself from the entrapment of the past.

~ *Focus on what you love and what you find beautiful in order to calm your fight-or-flight reactions.* Research by leading neuroscientist Dr. Richard Davidson at the University of Wisconsin has shown via functional MRI scans of healthy brains that a structure called the fusiform gyrus on the underside of the brain works in counterpoint to the amygdala, the primitive center that signals danger and the fight-or-flight response. The fusiform gyrus recognizes things we love and appreciate. The more we focus on what we love and value, the more enhanced the function of the fusiform gyrus and the calmer the amygdala. We become rewired for love, not fear.

~ *Create cardiac coherence.* Cardiac coherence comes when you smooth out erratic patterns of your heart rate so that your heart doesn't shift quickly from a relaxed state to beating quickly in response to perceived danger when there's no real threat to your safety. You can train your heart to be less reactive to emotional stressors so you don't regularly experience fight-or-flight responses to everyday life. One way to achieve cardiac coherence and an optimum heart rate variability (HRV) is by using a biofeedback device such as the emWave from the Institute of HeartMath. You can also meditate, practice mindful breathing, or, as I said, regularly think about what you value and love. Watch movies and listen to music that makes you feel loving and loved. Spend time looking at pictures of things you value: your kids, puppies, sleeping babies, fine art, nature scenes, or whatever. Over time, you can learn how to create this healthy heart state at will simply by tuning in to the exalted emotions associated with things you love.

~ *Listen to what is truly in your heart.* Change or
release old thought patterns and beliefs that no longer serve you. My chest pain is healed and so is my
heart. I'm perfectly comfortable and happy with my
life right now because I have learned to put the Divine first—not a man. Getting to this point has been,
quite frankly, harder than medical school, harder
than enduring several lawsuits, and harder than
going through a divorce. It has also been infinitely
more rewarding and exhilarating—and it's been the
work for which I was born. I have finally succeeded
in creating the sacred marriage of male and female
within myself—the *hieros gamos.* You, too, have a
heart that was designed to be whole, complete, and
healed, and this has nothing whatsoever to do with
whether or not you have a partner. Once your pain
has transformed and you have a solid connection
with the Divine Beloved within, you'll find that joy
and optimism are your natural state of being. Then,
ageless living is natural.

~ *Eat quality foods, especially vegetables, and also
healthy fats to support a healthy heart and express
love to it, but don't obsess about what's on your
plate.* Avoid processed foods, refined sugar, and trans
fats (hydrogenated and partially hydrogenated oils,
often found in snack foods and packaged desserts)
as much as possible. In the last 70 years, we have
increased the amount of these foods in our diets
while decreasing the amount of plant foods rich in
antioxidants. This dietary change coincides with the
rise of heart disease. The trans fats and sugars cause
oxidative stress that's toxic to the endothelial lining
of blood vessels unless you have enough antioxidants
in your system to counteract them.

~ *Experience the exalted emotions!* Schedule pleasurable activities into your life regularly, as this will
open your heart and help keep it fit. Dancing, going to movies and concerts, eating out with friends,
giving or receiving massages, playing with your dog

or cat—whatever makes you feel great, do it regularly. We tend to eat too much sugar or drink too much alcohol to quell painful emotions because of their opiate effect. Seeking pleasure and comfort is the pathway out. We humans are hardwired that way. However, importing chemical "pleasure" is not sustainable. It's addictive. Instead, treat yourself to activities that are inherently pleasurable.

~ *Move, and enjoy moving.* The body is designed to move so that your blood, lymph fluid, and oxygen can all circulate. Exercise promotes a healthy heart, but pleasurable movement is especially good for the heart. And remember, simply standing up 32 times a day if you sit at a computer can work wonders for preventing toxins from building up and cells from becoming damaged.

~ *Connect with Divine Love.* Your heart is fueled by this more than any other factor. Simply ask the Divine to help you feel your connection—and then, listen. Say "Divine Love now manifests in my heart. And now fuels my life."

CHOLESTEROL AND THE HEART

The same old myths about cholesterol and the heart continue to circulate even though research confirms that dietary cholesterol and high cholesterol are *not* risk factors for heart disease. In fact, your brain and nervous system are largely made of cholesterol, a vital substance manufactured in the body (which is why, when you eat animal products, you consume cholesterol). It's used to produce vitamin D and certain hormones, among other functions. In fact, when your overall cholesterol is too low, your body can't manufacture enough hormones to keep your system running efficiently. Depression often results, and the lower your cholesterol, the lower your testosterone and sex drive. Cholesterol is an important building block for hormones related to the libido. Molecules called LDL (low-density lipoprotein) and HDL (high-density lipoprotein) are actually cholesterol transporters that take this vital substance to cells that need it and transport the excess to your organs, which process and excrete it.

The role of HDL is to cart away excess cholesterol so the liver can process it. The job of LDL is to deposit cholesterol at receptor sites on the membranes of cells. LDL is only a problem when it becomes oxidized by free radicals. A free radical is a molecule that becomes unstabilized by losing an electron and seeks to steal an electron from another area to make up for the one that's missing. Traditionally, doctors have said that LDL is "bad cholesterol," but that's an inaccurate description. There's more than one type of LDL. LDL-B is dense and small and more likely to become oxidized than the other types of LDL, LDL-A and LDL-1. Oxidized LDL is big and sticky and doesn't interface properly with the cellular receptors seeking cholesterol. It holds on to the cholesterol and ends up sticking to the linings of inflamed arteries, forming the beginning of plaque. To counteract this process, you need to be sure you have enough antioxidants in the body to prevent LDL and the lining of your blood vessels from becoming oxidized. Dietary cholesterol doesn't cause the LDL to oxidize; free radicals do.

Aim for a diet that is free of trans fats, which both raise bad LDL and lower good HDL, and free of excess sugars that cause LDL to become oxidized. A diet high in sugars and low in fiber increases the amount of fat in your blood (the triglycerides), which then becomes stored in your body. And remember that even whole grains turn to sugar. Some people are far more sensitive to grains than others are, so pay attention to your body's response to them and keep an eye on your blood sugar levels.

Triglycerides (TG) are an independent risk factor for heart disease, and high levels are almost always related to eating a high-glycemic diet in which blood sugar gets spiked regularly. In general, TG levels should be 150 or lower, and on the cholesterol tests most doctors use, HDL is supposed to be above 45 (above 67 is ideal) and LDL at 130 or below. Your ratio of HDL to total cholesterol (total cholesterol divided by HDL) is a much more accurate predictor of heart disease than total cholesterol alone. If your ratio is 4.0 or under, you're fine. Don't let anyone put you on a statin drug just because of your total cholesterol number!

Today, though, there's an even more accurate cholesterol test available: an NMR lipid profile, which can tell you the number and size of your LDL and HDL particles as well as measure your level of triglycerides. Just as with LDL, not all HDL particles are the same. HDL-1 is smaller and denser than HDL-2, and it's more likely to become oxidized. What you want are the bigger, lighter particles—and you can get those from saturated fat in your diet. If you have a very high LDL count, it may be because you've got lots of the small LDL-B particles and not many LDL-A particles. A high LDL count may not be a problem because it may simply indicate that you've got a lot of big, light LDL-A. High HDL on a standard cholesterol test is equally misleading—if they're not the small, dense particles, then a high HDL is very good. Note that your physician will have to order this type of cholesterol test online (see Resources).

For a healthy heart, eat eggs and organic meats from fish and animals raised as naturally as possible. Whole grains, and sugars that aren't consumed with fiber in the form of whole fruit, are a problem. I advocate what's called a Paleolithic diet, which is close to what our ancestors ate before the agricultural era 10,000 years ago when grains such as wheat and rice became the staples of the human diet. Mostly, you eat plants, but you also have some eggs, meats, fish, and nuts as well as some healthy oils such as organic olive oil and coconut oil, and a small amount of natural sugars such as honey, berries, and stevia. And you can follow this type of diet even if you are vegan and want to avoid all animal foods. (All this will be discussed in greater detail in Chapter 8.) Even though eating a Paleo diet will increase the amount of saturated dietary fat you take in, it will *not* result in unhealthy cholesterol levels or harm your heart.

If you want to protect your heart, reduce cellular inflammation and damage to the walls of the arteries by cutting sugars and stress, expressing your feelings, and moving your body pleasurably. Regular exercise, meditation, and focusing on the causes of health will raise healthy HDL. If you and your doctor are concerned about your cholesterol, be ultra-cautious about using statin drugs, which are overprescribed. High cholesterol is not the cause of heart disease. Cellular inflammation is. Lowering LDL using statins won't prevent disease—in fact, half of all people who get heart disease don't even have high cholesterol! If your total cholesterol level is lower than 240 to 275 mg/dl, and your HDL is 60 or above, I certainly don't recommend statins to lower your cholesterol. They have serious side effects that include increased risk of breast cancer, dementia, muscle pain (known as myositis), and heart attack because they can deplete your body of coenzyme Q10, a vital nutrient that produces energy in the mitochondria of the cells. Also, keep in mind that statins are less effective in women than in men. And excessively low cholesterol, especially in women over age 50, correlates with early death, depression, and greater risk of cancer. If you don't have cardiovascular disease, lowering your cholesterol won't lower your mortality. If you do have cardiovascular disease, statins may reduce cardiovascular events, like heart attack, but not your mortality overall. In other words, if you have cardiovascular disease, start taking action to improve your heart's health—don't rush to get on statin drugs.[6] Bottom line: High cholesterol is not the cause of most heart attacks. And lowering cholesterol without addressing cellular inflammation and the longing of your heart is not very effective.

HEALTHY BREASTS

Did you know that National Breast Cancer Awareness Month was started by a company that manufactures and sells mammography machines? Let's change the conversation about our breasts from "how to avoid breast cancer and detect it early" to "how to have healthy breasts and enjoy them." How about a national breast health month when women make a point of expressing love to their breasts every day? And yes, lovers can help with this practice!

It concerns me that women feel pressured to think of their breasts as two potentially pre-malignant lesions sitting on their chests. Don't go on a search-and-destroy mission when you touch your breasts, or tell your daughters or granddaughters to do so. Instead, you might think of your breasts as "heart pillows" that are nourished by the energy field of your loving heart. When you touch them, do so with love. Give them a good massage from nipple to heart to lymph nodes under the arm. Affirm their ability to be healthy.

Breasts represent nourishment and the deep bonds love can create. They also represent the abundance of the Earth Mother, who always supports us and brings forth life and the foods we need for our bodies to thrive. Even if you weren't breast-fed or never used your breasts to feed a baby, your breasts carry the energy of love and nourishment. If you've cut yourself off from love, been betrayed, or withheld affection out of fear, these emotional experiences may affect the energy center of the heart, which affects the functioning of the cells and tissues in the breast.

There's a story I tell in *Women's Bodies, Women's Wisdom* that bears repeating here. I once had a patient who came to see me with two large fluid-filled cysts in her left breast that had manifested virtually overnight. When I asked her what was going on in her life in the areas of nurturing and receiving, she told me that her youngest daughter, her "baby," had just left home for college. Two days before that, her beloved 24-year-old cat had died. The night before the cysts appeared, she dreamed that she was nursing her infant daughter—the one who had just gone off to college. When I aspirated the fluid from her breasts, we were both astounded that it was milk! Clearly, her body had something to say about her need to nurture and in turn be nurtured after those two big losses. It was from this patient that I learned that what we call the "milk of human kindness" is more than a mere metaphor. Her body had literally manifested it.

When we move into the phase of our lives in which our mothering is no longer required in the same way it was when our children were young—or our relationships, businesses, or creative projects were just beginning—we have to figure out what to do with the milk of our kindness that is our gift to the world. To support ourselves and healthy breasts, we need new outlets for our nurturance. At the same time, we have to understand that loving involves reciprocity. If you give too much to others without nourishing yourself, or don't allow yourself to trust others and receive their love, you're likely to have an energetic blockage in your heart chakra—the energy center in your chest that's connected with your entire body's energy field and powerfully affects your breast health. A blockage in energy can lead to a physical manifestation if it remains there long enough.

Healthy breasts are breasts that are loved. Women have been taught to feel shame or embarrassment about their breasts. Often, the message is that to have power, you need to have big, bold, firm breasts that will attract men. That's one of the reasons why the number of women getting breast implants ballooned from 101,176 procedures in 1997 to 330,631 in 2012, according to the American Society for Aesthetic Plastic Surgery.[7] But it isn't the size or shape of our breasts that gives us true power or attractiveness. It's our relationship to our breasts and what they represent—our ability to give and receive nourishment and pleasure in a balanced way—that makes us beautiful, powerful goddesses.

If you're considering breast implants, that may be the right decision for you, but be informed about the downsides. Forty percent of women who get implants lose nipple sensation, and nipple sensation is a very important part of sexuality for most women. Also, if you don't regularly massage them, implants often become encapsulated in scar tissue that makes the breasts feel quite hard. The newer implants are not at risk for rupture and feel far more natural, but they are still foreign objects right above your heart that might be barriers to the loving energy of another. Breast implants also render a woman 18 times more likely to develop a rare form of breast cancer called anaplastic large cell lymphoma.[8] Most women, however, are very happy with their implants, and there is no shame in getting them. Every culture has had its favorite adornments to enhance beauty from time immemorial, whether it's tribal tattoos, rings around the neck to elongate it, or breast implants. You get to decide what makes you feel beautiful and desirable and then make a decision about whether to take action and change your body.

Regardless of their size or shape, here are some ways to love and appreciate your breasts.

How to Love Your Breasts

~ *Lovingly touch your breasts regularly.* When you touch your breasts, you're sending heart energy to them. In fact, back when you were an embryo, the tissue in your hands was connected to the tissue that went on to form your heart! Breast massage will increase the flow of lymph fluids and blood to the tissues and bring them oxygen and vital nutrients. Do this in the shower each day. However, don't do breast massage if you currently have breast cancer. Send love by placing your hands over your breasts and letting them rest there as you affirm the beauty and health of your breasts.

~ *Do the Female Deer Exercise.* The Female Deer Exercise is an ancient Taoist practice that has helped women achieve hormonal, uterine, and breast health for centuries. If done consistently, it can also vastly decrease menstrual symptoms including heavy flow and cramps. You can learn more about it in Stephen T. Chang's book *The Tao of Sexology: The Book of Infinite Wisdom* (Tao Publishing, 1986) or see it demonstrated in an online video, but the basic idea is this: You sit on the floor with the heel of one foot pressing into your pubic area. If you aren't flexible enough to make this contact, place a tennis ball by your pubic area and press your heel into that. Now rub both hands together until you feel tingling energy in them. Place them on your breasts for a few seconds. Then, with your palms, begin to make circular motions on your breasts with both hands. Circle for 50 to 100 times in whichever direction feels best to you. (Circling both hands inward tends to increase breast size. Circling in an outward direction can help dissipate excess energy in the breasts.) While circling, feel the energy in your pelvis rise up into your breasts and the energy of your heart sink down into your pelvis. Avoid overstimulating the nipples, because they can be quite sensitive.[9] It's nice to do the Female Deer Exercise first thing in the morning or last thing before bed using a soothing oil for the breasts. I personally like coconut oil. Pomegranate breast oil is also wonderful.

~ *Eliminate negative self-talk about your breasts, and avoid bonding with other women over how you don't like your breasts.* Groups of friends and family members affect each other's perceptions and behaviors. Be the first one in your family or group of girlfriends to reject the habit of complaining about breast size and shape. Instead, stand up and proclaim the following: "I have a magnificent set. I just love my 'girls.' How about you?" Stand back and see what happens.

~ *Open yourself to receive love, compassion, affection, and praise from others, and give it without resentment, jealousy, or strings attached.* Accept all compliments with a simple "Thank you" rather than denying or minimizing what the other person has just acknowledged about you. Admitting you have assets and positive qualities is not narcissistic!

~ *Acknowledge and express your feelings—honestly.* Notice when you tend to avoid the truth. Do you do it to make another person feel more comfortable, caretaking for their feelings but not your own? You'll learn more about releasing grief, anger, and fear later in the book, but for now, cultivate the skill of "getting things off your chest" regularly.

~ *Go braless as much as possible so your lymph fluids can flow freely.* If you have large breasts, it may be painful to go braless for too long or while you're exercising, but be sure you aren't in your bra all day long, much less at night. If you have daughters and granddaughters, teach them that freedom is good for breasts. There is no evidence that going braless causes breasts to sag earlier than they would otherwise.

Needing bras for "training" or "support" is simply a cultural myth—probably invented by some corset manufacturer back in the day. Bras are fashion accessories. They can be a most lovely addition to your wardrobe, but they are not a medical device!

~ *Pay attention to any breast symptoms that suggest the need for hormonal balancing.* Sore breasts are often a sign of suboptimal levels of iodine or estrogen levels that are too high.

~ *Sweat regularly.* Sweat is part of the body's natural system for shedding toxins and reducing cortisol levels. Exercise helps you to maintain healthy levels of estrogen and other hormones. Regular exercise decreases the risk of breast cancer, probably because it decreases total body fat and fat can produce excess estrogen. According to one large study, those women who were lean and exercised four hours per week had a 70 percent reduction in their risk of breast cancer.[10]

~ *Take vitamin D3, 2,000 to 5,000 IU a day, in supplement form or through sunlight.* Note that most women require a supplement in addition to regular doses of sunlight. Test your vitamin D levels first to find out where you stand, through your doctor or on your own using an online lab that can do a 25(OH)D test (see Resources). Optimal levels of vitamin D are 40 to 80 ng/ml (or 100 to 150 nmol/L), and research shows that a level of 52 ng/ml cuts your breast cancer risk in half compared to a level of 13 ng/ml.[11]

~ *Eat a healthful, low-glycemic diet with plenty of high-fiber vegetables and plant-based fats.* High-fiber vegetables include broccoli and cabbage, turmeric, garlic, onions, tomatoes, kale, and collard greens. Enjoy nuts and flax, hemp, or chia seeds. Eat fish or take fish oil supplements so that you get plenty of omega-3 fatty acids, because these antioxidants lower the risk of breast cancer. A high-glycemic diet causes insulin resistance over time and insulin resistance is a risk factor for breast cancer, so cut down on sugars and all grains while including healthy meats, fish, cheese, and eggs. Add healthy fats such as coconut oil, avocado, macadamia nuts, and flax oil. Don't worry about fats from healthy sources.

~ *Take antioxidants such as vitamin C.* I recommend 1,000 to 5,000 mg of vitamin C a day. (You'll find my specific supplement recommendations for everyone in Chapter 12.)

~ *Take coenzyme Q10 (ubiquinone).* Low coenzyme Q10 has been linked with breast cancer, and few of us get much of it in our diets. (Organ meats provide a significant amount of coenzyme Q10, but most women don't eat them.) Low levels can also cause breast pain in menopause. Take 10 to 100 mg a day, or 70 to 100 mg a day if you're at high risk for breast cancer. If you take a statin drug to lower your cholesterol, be sure to get your coenzyme Q10, because statin drugs reduce the levels of this important nutrient.

~ *Take iodine.* The breasts require about 3 mg of iodine a day for optimal health, and the body itself requires another 9 mg or so—you should take about 12.5 mg a day in supplement form. The safest food sources for iodine are kelp and organic eggs. Iodized salt, though better than nothing, isn't the best source because the iodine tends to evaporate out of the salt. To test whether you're low in iodine, you can buy Lugol's iodine solution from the pharmacist and put it on your inner arm; it will stain, and you should still see it 24 hours later. If not, you're low in iodine. If you have thyroid issues, increase your iodine levels slowly, ideally under the care of a health care practitioner such as a naturopath who is very familiar with iodine and thyroid conditions.

~ *Drink in moderation, if at all.* Drinking just one or more alcoholic beverages a day puts you at a 60 percent higher risk of developing breast cancer. The risks may be greater still for women taking HRT (hormone replacement therapy). Alcohol consumption inhibits the ability of folic acid, a B vitamin, to repair DNA. If you drink, take a B-complex supplement, and remember that health is about enjoyment, not addiction. Reaching for a glass of wine as a way to add pleasure to your meal produces an entirely different result than reaching for a glass of wine to quell anxiety or sadness.

~ *Don't smoke.* Smoking increases the risk of breast cancer. Like drinking, smoking is a behavior that tends to shut down the heart chakra.

BREAST CANCER SCREENING

Regular mammograms are considered the gold standard for the early detection of breast cancer, but it's important to know the truth about mammograms and breast health.

First, there's little to no evidence that getting a yearly mammogram starting at age 40 saves lives. This is why, back in 2009, the U.S. Preventive Services Task Force (USPSTF) published new guidelines, recommending less frequent mammograms for breast cancer screening.[12] While its previous guidelines had called for screenings every one to two years, starting at age 40, the USPSTF's new guidelines call for screening every other year for women ages 50 to 74. The American Cancer Society did not update its recommendations in response, so despite the USPSTF's findings, most women still follow the American Cancer Society's older guidelines and get a mammogram annually, beginning at age 40.

Second, *screening mammography is not benign.* In a groundbreaking study published in the *New England Journal of Medicine* in 2012, which I mentioned in Chapter 3, Gilbert Welch, M.D., a renowned medical authority on the risks of cancer screening, pointed out that routine mammography screening over the last 30 years has resulted in 1.3 million women being diagnosed with "cancer" because their mammograms picked up ductal carcinoma in situ (DCIS).[13] As I explained in Chapter 3, DCIS is not cancer but a type of cellular anomaly that women are more likely to die *with* than *from* because in the vast majority of cases, it will never progress to actual breast cancer. Autopsy studies of healthy women in their 40s who died in car accidents have shown that as many as 40 percent have evidence of DCIS in their breasts. Terms such as "cancer" and "precancerous condition" drive women and doctors to be overly aggressive in reacting to the presence of DCIS.

The problem is that once you find DCIS—especially with the newer high-resolution mammography that can pick up very early instances—there's tremendous pressure to do something about it. Hence, scores of women are having radiation, surgery, mastectomies, and chemotherapy treatments that are unnecessary. This is hardly benign! Plus, a recent study showed that having radiation of the breast increases your risk of heart disease down the road.[14]

Thankfully, a working group of the National Cancer Institute has recommended that DCIS should be renamed so that patients are less frightened and less likely to seek unneeded and potentially harmful treatments that can include the removal of the breast. The researchers suggested that these anomalies—along with the many lesions found in prostate, thyroid, lung, and other cancer screenings—should not be called cancer at all, but instead be reclassified as IDLE conditions, which stands for "indolent lesions of epithelial origin." Sanity at last prevails![15]

We don't need to be so aggressive about finding these IDLE conditions and addressing them because very often, the body simply heals itself. The data support this, which is why, in the spring of 2014, the Swiss Medical Board recommended abolishing all new mammography screening programs on the grounds that they do more harm than good. Its report in the *New England Journal of Medicine* stated: "For every breast-cancer death prevented in U.S. women over a 10-year course of annual screening beginning at 50 years of age, 490 to 670 women are likely to have a false positive mammogram with repeat examination; 70 to 100, an unnecessary biopsy; and 3 to 14, an overdiagnosed breast cancer that would never have become clinically apparent."

I realize this may be shocking to you, but it's important to look closely at the newest information and not make decisions based on old information and scare tactics.[16]

It has been very easy to sell mammography to women over the years because so many have been led to believe that early diagnosis via mammography saves lives. This was indeed the hope of many when mammography was first introduced. Unfortunately, like the use of Premarin and Provera in the Women's Health Initiative study to prevent heart disease, that hope simply hasn't lived up to its initial promise. Despite this, surveys still show that up to 70 percent of women believe that mammography saves lives.[17] In fact, it's better breast cancer treatments—*not* early diagnoses from mammograms—that are saving more lives than ever. It's time for women to make truly informed decisions about mammograms and the harm that can ensue from using them routinely. You can't be truly informed as long as you continue to believe these two things: one, that your breasts require constant surveillance to remain healthy, and two, that the benefits of mammographic screening outweigh the risks.

Recently, a woman asked my advice about continuing to get mammograms, which her ob/gyn was pressuring her about. She had developed microcalcifications along the milk duct in her right breast ten years previously after a rough year of taking care of others and neglecting herself (symbolically, the right side is the "giving" side of the body). A biopsy showed that the microcalcifications were benign, and they didn't increase for another five years or so. Then a screening mammogram she had during another particularly stressful year of caretaking for others showed that a few more microcalcifications had appeared. She refused a biopsy, which would have cost her thousands of dollars out of pocket, but agreed to more mammograms in the future to keep an eye on the condition. In the meantime, in a couple of deep meditation sessions, she noticed a dark, heavy spot in the energy field above her right breast and imagined drawing in pure love and exhaling it into that spot until she felt it dissolve. A session with an energy healer, who picked up on inflammation in that breast before the woman mentioned any medical conditions, further allowed her to influence the energy field that was affecting the cells. The next mammogram showed one new microcalcification, and in subsequent years, no more appeared. After ten years of worrying about her breast, being pressured to do more invasive, expensive tests that would put more radiation in her body, she decided she had had enough and was seeking my advice on whether she ought to say no to more screenings. She told me her heart, her head, and her instincts told her to continue the practice of loving her body and her breasts and being aware of any breast changes that she could detect. So far, she's had none. I told her that she should listen to her inner healer on this decision. Now that is an ageless goddess approach to loving and caring for the breasts!

BETTER BREAST CARE

There's a better way to screen for breast health. Unlike mammography, which involves exposing the chest and breasts to radiation, thermography detects heat in the breast tissue that may be due to cellular inflammation. It is a functional test: the results change as blood flow to your tissues changes. When blood vessels are being formed to support a cluster of abnormal cells with DNA mutations, the process releases heat that can be picked up on an infrared imaging camera. In essence, you're seeing potential problems long before they become actual diagnosable disease. You can respond to inflammation in the breast by taking action to improve your breast health and doing another thermogram three months later to see if the inflammation has reversed.

If you have dense breasts, a mammogram may show a problem where there is none simply because it's harder to get a clear mammogram picture of dense breast tissue, which is not the case with thermography. Thermograms are also completely comfortable since they do not involve breast compression of any kind. There are more than 40 years of research studies and more than 800 peer-reviewed studies supporting breast thermography. Using thermography can help you and your health care practitioner be proactive in improving breast health long before a problem in the breasts occurs. Of course, the very best approach is to work with someone who understands both mammography and thermography and knows the limitations and benefits of both technologies. One of the best resources for this is Dr. Tom Hudson, who is board certified in both radiology and thermography. He helps women all over the world interpret their results and has written an excellent book on the subject called *Journey to Hope: Leaving the Fear of Breast Cancer Behind* (Brush and Quill, 2011).

Paying attention to your breasts and caring for them is important—whether or not you have a history of breast cancer in your life or in your family. But please note that only 2 percent of all breast cancers involve an inherited gene mutation such as the BRCA1 or the BRCA2 (the first has a higher risk than the second). Mutations of both of those genes are associated with ovarian cancer too.[18] That said, if you have a strong history of breast or ovarian cancer but test negative for gene mutations associated with breast cancer, the family history may be a bigger indicator of your breast cancer risk than the gene is.[19] Our families' emotional legacies may be a factor in this discrepancy.

In discussing the risk of the BRCA1 gene mutation, the notion that it conveys an "87 percent chance of developing breast cancer" has been promoted often. If we look more closely at that figure, we can see it's a great example of our misunderstanding of the genetic connection to disease. First, the number 87 sounds frightening, because it is so large and so specific. A little research shows that the number is based on old estimates that have been disputed by the National Institutes of Health. In fact, a 1997 study showed the risk of breast cancer for variations on the BRCA1 gene to be closer to 56 percent, and only 16 percent for ovarian cancer. Also, the original figures of 84 to 87 percent at the highest were based on studies of women who had both the gene variations *and* a family history of breast or ovarian cancer *over two generations,* not just one.[20] Furthermore, we have no idea how many women in the original research had low levels of vitamin D (again, adequate levels can cut breast cancer risk in half), or were regular drinkers (which raises breast cancer risk), or exercised regularly, maintained a healthy weight, got enough iodine, or ate plenty of fruits and vegetables (all of which lower risk). The more carefully you look at the research, the more you realize that you can't simply assign a number to your risk of developing breast cancer—and you have to factor in lifestyle choices.[21] Even if you have had breast cancer in one breast, the odds of your developing it in the other, healthy breast in the next ten years are as low as 4 to 5 percent, especially if you don't have the BRCA1 or BRCA2 gene mutation. Again, you really have to look carefully at the statistics to get an accurate sense of what research shows your risk is.[22]

If you're considering genetic testing, think carefully about why you want to do so. As with any genetic testing, whether the results are negative or positive, there are no guarantees. Regardless of what your choice is, or what your results may be, the most powerful thing you can do for your breast health is to cultivate a loving relationship with them, make breast-healthy lifestyle choices, and, if you're concerned, monitor your breast health with an attitude of self-love and self-care, not a search-and-destroy attitude. If you want to find a practitioner who performs and interprets thermograms so you can monitor your breasts regularly as part of your plan for loving self-care, visit www.breastthermography.com; www.breastthermography.org; or the websites for the International Academy of Clinical Thermology, www.iact-org.org, or the American College of Clinical Thermology, www.thermology online.org.

THERE'S ALWAYS HOPE: CALLING IN DIVINE ORDER

There's nothing like illness to get your attention. The soul comes to us through our bodies. And the good news is that there's always hope, no matter what. Anita Moorjani, author of *Dying to Be Me,* quite literally was pronounced dead of cancer, with lemon-size tumors throughout her body. During her near-death experience, she discovered a loving reality awaiting her. When she returned to her body, she knew that she would be well. And indeed, all of her tumors disappeared. When asked if she still sees her doctors, she said in a recent lecture that she no longer sees them because they always tell her she's in "remission"—as though they are waiting for the cancer to return. Since she has already experienced dying, why worry? She also said she's not afraid of getting cancer again. There is a reality beyond what our physical senses can perceive, and when we are really "up against it," that reality becomes stronger.

I came across a story on Tosha Silver's Facebook page and was so moved by it that I contacted the poster to ask if I could share it with you here. It sums up this idea of surrendering to love and joy, not fear, very much the same as Anita Moorjani did. Here is what Annette Perez had to say about her experience with stage 4 breast cancer:

> I was diagnosed with stage 4 breast cancer, which had already spread to the lungs, liver, kidneys, spine, and brain, and given an "expiration date" of six months. I opted not to undergo chemotherapy and radiation treatments as the treatments would have been extremely aggressive and at that point, I was more concerned about my quality of life versus quantity of life. At the time of the diagnosis, I felt as if I had that illness pulsating throughout my body. I was experiencing all of the typical symptoms. As I have always done in life, I immediately began working on moving out of that dark corner, or what I often referred to as "the abyss." A month later, a friend sent me a copy of *Outrageous Openness* by Tosha Silver. I couldn't wait to dive into it! The wisdom in those pages was exactly the spark I needed to move forward through this latest challenge. At the onset of this journey, I knew I wanted to do battle and delved into researching what I could do to help myself as I began this challenge. As I spoke to others and did my research, I became overwhelmed and found myself taking action but in a frantic, frenzied way. But as I learned how to let go and move out of the way so that the Beloved Divine could work, beautiful moments and powerful opportunities began to happen. I let go and allowed the Divine to lovingly guide me as to what the next best step was for me and what action, if any, I needed to take. Information showed up for me, light was shed upon any new direction or action I needed to take, and people showed up on my path. Early on, I turned over everything to the Beloved Divine because this was just way too much for me to carry and it was not necessary that I carry it. Two months after my diagnosis, I was pain free and had energy, and all of the symptoms had vanished. I did have to undergo a mastectomy four months in, and I passed

through that challenge in an extremely effortless manner. I experienced three days of pain immediately following the surgery and after that—nothing. I had bottles of prescribed pain medication that went untouched as it was not needed. After I surpassed my six-month "expiration date," I continue to feel amazing, experiencing no symptoms of the illness, and have been able to get busy living! The oncologist and surgeon are amazed at my progress and beyond baffled that I am even able to get around. Most important, I am experiencing such peace, a peace that I have searched for all of my life and did not find, nor truly experience, until now. I continue to do well, long past my "expiration date."

Now *those* are words of wisdom and inspiration!

Hormones and Breast Health

As I've said, I believe the hormones you most need to be concerned with in midlife are your stress hormones. If you need some adjustments to your sex hormones, avoid synthetics and try plant phytoestrogens instead. But if you're taking synthetic hormones or those made from horse urine (such as Premarin) for menopause, be aware that the research shows you're at greater risk for breast cancer.

Plant-based phytoestrogens, on the other hand, do not increase breast cancer or ovarian cancer risk. And they work beautifully for many women. For those for whom plant phytoestrogens are not effective, bioidentical hormones may be an option.

Keep in mind that the Women's Health Initiative study that gave thousands of women HRT in the form of Prempro (Premarin, which is horse urine, and Provera, which is synthetic progestin) had to be halted suddenly in 2002 when researchers discovered that menopausal women taking these hormones had higher rates of breast cancer and heart disease. Unfortunately, researchers don't always distinguish between the three types of hormone replacement—synthetic, bioidentical, and plant phytoestrogen. What's more, many doctors and health care providers do not understand the differences.

Hence, women are often needlessly scared away from the very thing that can give them relief.

Thankfully, some exciting new research is finally confirming the fact that bioidentical hormones are far safer than synthetic ones. Researchers from the Karolinska Institute in Sweden led by Professor Gunnar Söderqvist found that different types of HRT a woman takes and the way they are administered can have a wide range of effects on genes associated with breast cancer. Their studies of gene activity in the breasts of healthy young women found that synthetic Provera and Premarin (the kind used in the Women's Health Initiative study) were far more likely to cause gene expression associated with cancer than bioidentical estrogen gel applied to the skin along with oral bioidentical progesterone. This finding, presented at the World Congress on the Menopause in Cancun, Mexico, in 2014, opens the way to identify which forms of HRT have minimal effect on breast cancer risk. That is very good news.

THE SEAT OF YOUR CREATIVE POWERS

The pelvic bowl and the muscles, connective tissue, and organs cradled in this area (uterus, ovaries, bladder, urethra, female erotic anatomy, pelvic floor muscles, and large bowel) make up the body's creative center. This is the place in our bodies from which all creative energy arises. Although some women will use this creative center to give birth to babies and others will not, we all access its life-force energy to birth new ideas into new projects and create new perceptions of who we are and what we would like to contribute while we're on the earth. The pelvic bowl is associated with the second chakra, the body's energy center that is governed by our relationships with money, sex, and power.

If you haven't severed your mind from your body and developed a sense of disconnection from your lower half, you're probably aware that pleasurable thoughts, actions, and activities increase blood flow and feeling in your sex organs and pelvic bowl. Our souls come into our bodies through our hips at the back of our pelvic bowl, where the sacrum—or "sacred" bone—is located. This is the place in the body that physical therapist Tami Lynn Kent, author of *Wild Feminine* (Atria Books, 2011), calls the "spirit door." It's the entryway into the "birthing field": the place where energy becomes form. Your pelvis and genitals are your sacred center, the area in the body where you access the energy to create everything—whether it's a book, a relationship, or a baby.

When we listen to the call of our pelvic energy to live with greater creativity, take more risks, feel more pleasure, and not be afraid of what others might say or think, we are honoring the creative female force within us. If we don't listen to this call, it's likely that we'll experience symptoms of imbalance and disruption in the pelvic area. Fibroids and prolonged heavy bleeding can be Mother Nature's way of saying, "Pay attention! Are you directing your creative energy into a dead-end job or relationship? Are you abdicating responsibility for your own creative expression to something or someone else while resenting them for holding you back? What needs to be born through you?"

I once heard Esther Hicks tell the story of admiring a gorgeous painting done by an artist friend. Esther asked her, "How long did it take you to paint that?" The woman answered, "Seventy-six years." Our creative expression is like that. Each year that we walk the earth, we become more creative—*if* we allow ourselves to connect to this life force. And those who open themselves up to creative channels tend to live very joyful and happy lives. That's why orchestra conductors tend to live a long time, even though they have heavy travel and rehearsal schedules. In his 80s, comedian George Burns, whose career was rejuvenated when he was in his late 70s, would tell people he had to live to be 100 because "I'm booked." When you have a mission of living creatively, expressing yourself and your ideas to the world, when you let joy and humor flow through you, you'll find you're booked. (Yes, George Burns did make it to 100, in good humor and good health. And his cigar habit was one of the "pleasurable rituals" that was obviously part of his health plan!)

Too often, we women repress our creative urges because we don't trust ourselves or don't want to bring attention to ourselves.

One of the reasons our culture has such an ongoing love affair with famous actors, musicians, performers, and celebrities is that these people perform the function of being willing to get up on stage and do what so many of us don't have the courage to do: risk failing in public and being humiliated and judged for our contribution. Celebrity women, whether they're performers or speakers and cultural innovators, have great courage and enormous self-esteem to keep putting themselves out there year after year despite the shaming they face as women in a culture that is uncomfortable with bold, creative expression by women. Believe me, they aren't doing it for the money. It's so easy to stand back and take potshots at those who are willing to play full out and get on a stage or a television screen. But it's far healthier to, in the words of Theodore Roosevelt, "Dare greatly." Have the courage to live creatively from your own center.

At some point in our lives, perhaps when we're finished with up-close-and-personal mothering, we need to access and channel our creative energy in ways that give us pleasure and inspiration—writing a book or poetry, learning how to paint, learning how to dance. The creative urge can also express itself in coming up with new ideas, new business models, or new ways of working with technology. The possibilities are endless. The older we get, the more direct access we have to our creative energy flow.

There are times when a woman wants to honor her creative urges but is stopped in her tracks by fear. How can she spend time innovating and inventing when her retirement accounts are underfunded? The unmet callings of our spirits are often due to playing it safe and being afraid to say no to loved ones who think we should have different priorities. The only way out of this dilemma is to name your fears and then learn the skills of standing up for yourself—even when your children, spouse, or boss has other ideas about how you should spend your time and energy.

Fibroids, cancers, and pain in the pelvic bowl are all indicators that you should explore your longings to live more creatively and authentically with less fear and more adventure. And much of what I've already discussed about cancer risk and screening applies in this area of the body as well. The pelvic bowl houses our "low heart," if you will. Have you been raped, or felt violated to the point where your sense of security was shattered? If so, it will show up in your pelvis. The health of your pelvic organs is also related to how well you have learned to negotiate the creative energies embodied in money, sex, and power. Ovaries are, quite literally, your female balls—the organs associated with your drive to go after what you want in the world. Quite often this drive has been routed through a man—or through the masculine aspects of ourselves—and pelvic disease is often the result. At the very least, you want to make sure you keep your ovaries. They are removed routinely far too often when women have hysterectomies for benign disease. Ovaries are necessary for hormone production throughout your life, and the risk of removal in terms of overall bone and brain health is far greater than the risk of ovarian cancer in the vast majority of cases. For very extensive discussions on these points, please see *Women's Bodies, Women's Wisdom* and *The Wisdom of Menopause*.

If you're reading this book, you have the ability to connect with your birthing field and bring in the resources and support you need to create heaven on earth for yourself. Just ask Spirit to show you exactly how to do this. And be sure to read the chapter on sexuality in this book so you can learn even more about your pelvic bowl and its relationship to your power and sexuality—and more about the psoas (pronounced SOH-us) muscles connected to it.

PELVIC FLOOR MUSCLE TONE

Being disconnected from our pelvic bowl correlates with our ignorance of our pelvic floor muscles. I'm willing to bet you weren't taught about these muscles in health class back in school!

The pelvic floor muscles involve several interconnected muscles that support the internal organs of the pelvis. Together, they're like a trampoline or hammock that stretches from your tailbone to your pelvic bone. These muscles lose tone when they are not used properly and regularly, which is the case with most women who sit too much and almost never squat. They stop working together as they should, creating an imbalance. If the pelvic floor muscles lose too much tone, you can even experience prolapse, which is when the organs the muscles support actually fall through what is called the pelvic diaphragm. Prolapses are usually treated surgically, but it's better to go to a women's health physical therapist who knows how to rehabilitate your pelvic floor—or use classical Pilates training for rehabilitation.

Weak pelvic floor muscles may result in stress incontinence (urine leaking upon sneezing, laughing, or moving) or urge incontinence (the feeling that you have to urinate right now or you'll have an accident). Both these forms of incontinence can get worse over time if the root cause, a weak pelvic floor, isn't addressed. In the U.S., urinary incontinence is a major reason older women are admitted to nursing homes, but no one wants to talk about how Mom needs help going to the toilet. About one in four women experiences stress incontinence. It's time to put an end to the shame and secrecy and get serious about this very preventable and treatable problem that, left unchecked, is likely to lead to urinary incontinence down the road!

Women will say, "I have a small bladder," or "ever since I had babies, I have to 'go' all the time," but neither is an accurate description of urge incontinence or stress incontinence. Both are very treatable conditions that women experience when their pelvic floor muscles aren't toned. Physicians are likely to recommend pads and adult diapers, surgery, and pharmaceutical drugs. The drugs block the nerve endings that affect the muscle that keeps the bladder from releasing urine, and they are effective. But they can have side effects such as dry mouth, and they don't address the underlying problem of low tone in the pelvic floor muscles.

Why is low tone in our pelvic floor muscles so common? Our bodies are designed for continual movement and for squatting: for hundreds of thousands of years, women spent much of their time squatting as they prepared meals, cooked, gathered roots from the earth, socialized, defecated, urinated, or gave birth vaginally. But we're always standing, sitting, or lying down, which causes our pelvic floor muscles to lose tone. The situation can worsen after childbirth or abdominal surgery such as a C-section or hysterectomy, but this risk has been overstated. Even teenagers and women who have never given birth can have low pelvic floor muscle tone. Whatever your age, you can train your muscles and bladder to feel the urge to urinate, and go, every three to four hours during the day and once, if that, at night.

How to Support Your Pelvic Floor

~ *Drink plenty of water.* You need to be well hydrated to be healthy, so even if you experience urge or stress incontinence, don't make the mistake of not drinking enough water in the vain hope that this will solve the problem. The bladder actually holds 16 ounces or about two cups of liquid, so even if you're drinking eight glasses of water a day, you shouldn't feel the urge to pee every two hours. The bladder feels the urge to go when it doesn't actually have to be voided because it's confused by signals from the brain, which originate in the pelvic floor muscles and the muscles that hold the bladder closed. When you actually need to urinate, the pelvic floor muscles should signal the brain, which signals the bladder muscle to contract so that the opening to the bladder widens and urine flows out naturally. If your pelvic floor muscles are weak, they will send this signal when it's not needed, your bladder muscles will contract, and you'll have to consciously try to prevent yourself from letting the urine flow.

~ *Exercise your pelvic floor muscles regularly.* Many women have learned how to do Kegel muscle exercises, which were invented by a gynecologist named Arnold Kegel back in the late 1940s. His exercises, commonly called Kegels, involve the building up of one pelvic floor muscle, the PC (pubococcygeus), which is used to stop the flow of urine from the bladder. Dr. Kegel was on to something, but building up just one of the pelvic floor muscles is incomplete. The idea isn't to make one muscle strong, because that allows other muscles in its muscle group to remain weak. For overall pelvic floor tone and functionality, you want to get a feel for where your pelvic floor muscles are so you can exercise all of them properly. Simply standing up 32 times per day, then sitting back down at your desk, will apply gravity to your pelvic floor. That alone will help. Another effective pelvic floor toner is to lie on your back with your knees bent and your lower back resting on the floor. Insert your middle finger into your vagina. Squeeze your vagina so that you feel pressure against your finger. Don't tighten other muscles such as the muscles in your buttocks. Just squeeze your finger inside your vagina. Do a series of quick and long squeezes at least once a day, building to the point where you can feel a difference in the pressure against your vagina and you're experiencing less stress incontinence or urinary urgency.

~ *Squat!* Squatting supports the natural stretching and toning of all the muscles. Whenever you take a shower, squat to urinate. The butt muscles you use to help you balance in this position will support the toning of the pelvic floor muscles. Your urethra will be pointed downward, allowing gravity to help you naturally release urine. Squat when you can during the day too.

~ *Use your toilet time to build your pelvic floor muscles.* One habit all of us should change is how we use a toilet. Women tend to sit up straight like proper ladies instead of leaning forward or putting our feet on a stool to raise the knees. Whether you're sitting to urinate or defecate, lean forward and place your elbows on your knees, or put your feet up on a step stool to raise your knees above your waist. This squat-like position supports the toning of pelvic floor muscles. I like to use the Squatty Potty toilet stool for this purpose, which you can find online. See if using it regularly doesn't reduce the number of times you have to urinate during the day and night.

~ *Squat regularly to strengthen your glutes.* Understand that most pelvic floor problems are the result
of misalignment, not the aging process. Check out
the work of Katy Bowman, who has a wonderful
series of YouTube videos available to teach you
proper pelvic alignment: www.youtube.com
/watch?v=OrMU2tQ2SUk.

~ *Relax, don't push, when you urinate or defecate.*
Because we want to please other people and stick
to our hectic schedules, we develop the habit of
retaining our urine in our bladders until we get
a chance to sit on the toilet, where we push so
we can quickly get out all the urine. The pushing
builds muscles that take over for weak pelvic floor
muscles. Stop worrying about the next person in
line for the ladies' room and take your time!

~ *Stop the urge to pee unnecessarily.* There's a simple
trick to get rid of the false urge to urinate when
you feel you absolutely have to go but know you
didn't drink enough liquid to justify another trip
to the toilet. Squeeze your pelvic floor muscles and
hold them tight for five seconds before releasing
the muscle tension. Do this five times. Then, take a
couple of deep, slow breaths. The urge should have
been greatly reduced. You might need to repeat this
exercise to reduce the feeling that you must urinate
immediately.

This list is a very simplified version of how you can retrain
your pelvic floor muscles. You can find more ideas and specific
exercises for pelvic floor muscle health in the book *The Bathroom
Key* by Kathryn Kassai and Kim Perelli, and use their website to
find physical therapists specializing in helping women overcome
incontinence and weak pelvic floor muscles.[23]

Also, I recommend authentic Pilates, which is great for developing pelvic floor muscle tone. Pilates is part of the treatment

many women's health physical therapists use for strengthening our stabilizing core muscles, which respond so well to gravity. (The core is the part of the body that would be covered by a 1940s one-piece bathing suit.) And it's worth mentioning that all of this strengthening and toning does wonders for a pleasurable sex life.

Perhaps the most important piece of information you can have about your body is this: no matter what is going on in your body right now, you can always access your ability to self-heal and be healthy. Support your well-being through habits that nourish and delight you instead of habits rooted in old defense mechanisms or shame. Addictions, avoidance behaviors, and people pleasing are common behaviors that become habits for too many women who are afraid of or uncomfortable with the regular expression of difficult emotions. We can push feelings like grief, resentment, shame, and rage back so far into our subconscious that we have no idea what we are holding on to. And these emotions secrete inflammatory chemicals into our bloodstream day in and day out, which causes aging. For a goddess to enjoy vibrant health, she has to learn how to grieve and rage without apology and then commit to experiencing more exalted emotions and experiences. That's how these old, stale, and destructive energies can be released. And that is how we remain ageless, which is our birthright.

CHAPTER FIVE

GODDESSES GRIEVE, RAGE, AND MOVE ON

Your pain is the breaking of the shell that encloses
your understanding . . . And if you could keep your
heart in wonder at the daily miracles of your life, your
pain would not seem less wondrous than your joy.

— KAHLIL GIBRAN

Several years ago, I developed what we call "frozen shoulder." It's very common in midlife women and, like just about everything else, it's believed to be related to hormone levels and menopause—but I knew that wasn't my problem. The pain started one day, seemingly out of the blue, while I was picking up a piece of wood to place in the wood stove. I developed immobilizing pain in my left shoulder, dropped the wood, and actually fell to my knees. The next day, I could not stretch my left arm behind my back very far without wincing in agony, and the pain continued day after day. Because I hadn't suffered an injury, I felt that the cause had to be emotional, and that the pain and immobility, real as they were, were ultimately rooted in unresolved emotions. The brain doesn't recognize the difference between emotional pain and pain caused by a physical injury. In fact, brain studies have demonstrated that emotional pain registers in precisely the same areas of the brain as physical pain.

Because of my work with thousands of patients and my personal experiences with emotions and illness, I have long known that at their core, all illness and physical ailments—including those seemingly caused by accidents or viruses—have an emotional component. If we knew what the emotional issue was, we wouldn't have to manifest it physically! So I was certain there had to be some old, unprocessed emotional wounds in the area of my heart, ribs, and shoulders, all associated with the fourth or heart chakra. Despite my intellectual understanding, though, I didn't know the cause— and despite knowing my pain had to be psychosomatic, I didn't get relief. With the help of a holistic chiropractor and my Pilates teacher, I spent months trying to open up my rib cage and move my shoulder, which helped ease the pain and expand my mobility slightly. But I knew that the key to complete recovery lay in releasing the blocked emotions related to my heart.

For several years, I had been romantically involved with a man I loved deeply but who was not emotionally available to me. I desperately tried to fix the relationship, which in many ways mirrored my failed marriage. Because I couldn't get this relationship to meet my needs, I was doubting my desirability as a woman—an old issue for me. Could it be that my shoulder pain (and the occasional chest pain I had had about once a year for a decade) had something to do with my relationships with the important men in my life?

Much as I idolized my father when I was growing up, he was busy taking care of my mother and her needs, as well as earning a living. It was a time when I needed my desirability validated by the number-one man in my life: him. I remember one day when I was around middle-school age, I was waltzing in the kitchen with him, trying to learn this skill. My father was a good dancer, and as we ended our dance together, I asked him what he thought, hoping he would approve of my moves. He replied, "You'd do okay if it was dark—and the man was drunk." My Scorpio dad's barb hit me very deeply, right in the heart. He made similar criticisms of my tennis playing even though I practiced for hours and tried so hard to please him by being a good player. He didn't take the time to teach me or arrange for me to take lessons from someone else, but simply criticized me in his forthright way.

I'm sure his comments were the result of being irritable from overwork, or simply thoughtless in the way all of us can be at times. And I know many women have suffered far worse things than I did. But that doesn't mean I should have made excuses for him or downplayed the emotional impact on me—"Oh, for heaven's sake, that was decades ago! Are you still holding on to *that?* Just get over it!"

No matter what happened to you—or how long ago it happened—you must do the healing work that only you can do. Failure to do so just perpetuates pain and dis-ease. My father's insensitive jokes and comments had created a wound that became buried in my tissues. Now that the old theme was playing out in my adult life, all these years later, the old emotions I had felt as a child were expressing themselves as pain and immobility in my shoulder. My body was telling me to heal the old hurts.

I didn't realize this right away, however. It began to dawn on me during a session I had with Doris E. Cohen, Ph.D., author of *Repetition: Past Lives, Life, and Rebirth* (Hay House, 2008). Dr. Cohen has been a clinical psychologist for 40 years and also works on the spiritual level and with dreams. For a few years now, she had been suggesting that I look at my father issues, but until this point, I hadn't been ready to face that possibility. It took the repetition of the original heartbreak with my father—in the form of an adult love relationship—to bring the issue to the surface by bringing on physical pain. The severity of my discomfort made me willing to look again at my emotional issues surrounding my father and begin a program of healing, as Dr. Cohen suggested to me.

For three days in a row, I set a timer for 15 minutes to do an anger and grief release session. During the first five to ten minutes of each session, I imagined my father sitting in front of me and let my rage fly. I just let him have it! I shouted at him for making those thoughtless, hurtful comments years ago. I swore at him, crying, "How the f--- could you talk to your daughter like that? What were you thinking, you bastard?!" In addition, I took a hand towel and snapped it against some sturdy woodwork, all the while yelling expletives of rage until I felt spent.

After these sessions—and sometimes, just a few minutes into them—I often found myself lying on my bed, curled up in a fetal position weeping and crying out, "I want my Daddy." It was the cry of a little girl whose broken heart had been running her relationship life on some level for decades. My level of grief surprised me. But underneath anger there is nearly always hurt. My ever-present "witness" self stood watching while I went through these steps of releasing pure, unfiltered anger, getting in touch with my grief and letting it out, and nurturing myself and my body afterward. After this process each day, I took a bath with Epsom salts. As I sat in the warm water, I imagined all of the toxins in my body and mind leaching out of me and down the drain.

For three consecutive days, I used this anger and grief release process, and then I spent five to ten minutes a day for the next two days doing "active imagination" work, imagining exactly how I wanted my father to have responded to me during the times when he was so critical. I imagined him dancing with me in the kitchen, praising me for my beauty, grace, and skill as a dancer. I imagined myself glowing with pride, awash in his praise of my desirability.

Having cleared out the toxins from my cells, I was now reprogramming those cells with a new story. It was like removing the rocks from the soil and cultivating it before planting new seeds. I also did some of that towel work and raging to express my frustration, anger, and grief about the emotionally unavailable man in my life. Within about two weeks, the shoulder pain and limitation were nearly gone. It took about another month for full range of motion to return and all pain to completely resolve, but then I was pain-free even during my Pilates sessions.

One of the insights I had during my healing process, which I developed over the course of a few months, was that the imprint of lack of love toward myself was being mirrored in some of my closest relationships. People were reflecting my own beliefs about myself back to me! My well-developed intellect wouldn't let me see that at first. But working with my dreams, with Dr. Cohen, and with exercises for releasing my feelings about my father, I came to appreciate my role in keeping myself stuck in old beliefs and behaviors that no longer served me. Notice I didn't say I had no right to my old feelings, or no right to see my father as cruel in some ways, or no right to my defensive behaviors and choices—such as getting and staying involved with an emotionally unavailable lover. I said I rid myself of what was *no longer serving me*. I stood up for myself and my own worth. I declared that I deserved to be treated better, and that had to start in the only place I have any control over: how I treat myself. The fact that you are entitled to your hurt, grief, and defensiveness doesn't mean it's working for you. You get to decide whether the payoff of holding on to all that is worth jeopardizing your health, feeling lousy, and pushing away new opportunities because of your distrust, or cynicism, or avoidance behaviors. It's up to you to make the choices. I'm just advising you to let all that crap go so you can flourish.

Healing is always a combination of emotional, physical, and spiritual work, and we all have our unfinished business with our parents or other important figures from childhood that has to be resolved. These patterns set the stage for our health and relationships for our entire lives because our early years are when our core beliefs about the world in general, and our self-worth in particular, are formed. As children, we don't have the capacity to emotionally or mentally process our painful experiences. We may think that the harsh words of others have rolled off our backs, or that we've worked it all through in therapy or by writing in our journals. But then a physical ailment or an emotional crisis arises—or both do. That's when we realize that there's some old stuff buried within us that has to come up and out the way it went in: through our bodies' energy fields and tissues.

Our bodies love us so much that they will do anything necessary to bring us to a place in which we recognize and release our unlovingness toward ourselves that's causing us deep heartache. The message of illness and pain may be "It's time to bring healing love into your energy field. You've been in emotional pain long enough. Let me turn up the volume by creating physical pain so you'll pay attention and take care of your heart."

WHERE EMOTIONS GET STUCK

When you don't feel and release emotions regularly, they get stuck and eventually create illness. The older the trauma, the more deeply buried that trauma will be. We learn to wall off our pain and "soldier on," and after a few decades, most of us are very skilled at this and have a lot of very old emotions stuck in us. Our culture doesn't teach us how to release our emotions as they come up, much less when they've become buried.

In my teen years, when I was going through a breakup with my first boyfriend, my father hugged me and said, "Feelings are facts. And sometimes you just have to get them off your chest." Much of what is required to truly flourish is embedded right in our everyday language. To "get something off your chest" means to free up your heart, your lungs, and your shoulders from the burdens of feeling unloving and unloved. Grief, rage, hurt, and resentment are all forms of being unloving toward ourselves and others. And though we are sometimes visited by a divinely inspired moment of grace and insight that quickly and easily lifts this burden of "unlovingness," most often the burden is not lifted until we are brought to our knees by the weight of it. We don't have to wait until that moment to free ourselves! We don't have to create illness to awaken to our need to heal.

I loved my father dearly. We were a lot alike, and I looked up to him. He was a pioneer in what we would now call holistic dentistry. My dad often said that you could tell the state of someone's health by looking in that person's mouth. His philosophy of health and disease, in direct contrast to that of his sister and brother, who were conventional physicians, became the basis of my own holistic medical practice. My father could do no wrong in my eyes. But long after his death, I was stunned by how much resentment lay buried deep in my mind and body. I thought that everyday misunderstandings and the ordinary mistakes our mothers and fathers make in the course of parenting couldn't possibly cause wounds that can remain unhealed for a lifetime.

We can love our family members dearly and make a conscious choice to forgive them for whatever hurts they have caused us. In fact, this step in our healing is crucial. But it's not enough. We still need to clear old hurts, anger, and grievances from our bodies. The health benefits of this are immense.

When the pain of staying stuck is greater than the pain you have to go through to get free, you have the opportunity to let go of the heartache of the past and be free to bloom. Once you get to the point where you're ready for the breakthrough, the emotions will appear one way or another. If you ignore them or repress them again, they'll come back up. And the longer you wait, the more likely they are to come up accompanied by physical ailments meant to awaken you to the need for healing.

There are four crucial truths about stored emotions that you must know if you want to be an ageless goddess:

- We store our emotions in our energy fields and tissues, where they can remain for years, suppressed and waiting for us to have the courage to express them.

- Unprocessed emotions of anger, grief, sadness, and shame are a serious threat to health and well-being. They cause the body to create and hold on to stress hormones that lead to cellular degeneration, inflammation, and all sorts of physical ailments we associate with aging, as you've seen.

- You must process your emotions. You do that by learning what need they signify and then releasing them through movement, sound, and tears. It can take a lot of repetition—using techniques like the ones you'll learn about in this chapter—to bring the emotions up and out of you. I know that letting yourself feel and release so-called "negative" emotions is easier said than done. Shame is endemic in our society, and we're taught to feel ashamed of ourselves and our strong emotions that make others uncomfortable, especially our anger. As shame researcher Brené Brown says in her book *Daring Greatly,* "We're all afraid to talk about shame. . . . The less we talk about shame, the more control it has over our lives."[1]

~   There's no need to fear the emotions that come up, because they won't last forever or overwhelm you— though at first you may think they will. The good news is that we're designed biologically to feel and release emotions regularly and easily.

Many of us were taught that as long as we mentally acknowledge that we're ticked off, or sad, or jealous, or embarrassed, or ashamed, and we think through why we feel that way and make some conscious choices about our thoughts and behaviors, that's the end of it. Wrong. Emotions have an energetic and physiological reality that doesn't magically disappear when you think to yourself, *I don't want to be mad at my mother anymore, so I'll just go along with her holiday plans and try not to let her get to me.* They don't disappear simply because you've cried a few times, or shouted at someone, or talked to your therapist. Shifting your thoughts is very important, but it's not enough. You have a lot of emotional energy to release too. As Dr. Joe Dispenza says, "Emotions are the language of the body. And they are also a record of the past." We can't change our bodies or our health simply by changing our thoughts. True transformation involves changing both our thoughts and the emotional connections that keep us stuck in the past.

The *only* way to get rid of your anger, guilt, shame, grief, or fear thoroughly so that it doesn't affect your health in the long run is to start a process of emotional release. Learn what you can from your experiences. You might want to do this with the help of a coach or therapist—there are many who incorporate emotional release work into their sessions. However, after you've gleaned what you need to know about the origins of your feelings and behaviors, don't talk about your childhood traumas over and over again in lieu of doing emotional release work. As author Anne Wilson Schaef said to me once, "We take our shit and we put it on an altar and worship it!" And unfortunately, we expect everyone else to worship it too, which is why "victims" can be so manipulative. How many of us have been taught to repress our inconvenient feelings and walk on eggshells around others who have unfinished business that may have nothing to do with us? Maybe you were told, "Don't talk about that in front of Aunt Mabel. You know that she lost a daughter in the past and has never gotten over it!" It's always important to be kind. But worshipping the family wounds for generations is just not healthy!

All of us are given a certain amount of crap to compost. Get it out of you so that you can mix it into rich soil and create something new. Learn from it, write a poem expressing it, and dance or cry it out of you to heal yourself. Create something better from the crap so that it doesn't define your life or make you sick. And while we're composting, let's throw onto the compost heap the old belief that suffering is redemptive. You are not getting a ticket to the VIP seats in heaven by torturing yourself on Earth today. The atonement archetype has to go. And it's deeply embedded in most of us.

When it comes to painful emotions, it's important not to indulge their inherent drama. There's a difference between bringing emotions to the surface of your awareness so that you can release them and artificially keeping these emotional experiences alive in you. Don't be fashionably cynical. Don't identify with your depressive feelings and tell yourself that the world is out to get you so you might as well anticipate the worst. Better to indulge in "pronoia," which writer and astrologer Rob Brezsny defines as "the belief that the world is conspiring to shower us with blessings." Now *that* is a mind-set that supports health.

So stop waiting for the moment when it's okay to be happy— when you've lost the weight, stopped making financial mistakes, or achieved whatever goalpost of perfection you set up for yourself. Put on the music and dance *now*. Your unrestricted, luscious, rich joy serves not only you but the planet. So move those lower chakras, open your heart, and let your life force express itself like the most succulent, juicy fruit, the most redolent and colorful flower, or the loudest and most raucous song. After that, make a commitment to getting rid of all the old emotional toxins that have become stuck inside you so you can live freely and agelessly.

Let's look at the emotions you hold on to, how they affect you, and how to get rid of them when they're no longer serving you so you can bring in the healing forces of love, laughter, pride, and sheer delight in being alive on earth.

LEARN FROM YOUR EMOTIONS

By midlife, you've had your heart broken at least once, and probably more, by someone or something. Heartbreak is how your heart becomes wise, because it has to be cracked open for you to experience your divinity. The more you try to avoid heartbreak and dull the pain through drinking, smoking, eating, or denial, the worse the pain gets and the deeper it buries itself. Fortunately, the heartbreak you've survived gives you the strength to face the emotions you've been encouraged to avoid.

Anger, fear, sadness, betrayal, abandonment, and shame are the more challenging emotions we tend to avoid, to our detriment. Shame is the most painful because it stops us from facing the other emotions. There really aren't any "negative" emotions because all emotions have a function. They serve as our innate guidance system, alerting us to what we truly need and what we need to change. Anger and fear—and those are closely related—are experienced in the primitive limbic brain system that evolved to help us avoid danger. When faced with danger, the limbic brain begins a process of reaction that involves anger, fear, and the urge to fight or run away. But we also feel anger and fear in response to thoughts, and to situations or people that aren't actually dangerous.

It's good that we have a fear response, because fear and anger can remind us to slow down and sort out what we think and feel before saying yes to whatever's being asked of us. However, fear and anger aren't supposed to be a way of life. As Stephen Covey wrote in *The 7 Habits of Highly Effective Families* (St. Martin's Griffin, 1998), quoting Viktor Frankl, "Between stimulus and response, there is a space. In that space is our power to choose our response. In our response lies our growth and our freedom." Agelessness happens in that space where we choose to step into joy and possibility rather than remain stuck in a vicious cycle of anger, fear, and grief. This experience can also be called wisdom—which Dr. Joe Dispenza brilliantly refers to as "memory without the emotional charge."[2]

Grief is a little different from anger and fear. It tends to have less energy—in fact, it zaps us of energy. Becoming sad is a part of life, but if you carry your grief for too long, it will age you very quickly. Don't suppress your grief because you feel pressured to keep your tears to yourself. What's the first thing you do when you see people crying? You probably tell them not to cry and try to talk them out of their sadness. And chances are you also hug them—as a way to stop their pain. Then they feel obligated to stop crying because it's making you uncomfortable.

There's a happy medium here. One mother says to her sensitive daughter after a good ten minutes of her daughter moping on the living room couch, "I know you're sad about this and I'm sorry you feel that way. Maybe you should take some time in your room to cry." She's not banishing her daughter, or saying her daughter is being too sensitive. She's just teaching her that sometimes it's best to be alone with your tears. Now, this mom checks in after a while to make sure her daughter hasn't gotten stuck in her mood, but she gives her daughter room to be sad. Wouldn't it be marvelous if we all encouraged each other to let it out but not indulge sadness to the point where everyone feels the need to flop in a chair and begin weeping?

Thoughts and beliefs can fan the embers of sadness just as they can rekindle any emotion, so it's important to look at any depressing, pessimistic attitudes and stories you have about your life and decide whether you want to replace them. Recently I had some old slides that I hadn't looked at in decades scanned into jpegs. And I was utterly astounded by how lovely I looked in the early years of my marriage. But back then, I didn't feel beautiful at all. It didn't help that the man I was married to was always happy to tell me that I could stand to lose weight. I spent many years certain that I was too fat and not desirable as a woman. Those beliefs—and the shame and grief that were part of them—eventually showed up as a frozen shoulder, chest pain, and a large fibroid in my uterus. I have reversed all of these conditions through bringing the beliefs and the feelings associated with them to consciousness to be felt and released. And with each layer of the onion that I've shed, I have become healthier and happier—which is really the body's natural state. What old beliefs and feelings do you need to release? What sadness are you holding on to?

I don't mean to minimize how strongly you can be affected by anger, fear, or sadness. It's incredibly scary to contemplate the end of a relationship, losing your job or your home, and so on, and those things can happen, forcing you to accept that change is a part of life. You can't freeze your circumstances and avoid future suffering, but you can choose to live in fear or live in faith. Most of what's called security is an illusion anyway. You can create a sense of security even when you're in a transition or your circumstances aren't what you would like them to be. Your inner power to generate emotions such as confidence and faith is incredible. And the ability to do so literally rewires both your brain and your body. But to do this, you first have to connect with the Divine.

The actual problem isn't what we fear so much as the emotion of fear eating away at us. Many women, myself included, share a primal fear that somehow we'll end up homeless and living alone in a cardboard box on the street. (I shared this scary daydream with a friend recently and she quipped, "You had a box?" Apparently in her version of the daydream, she didn't even have that!) This fear of being completely helpless and broke is irrational for most of us—but there it is, seeping up from the collective unconscious. In general, we humans tend to look out for each other, and support can come from unexpected places when you turn your life over to the Divine Beloved. To live as an ageless goddess is to release fear and strengthen faith.

Name your fear and transform it instead of hanging on to it. One of my favorite prayers to heal fear goes like this: "Divine Beloved, please change me into someone who trusts that the perfect outcome to this situation has already been chosen. Change me into someone who can relax and let go." Say this prayer (or something in a similar spirit, such as the Twenty-third Psalm) when your fear of the future or the unknown has you in its grip. Over time, it will become a habit. Letting go and letting God is a learnable skill.

MANY FORMS OF SHAME

Fear and anger are like weeds that feed on shame—and shame is a toxin we need to release if we want to be ageless! Again and again, we get the message that our needs aren't important and that we're being selfish and bad if we take care of ourselves. No wonder we're afraid to feel our emotions. A patient of mine once told me, "In my household, I was so certain I wasn't wanted, I was afraid of breathing deeply because I might take up oxygen other people needed." Guilt serves a purpose, waking us up to something we need to correct, but shame is downright poisonous. Brené Brown distinguishes between guilt and shame this way: guilt is feeling you *made* a mistake while shame is feeling you *are* a mistake. That said, *healthy* shame serves the purpose of alerting us when we've truly been selfish and even cruel. It creates good boundaries between people and leads us to create a balance between our needs and those of the people around us. Our conscience makes us feel ashamed when we've acted shamelessly, oblivious to anyone else's feelings and needs.

However, unjustified shame is very different. It is hands down the most destructive and painful emotion that we humans are capable of feeling. It drains us of life force and creativity. Our energy goes to hating ourselves instead of to self-correcting, and we forget that, like everyone else, we deserve love and acceptance. Too many women are terrified of taking risks and making a mistake, socially or otherwise, because they fear other people shaming them. And no wonder—it happens all the time.

Women are shamed for just about everything. They are especially shamed for not being perfect: being too thin or too fat, too beautiful or too plain, too bubbly or too serious, too emotionally expressive or too cold, and of course, too sexy or too unsexy. You can't win if you're trying to please the perfection police!

Mary Pipher, author of *Reviving Ophelia: Saving the Selves of Adolescent Girls* (Putnam, 1994), and others have pointed out that as teenagers, girls start to realize they can never achieve that balance of perfection that's expected of them and their self-esteem plummets. It seems no matter what we do, there's plenty of public shaming to keep us from flourishing.

We're even shamed sometimes just for feeling happy. A woman was telling me the other day that at her meditation center, the group was instructed to meditate on equality in honor of some civil rights legislation breakthrough that had just occurred. Afterward, the meditators shared their experiences. One of the men said he had meditated on all the work that still had to be done, and expressed how depressing and upsetting it was for him to hear people celebrating the new law when its scope was so limited. He was, in essence, shaming those who were looking on the bright side. "How dare you feel happy when there's still so much more to be done!" This was a blatant example of what I call the "moral superiority of pessimism"—making everyone feel as though they had no right to celebrate while others were still suffering. Happiness shouldn't be shamed!

It's crucial to your health and happiness that you learn to spot this kind of manipulation the moment it's happening and not allow yourself to get sucked in. Let's look at the logic here: you can't actually get sick enough to help those who are sick, you can't get sad enough to help those who are sad, and you can't get poor enough to help those who are destitute. The belief that suffering somehow makes us holier or superior is rooted in what is called the "zero-sum model" that runs most of Western culture—the system that says, "Resources are limited. So if you get more, someone else will have to go without." This is simply not true when it comes to the currency of health and happiness!

SHAME HOLDS YOU BACK

Shame is toxic not just to your health but to your creativity, learning, and growth. In the medical and research professions, the one thing you can count on is this statement at the end of just about every research paper that presents new, sometimes helpful

information, such as the health benefits of vitamin D: "More research needs to be done." It's become a mantra to let the doctor
off the hook of taking a position. After all, if she's wrong she will
be shamed. In the early days of being an ob/gyn, I read many research studies showing that if you prescribe folic acid to pregnant
women, you reduce the risk of the baby developing spina bifida,
so I went ahead and prescribed it. Despite all the research, it took
the American College of Obstetrics and Gynecology 15 years to
officially recommend this intervention. How many babies were
harmed in the meanwhile because shame and fear held doctors
back from doing the right thing? We're still awaiting official permission to get rid of fetal monitoring, which has never improved
outcomes for mothers or babies but does increase the risk of C-
sections. Current research shows very clearly that having optimal
levels of vitamin D in your blood can cut your risk for breast cancer in half and substantially lower your risk of other cancers, such
as colorectal cancer. And giving enough vitamin D to pregnant
women drastically reduces a child's chance of developing type 1
diabetes, which should be mainstream knowledge. But almost no
one wants to make the first move for fear of being wrong.

What are you afraid to change in your life because you think
you might be shamed for making a mistake? Is the desire to be
seen as perfect keeping you from expressing yourself? You have
to take risks to be adventurous. Not every risk turns out to be
a good one, but we can only learn and change and bring about
something new if we let ourselves be clumsy, unskilled novices
who screw up here and there. Repressing the need to grow and
try something new is disastrous for health and well-being. Remember, creativity *is* the life force. Cut it off, and you cut yourself off from the Source of everything.

Let's face it: shame can get us stuck in every sort of emotion
and behavior that can hold us back. Because we're often afraid of
being shamed for not being a "good" person, or for being disloy-
al, we don't prioritize our desires and instead focus on pleasing
everyone else. Because our culture doesn't agree on what constitutes "appropriate" grief, we get shamed for being too sad after
a loss—or not sad enough. You might find yourself holding on to
grief to prove what a good spouse, parent, or daughter you are.

You start feeling like Scarlett O'Hara in mourning, desperately wanting to dance but instead feeling compelled to look every inch the bereaved widow in head-to-toe black.

On the other hand, you might be encouraged to "get over it" when you haven't had the chance to express your grief fully. Grief is a process, not an event. An acquaintance of mine lost her son in a car accident. A year later, her husband told her she should be "over it" by now. But each of us has our own timeline for recovery from loss. How can you decide for another person when grieving should end?

Sometimes people will shame you because they're jealous and think, *I should have had that opportunity she had! It's not fair!* Many people have what author Gay Hendricks calls an "upper limit problem," meaning they have internalized an upper limit to their joy, their success, their happiness. This upper limit of what is possible is generally set in place by age 11 or so. We learn in childhood what we can expect in love, success, and freedom. And when we surpass that "upper limit" with more success or love than we thought possible or thought we deserved, we tend to get sick, pick a fight, or have an accident in order to bring ourselves back below that subconscious limit.[3] Paramahansa Yogananda said, "Everyone has self-limiting idiosyncrasies. They were not put into your nature by God, but were created by you. These are what you must change—by remembering that these habits, peculiar to your nature, are nothing but manifestations of your own thoughts." Don't be afraid to transcend your limits!

RELEASING SHAME

Life is too short to live in shame and limitation, leading a vitality-sapping existence of anxiety and depression as we scramble in vain to hit that sweet spot of perfection where no one will criticize or shame us. The truth is that the sweet spot doesn't exist. To move beyond shame, we have to learn to consciously feel our shame fully and eventually learn to laugh at it—and at ourselves. Happiness researcher Robert Holden points out that shame cannot continue to exist when the energy around it is lightened up with laughter.

People whose lives are shame based live with the mistaken idea that the harder they are on themselves, the better human beings they'll be. Western civilization and many religions have sold us on the idea that suffering buys us something and that we have to atone for our very existence.

Our biology takes its cue from these beliefs and responds accordingly, making our physical experience mirror what we believe. Dr. Mario Martinez has studied numerous cases of stigmata, the phenomenon of bleeding from areas in the hands and feet associated with Jesus's wounds on the cross. The wounds don't become infected but they don't heal, and they're quite painful. Dr. Martinez's cases include the famous Padre Pio, and he has even been hired by the Catholic Church to carry out his research. In working with some of these individuals, Dr. Martinez has helped them heal and recover from pain simply by offering them the understanding that suffering is not necessary in order to serve your community.[4]

Like stigmata, illness and accidents are often the result of culturally supported beliefs about the need for suffering and atonement. Unlike the placebo effect, which is the belief that good things will happen, illnesses and accidents can be a kind of cultural nocebo: a belief that something bad will happen or needs to happen. The more critical and unforgiving we are toward ourselves, the more miserable and sick we're apt to be. The body has a remarkable ability to manifest shame as illness or physical problems, because the hurt of shame registers in the brain in exactly the same way physical pain does—and it also produces inflammatory chemicals in the body that set us up for illness. This is why, in the famous CDC-Kaiser Permanente study of adverse childhood experiences (ACE), it has been documented that those who experience adverse events in childhood generally associated with shame, abandonment, and betrayal are far more likely to experience health problems and die prematurely than those who didn't experience these things.

Fortunately, there's an alternative. Shame researcher Brené Brown discovered that it's possible to become shame resilient, or what she calls "wholehearted." She says the only difference between those who are wholehearted and those who are shame based is—get this—the belief that they are worthy of love and connection. That's it. Nothing else. Wholehearted people can be found in every socioeconomic group, and they lead healthy lives and have rich emotional connections to others. And becoming wholehearted is a learnable skill. It begins with simply accepting where you are now, having compassion and understanding for yourself, and rejecting the cultural belief that self-care is self-centered and wrong.

How many of us are holding on to anger, sadness, and hurt over the false belief that we missed our big chance or someone else stopped us from living the life we wanted? Limiting beliefs can keep old, destructive emotions alive inside us like a cancer that refuses to die. Dissolve it with Divine Love and understanding the minute you become aware of it! Or spend a couple minutes each morning or evening using Gay Hendricks's Ultimate Success Mantra: "I expand in abundance, success and love every day, as I inspire those around me to do the same." The subconscious mind is very receptive to the word *expand,* and that word and the feeling of expansion help you release from your body beliefs about what your upper limits are.

LETTING IT OUT

Letting your emotions out isn't pretty: You aren't going to look like the flawless-skinned Hollywood beauty in a 1940s movie with one perfect tear trailing down your cheek as your moist eyes glitter with light. You're probably going to be a ruddy, honking, snorting, sobbing wet mess of raw emotion, and so what? Let it out. It's not frowning that causes your face to develop jowls and frown lines, but the slow death that comes from stuffing your emotions and keeping them tamped down by drinking, smoking, and worrying about what people will think of you if you're honest with them. If you want to make your cells sick, hold on to shame and guilt. But if you want to be a goddess who never ages, release those emotions.

According to traditional Hawaiian spirituality, the goddess Pele causes volcanoes to erupt because she's enraged that she can't be with her lover. She yearns for sexual pleasure and release, and if she can't have it, there will be hell to pay! But let's not forget that it was volcanic eruptions that created the islands of Hawaii—a process that continues every day. Since its eruption in 1983, Mount Kilauea in Hawaii has created more than 540 acres of new land on planet Earth. Anger can be a force for creation and positive change if you stop fearing it and start expressing it appropriately. Think of your anger as your own personal volcano—creating acres of new choices, new cells, new relationships, and new opportunities from your own bone marrow!

When I was releasing my anger toward my father, I suspected my emotional release process would not only cure my frozen shoulder but free me up to let go of my fear of not being desirable. I wanted to reclaim my womanly attractiveness—my belief that I am one hot, luscious woman that any man would be lucky to be around. I couldn't do that until I released the emotions that were holding me back. I couldn't create my new life while I was still hanging on to anger and grief from the old one.

Exercise: Snapping Out Grief and Rage

In her Seven Sacred Steps workshops (www.theseven sacredsteps.com), Unity minister Jill Rogers suggests a method for releasing the intertwined emotions of anger and grief that create pressure in our cells. This is an exercise I used in my own release of anger and grief about my father. You can use it for releasing these emotions about anyone you've been close to. You'll find that at the core of your anger at that person is actually your grief and rage about the fact that their heart was (or is) closed to you. To do this exercise, you'll need a timer, a towel (a terry cloth hand towel will work perfectly), and an empty chair that you place in front of you.

Set the timer for five or ten minutes, no more, in order to contain your expression of grief and rage so that you don't become overwhelmed by your emotions—or the soreness in your arm, because you'll be whacking a surface with that towel and giving your arm muscles a workout! Now, facing the chair, imagine that the person you are angry with is sitting there. Then start letting that person have it. As you do, turn and snap the towel against a hard surface, such as a sturdy wall, a door, or the frame around a door. Make sure that the surface can take it. As Jill suggests (and I have to agree), it's the snapping of the towel along with the yelling that is so satisfying.

Really let it rip, expressing your rage and anger at the person whom you're imagining in that chair. Speak your truth and tell that person exactly what he or she did that makes you mad. Use the worst swear words that can come out of you! Remember, even if you have done the psychological work of forgiving this person, the child within you who was hurt is holding on to anger. It's not your adult self who is getting healed here. It's that angry and wounded child self who is still running your endocrine, immune, and central nervous systems. Let her have her say!

After a few minutes of towel snapping, cursing, and shouting, you may be ready to declare, "I hate it when your heart is closed to me!" If not—if you're too caught up in your rage—leave it for your next session. But don't skip this step! When we're really furious with someone, it's often because we wanted to be connected to that person in love, but for some reason, the person couldn't connect with us. Saying, "I hate it when your heart is closed to me!" acknowledges and releases grief along with the anger that you weren't able to have the experience with this person that you wanted, needed, and deserved.

When doing this exercise, don't try to be "spiritual" and compassionate toward this person—who isn't actually there anyway! Don't forgive him or her too soon. Otherwise, you'll block the healing. Once you begin to release the anger, the hurt, and the resentment with movement and tears, you may actually be able to feel the pressure in your cells release. Tune in to how it feels in your body and energy field afterward. If the person is still in your life, notice whether you feel a shift in your response to him or her the next time you get together.

Emotional release should be followed with healing work (see the suggestions that follow shortly). It should be repeated regularly until you feel a shift in yourself. But don't think you can skip the release part and go straight to the healing. There are no shortcuts or detours around the pain.

Forgiveness isn't an intellectual exercise. If you attempt to mentally forgive someone who hurt or betrayed you but don't release the anger, resentment, and grief, it's like snipping off the top of a dandelion and leaving the long roots in the earth. Forgiveness is a process and it must involve emotional release that occurs in your body and mind simultaneously. Don't be distracted by the other person's emotional issues, which aren't yours. *Your feelings matter.* Remember, this process is for healing and freeing *you.* You don't have to discuss it with the other person—ever! Nor do you need that person to apologize to you. You don't need to reconcile with or even see that person ever again. That's not the point. You don't want to remain angry, of course, but you have to let your true feelings arise and be experienced and expressed. Then, after you feel your grief or rage starting to subside as you do the work of releasing it, you can look at your past more objectively and sort out what belongs to you and what belongs to someone else. Forgiveness isn't condoning what the other person did. It's deciding to release the toxic feelings that remain and to set firm boundaries for yourself so you don't get hurt again. Dr. Mario Martinez refers to forgiveness as liberation from self-entrapment. It is a process of reclaiming the worthiness and self-love that you inadvertently gave to the person who hurt you. Forgiveness is about loving and freeing yourself in the present. Releasing your old emotions and replacing them with loving kindness toward yourself is like climbing to a mountaintop and breathing clean fresh air.

THE PAIN THAT ENDS THE PAIN

It's incredibly painful when people betray you, dismiss you, or harden their hearts to you. It's as if you have a boil that needs lancing, or a sliver that is trying to work its way out of your skin. When your body creates inflammation, it sends fluids to surround the foreign substance or object that needs to be removed, which causes an exquisite sensitivity. The pressure is intense. Blood can't get to the area to wash out the foreign body or toxin. If you cut into the boil or pry out the sliver to release the pressure, it will be very painful at first, but then the fluids will flow, cleansing the area. Tears, sweat, urine, mucus, and blood escaping through the skin all remove toxins, which is why your eyes itch and your nose runs when you've got a cold. All of this can be seen as a metaphor for our need to let our emotions flow forth and wash out of us. As meditation teacher Stephen Levine says in his book *Healing into Life and Death* (Anchor Books, 1987), feeling challenging emotions is "the pain that ends the pain."[5] Intuitive Llorraine Neithardt recalled her mentor Reverend Phyllis Woodbury telling her, "My dear, the only way to heaven is through the gates of hell."[6]

Simply allowing yourself to have a good cry can be cathartic and healing. It energetically releases stagnant emotions of anger and grief. This is why the famous writer Isak Dinesen wrote in *Seven Gothic Tales* (Random House, 1934) that the cure for everything is salt water: "Sweat, or tears, or the salt sea." Movies and music that make you cry can also help you get in touch with and release your blocked emotions. A movie like *Beaches* or *The Notebook* primes the pump so your own feelings can come up and out. My daughters and I watched the 2012 movie *Les Misérables,* and the sequence where Anne Hathaway sings "I Dreamed a Dream," channeling every feeling of abandonment, sadness, and hopelessness any woman ever experienced, is so powerfully cathartic that the short clip should be sold separately for any woman who needs a good cry! The three of us sat together in the theater, awash in tears.

In fact, weeping in order to let out your feelings is crucial for your health. If you find tears welling up at an inconvenient time, I suggest you silently say to your emotions, "Don't go away. I'll get back to you. Please come up again." Then, as soon as you can, get to a place or into a situation where you can let your body release those tears along with the sounds and movements that go with them.

Releasing your emotions shouldn't involve force. Just as pulling out a baby with forceps can cause damage, trying to force out emotions before you have the strength to deal with them is not wise. The body knows how to heal. You can assist a little as the head is crowning, but you have to work with nature and not be too aggressive. Don't go digging for buried pain; gently allow it to arise. A *New York Times* blog cited research showing that soldiers who have suffered PTSD may avoid therapy out of fear that they'll be pressured to talk about their trauma in detail before they're ready to. These soldiers may instinctively sense that directly confronting deep trauma can be too painful an experience for them in the early stages of their recovery.[7]

You can also let emotions surface by doing meditation, Reiki, or bodywork such as massage, all of which still your mind and allow your body and energy field to bring to the surface feelings that need to be released. If you're working with an energy healer or a masseuse, be sure they know that the best way to support you in emotional release is through encouragement—words such as "Good job! You're doing great! Let it out!" are helpful.

Another way of releasing emotions is through movement. Indigenous people danced, sang, and chanted for healing. Eve Ensler, author of *The Vagina Monologues,* organized the global movement called One Billion Rising to draw attention to the fact that one in three women—that's one billion people on the planet—have experienced being raped, sexually abused, or physically assaulted. Instead of the usual angry protesting, Ensler used a far more celebratory—and effective—approach to healing: strike, dance, and rise. She urged people to leave work, dance with passion, and rise up as one to end violence against women. What a great way to honor the joy of living rather than dwell on pain! Recognize the grief and anger, and then move your body into a primal space of healing.

Singing and chanting give voice to emotions too. Sing on your own or in a choir, or start a sing-along with others. I know some women who sing old camp songs from their Girl Scout days, complete with hand motions, every time they get together. Their husbands and kids have learned to join in because they know there is no stopping the sing-along when the "girls" gather with their families. It is a celebration of the friendship and love they have shared for years, and the strength they've received from each other and given back to each other. Don't you love how women—particularly sisters and good friends—tend to giggle whenever they get together?

RELEASE AND RELIEF

When you let any emotion flow, it makes it easier to get out of that numb state and let all of them flow. I look back now at videos of myself from 20 years ago, before my divorce, and I'm shocked by how shut down I looked and sounded. None of my feelings flowed freely because I didn't want to face my fear, pain, or anger. I was too busy trying to keep my marriage and family together, look like a professional, and reinvent the language of women's health for the sake of my patients, for whom I felt responsible. The burden of this was huge.

When you do finally allow yourself to feel your emotions fully, you may be surprised by how quickly they move through you. They rise and subside naturally, even though it may seem you'll never stop crying or raging when you first let your feelings surface. Look at how children will wail and tantrum but then allow their feelings to subside. They'll sniffle and then run off to play. They don't brood and hold on to the anger or sadness.

That said, you don't want emotions to get so intense that you end up believing you can't handle the experience—that the tears will never end and you'll fall into a never-ending abyss of sadness. That fear-based belief can shut you down all over again. Create a container for releasing your emotions by using a grief or anger releasing ritual (see page 139).

After a release of emotions, you will feel a sense of relief. Your muscles will relax and your entire body will feel cleansed. And you may well end up laughing. Then you can enhance the healing by further shifting your energy. I like to dance, watch a funny movie, or read something inspirational that redirects me to turn everything over to the Divine. Reward yourself for doing the hard work of feeling your old, painful emotions to get them up and out of you.

After an emotional release session, you can also do an Epsom salts, mineral salt, or sea salt bath, which will relax your body and release toxins. Baths can be a marvelously soothing form of self-nurturing. While in the bath, or out of it, you can close your eyes and do affirmations or a Divine Beloved prayer. To heal yourself further, you can also do what I did with my father, as I explained

How to Do a Releasing Ritual

Ritual is incredibly powerful because it gets us out of our heads and right into our bodies. Set aside 15 to 30 minutes to do this ritual.

Gather a pen and paper and be ready to play some recorded music that touches your heart.

Light a candle and say a prayer or set an intention for releasing your feelings. You can say something like "I invite my spirit to join me now to assist me in releasing my anger or grief concerning . . . (fill in the blank). I also invite in my guardian angel, my guides, my teachers, Mother Mary (or whatever Divine beings you feel comfortable calling on). For the next 30 minutes, please assist me in releasing whatever needs to be released." Note that the words aren't as important as your intention to be healed through the release of old emotions.

Start the music.

Take one deep breath and then begin writing a letter to the person who has hurt you. Pour out all your feelings on paper.

After 15 to 30 minutes, read out loud what you wrote. Feel the emotions as they arise. Take time to cry if necessary.

Burn the paper. Shut off the music. Thank your guides and blow out the candle.

Repeat this ritual as needed. Releasing grief and rage can be like peeling an onion. There are layers. And they tend to get released one layer at a time.

earlier, and reimagine that painful scenario of your past playing out differently. I imagined dancing with my father and seeing him respond with encouragement and compliments, and imagined myself glowing with pride under his approving gaze.

Humor raises your vibration and makes you feel good again, so go ahead and laugh at yourself or your situation. Crack a joke as you reach for a tissue. You can't sustain shame, fear, and sadness when you're laughing.

You can also say a prayer, such as "Divine Beloved, please change me into someone who loves myself fully and sees how desirable, smart, and wonderful I am." Make sure you say this out loud daily for 21 days. Affirmations train your brain and mind to feel comfortable with a new reality you're choosing for yourself: a reality in which you are strong, able to love with an open heart, and so on. Say your affirmations or prayers with feeling until you sense an energetic shift in yourself. The shift begins inside you and then is mirrored outside of you. As I've heard Agape minister Michael Beckwith say, "Affirmations don't make something happen. They make something welcome." So true!

I also recommend the At Oneness Healing System created by Robert Fritchie, founder of the World Service Institute and featured in his Healing Yourself from Within webinars. Bob, who wrote the marvelous book *Being at One with the Divine* (World Service Institute, 2013), teaches the power of Divine Love to people all around the world and has spent decades documenting the healing power of this energy.

To truly heal from emotional, physical, or spiritual wounds, you first need to connect with Divine Love—and this love is available to everyone, but we have to ask for it. Making this connection is the most important part of living like an ageless goddess! Bob has created a type of prayer called a Divine Love petition for just this purpose. You can learn more about his incredibly helpful program on his website, but even just doing a Divine Love petition of your own can be very powerful.

Exercise: Divine Love Petition

Bob Fritchie's Divine Love petitions are prayers that use the power of your spirit to connect with the Creator. Here's an example of a petition: "With my Spirit and the angels' help, I focus Divine Love throughout my system. I ask my

Spirit to identify any beliefs I have about being unworthy or unlovable. And I ask that these be dissolved and healed with Divine Love, according to the Creator's Will."

After stating the petition, inhale through your nose. Hold it for a few seconds. Then exhale it through your nose in short bursts. The inhale draws your energy within. The exhalation through your nose sends the intention back into the universe.

Continue to be fully present in the moment, mindful of your breathing, your thoughts, and the bodily feelings that come to you after you've said this petition out loud. Afterward, you might want to ponder what came to you when you were doing the Divine Love petition and journal about your experience.

The words aren't important. The intent is. And when you add "according to the Creator's Will," you are acknowledging the biggest possible picture—and that there might be reasons for your current situation that are far bigger than your intellect can appreciate.

(For more information on Divine Love and to access the free Divine Love healing program, see the website www .worldserviceinstitute.org.)

PRACTICES OF AWARENESS

Meditation, prayer, or any mindfulness practice can help you get in touch with your emotions and remain present with them so that you can release them. Sometimes if you just stay present with bodily pain and ask that it be released to Divine Love or to God, it simply dissolves in the light of your love and consciousness. The same is true of emotional pain. Buried emotions and unresolved issues can reveal themselves in dreams too. Don't ignore any dream that produces a strong feeling in you, whether or not it's a nightmare. Pay attention to symbols, particularly how you feel about them in the dream. Doris E. Cohen points out that women will often dream about their homes (which represent themselves) or toilets (which represent the need for cleansing when you're feeling pissed off or in need of getting rid of emotional crap). And pay attention to the specific qualities of the symbols. If you dream of water, is the water cold? Polluted? Part of a deep mountain lake? Leaking from pipes? Full of debris floating by? The details can help you understand what it signifies.

As you're writing down your dreams, allow other images, thoughts, emotions, and impressions to arise, because they will be part of the message of the dream. She also suggests you give the dream a title, as though you were reporting for a newspaper. The title generally nails the issue. For example, you might name it "Filthy toilets and company's coming" or "My childhood home is for sale" or "Basement floods: Everything must go."

Keep a journal in which you record your dreams. You can also record them in the voice memo section of your phone and listen to them later. That way, you can correlate your waking life with your dream imagery. Over time, themes will arise. For example, this past year, I've had recurrent dreams about water—rivers, lakes, bathtubs, flooding living rooms, and so on. Water represents emotions and cleansing as well as spiritual power and abundance. I have gone through a huge amount of emotional cleansing in the past couple of years, and now I can feel how this process has been preparing me for the next phase of my life.

Journals can also be a great container for your feelings and help you break the habit of unproductive ruminating. They are an excellent tool for helping you reflect on your life, which is important when you consider how much pressure women are under to keep their focus on everything and everyone except themselves! I like them because you can go back to earlier entries and see how far you've come in processing your experiences and moving forward in your healing. I keep all my journals in the basement of my house (akin to the subconscious!). They are labeled with dates so I can easily look at what I was thinking, feeling, experiencing, or intuiting at a certain time. I also like to correlate them with astrologic cycles such as Jupiter or Saturn transits. Over the years, this has shored up my faith in the Divine and a Power and plan much bigger than I can imagine.

A LIVING, JOYFUL, PRESENT ORIENTATION

Emotions don't have to get stuck in the connective tissue and energy system of your body, burying themselves ever deeper with the passing years. You can release them as they come up even as you're working on releasing the old ones. If you adopt a living, joyful, present orientation, you can end the habit of letting unprocessed emotions adversely affect your health and well-being. Dwelling on the past and keeping the old stories alive by retelling them as stories of sadness and loss will age you quickly. You don't have to be the grieving widow, parent, sister, or daughter anymore. Maybe you're ready to stop going to the cemetery or to the school where they annually present a scholarship in memory of your late loved one. It's okay to move on.

First come the grief and anger. Then comes the party to celebrate everything that was, is, or will be good. The party has already started and it's called life, so put on your dancing shoes. I currently have about eight pairs of dancing shoes, and I keep them on an altar—with candles! It's really just a display, but I feel it's a tribute to the goddess of dance who lives within me and whom I have wanted to welcome my entire life!

Having a living orientation means paying attention to the goodness in this moment right now. Every time I sit down to have a meal with friends, we join hands and I say an impromptu prayer—I bring Divine Love into the food, I praise whoever is sitting at the table, and many times, I comment on whatever pleasure or good has shown up that day. This raises the vibration of the whole gathering and helps keep attracting more happiness, great people, and wonderful situations. You can do the same.

Speaking of shoes, whenever you see someone wearing a great pair, tell her or him, "Those are gorgeous shoes." Compliment and thank people whenever you can. Share a joke and a burst of nitric oxide. Spreading joy in the moment is a spiritual practice—and so is saying yes to life by allowing yourself to ask for, or go for, whatever it is you want rather than giving in to fear and shame ("Who am I to ask for what I want?"). A couple of years ago, I asked my tango teacher, Paul, to come down to New York City from Portland, Maine, with me so we could dance together at the opening of men's night at Mama Gena's School of Womanly Arts. He said yes. I was shocked—and thrilled. When I thanked him afterward, I said, "I can't believe you came down. You're such a great dancer!" His response was, "Well, I can't believe you didn't ask me before. Why wouldn't I want to come down and dance with you in New York?" Even though I believe we should always go after what we want, I had convinced myself he wouldn't want to dance with me because I'm not a master, like he is—and that it would be too much to ask of him to perform with me as his partner. As it turned out, I was completely wrong. He felt it was an honor for him and, in fact, the experience led to an entirely new career for him both in teaching tango and in writing about what this dance has to teach men and women about relationships and pleasure. The lesson is that you can't get what you want if you don't ask. And if your desire is genuine and coming from your heart, you will find that the fulfillment of that desire has the power to transform everyone who assists you in fulfilling it.

Discard the past and the old ways of doing things. You can create rituals around saying good-bye to the way you used to experience life as a struggle, or to your identification with something that happened long ago that you don't want to keep breathing life into. Write a letter to the person or situation that you want to release. Read the letter out loud to a trusted friend—or just into the ether. Then burn the letter, letting the smoke rise into the night as a symbol of your transformation. Do this ritual as many times as you need to completely free yourself.

RELEASE THROUGH DECLUTTERING

Discarding the past can take a very literal form too. Possessions carry emotional energy and constantly talk to you, so let go of objects that you don't love *even if they're practical*. If you keep that ugly dresser that your mother gave you because it seems foolish to get rid of it, even though every time you look at it you remember how your mother used to harp on you about your clothes, you're keeping alive all of that negative energy associated with your relationship with your mother. You're not storing sweaters in that dresser—you're storing grief, hurt, frustration, and disappointment! Pitch the dresser and release those emotions. In fact, when you're feeling stuck or depressed, often it's empowering to clear out a drawer or closet, shine your sink, or even paint a room or a wall.

Clutter isn't just draining. It can accumulate dust, mold, and mildew and cause respiratory illnesses. You'll literally have trouble breathing because of all the old stuff you've been carrying around. That's why it's very important to let it go—along with any old emotions attached to it. Invite chi, the life force of the Divine, to flow freely through your house. Don't create obstacles for the flow.

As an ageless goddess, you deserve a home that's a haven from the outside world, a place where you can replenish yourself. I like to use feng shui to help me create sanctuaries within my home. Feng shui is based on the idea that by using elements of nature and arranging the objects in our physical space in ways that allow chi to flow freely, we become rejuvenated. My home hugs me now after years of working with feng shui. Your home ought to be your haven too, even if you live in a studio apartment. It's difficult to feel happy, sensual, and sexy when you're tiptoeing through clutter or your space says to you, "Take care of others but not yourself," or "You haven't followed through on your intention to fit in those clothes, or worked out on that exercise equipment, or lived up to the financial success of your parents or your ex." Who needs that in her space?

You might think of your storage areas as the "colon" of your house. If these spaces are stuffed with old, unused materials, chances are good that your body will be too. Our physical surroundings are a reflection of our bodies. And like our bodies, they require regular purging and circulation. I hired a personal organizer a while back because I had renovated a bathroom and didn't want to move into it with all my old stuff. What started with just one bathroom eventually became a cleansing of the entire house. Yes, it was exhausting, so I devoted an afternoon at a time to purging. But within two months I finally had the kind of physical space I had always longed for: neat and organized (for the most part). I no longer come across a stash of toothbrushes I bought on sale and forgot about. I don't feel weighed down by too much "stuff." Better yet, I know where everything is for the very first time in my life! (I'm not kidding.)

Once you've created a haven-like home, establish routines to keep up your beautiful, replenishing space so it doesn't become cluttered again. Do this even as you continue your emotional release work and it will be easier to let go of things you feel you ought to hang on to "just in case." Every time you bring something new in, take something old out. Feel the pleasure of letting go of the junk and the emotions like guilt and shame attached to it so you can restore the flow of chi. And if you want to retain a sentimental memory, take a photo or digitalize your pictures and videos so you can go back and reminisce without having a basement stuffed with storage bins.

If you find yourself overwhelmed by clutter, try the following exercise for restoring order within and without.

Exercise: Decluttering 101

The amount of time it takes to sort through and get rid of clutter can feel overwhelming and cause you to put it off. Here's a great way to tackle clutter 15 minutes at a time.

First, set your intention by saying aloud, "Divine Beloved, please change me into someone who is organized and whose surroundings are beautiful. Show me what needs to be released." Then set a timer for 15 minutes and clean out and organize one drawer or shelf. As you toss things, offer the process to the Divine. Make a ritual of clearing and sorting out your own life—drawer organization as spiritual practice!

You have to choose a small, contained space or the 15 minutes will be up and you'll feel you have a bigger mess than before. When you've finished throwing out what you no longer need, cleaning anything that's become soiled, and rearranging the items you're keeping, stop for a minute or two and take in how good it feels to have that much decluttering done. Repeat this process again tomorrow—and the next day, and the next.

You can also follow the instructions of The Fly Lady (www.flylady.net). Walk around your home with a large bag and collect 25 items in it to either throw away or give away. When you have 25, toss the garbage and put the rest of the items in your car immediately so that they're out of the house. Schedule a trip to a secondhand store or arrange for a charity to pick up the bag. In fact, get on their call list so they remind you to grab a bagful of things to get out of your home.

If you have trouble parting with possessions and might be tempted to pull that bag out of your car trunk because you're struck with "declutterer's remorse," here's a trick. Imagine someone receiving your old possessions and being thrilled by them. Feel the excitement as you picture someone putting on the sweater that never really looked good on you anyway, plugging in the appliance you only used once a year (if that), and being grateful for this treasure. When you know someone else will get joy from something that you really don't need anymore, it's easier to let go of it.

To further make your home a haven and let the chi flow, bring nature indoors through nature sounds, fish tanks, natural light, plants, photographs, and window views of nature—all of which have been shown to reduce stress.[8] Decorate your living space with natural scents and flowers, or pinecones or stones from the beach, or whatever makes you feel a connection to the Mother Earth energy of nature. Bring in the sounds of nature: you can get apps for your computer or devices that play the sounds of birds singing, waves lapping against a shore, and so on. Design your home as if it were your goddess palace, a refuge and a foundation where you can replenish yourself.

No matter how small your space, no matter what limitations you feel you have in your life, open up to possibilities by letting your grief, anger, and shame flow out and your joy flow in. Emotional release and physical decluttering open you up for living agelessly, with a renewed sense of vigor and enthusiasm. In the next chapter, you'll learn about an important part of ageless goddess living that is easier to reclaim once you've purged the old emotions of grief, anger, and shame: your sensuality and sexuality.

CHAPTER SIX

GODDESSES
ARE SEXY AND
SENSUAL

Sex begins long before women enter the bedroom
and reverberates long after.

— GINA OGDEN, PH.D., *WOMEN WHO LOVE SEX*

Awoman named Charise went to a community picnic
where she began chatting with two World War II vets
eager to flirt. Charise was lapping it up as these older
gentlemen tried to one-up each other to impress her. "I felt like
a French village girl sharing a bottle of Burgundy with a couple
of hot young Allied soldiers," she said, "which is strange when
you consider both these fellows were several inches shorter than
I was, and one even had to lean on a cane! I mean, they were in
their nineties but I swear, they were making me hot! And I forgot

my insecurities about the weight I've gained and felt like I was in my sexual prime too."

Charise's delightful experience of flirting and feeling turned on in the presence of vintage masculinity is a perfect example of a profound truth. As long as we're in physical bodies, we are sexual creatures—whether or not we ever end up taking off our clothes with another person. In the absence of undue shame, we're drawn to sexuality as naturally as bees to flowers. Flowers are simply the sex organs that plants use to attract the bees that pollinate them and keep them fertile, but they're so much more than that: they're part of the joy and beauty of life on planet Earth. Women's sexuality doesn't exist solely for procreation. We don't stop being deliciously alluring just because pregnancy is no longer possible.

We're wired for sensual pleasure from the start. Our physical bodies were formed through sex. Human life itself is, in fact, sexually transmitted. It's even possible that the entire universe came into being through one big orgasmic bang. Who knows? What we know for sure is that for most of us, our bodies were conceived in a moment of mutual pleasure—at least, that's how it's supposed to work. On a primal level, our cells remember the energy of creation: the pleasurable life force that keeps us alive and makes life worth living. This life force is transmitted through nitric oxide, beta-endorphins, and all the other neurochemicals of joy and pleasure. It's important to realize that sexuality is about far more than just sexual acts. It is about life renewing itself! Sexual educator Layla Martin says the key to a woman's happiness lies in a positive relationship with her vulva. Pure and simple. And I agree.

Earlier, you learned that your soul enters the body through what Tami Lynn Kent calls the "spirit door." This is a portal into the "birthing field," where energy becomes form. When you become aware of the profound connection between your sexuality, your spirituality, and your creativity, you will have discovered a powerful and renewable resource with which to source your life.

What Charise experienced at the picnic that day was two men who knew how to connect with their own masculine life force while also connected with their hearts—and that lit Charise's "pilot light," if you will. I've had the same experience dancing Argentine tango with men who make exquisite partners regardless of how they appear at first glance. They may be balding or short or a little paunchy, but boy, do they know how to move with their own sensual, emotional energy, making it both safe and enjoyable for their partners to respond in kind. When both partners are dancing in full communication with each other's hearts and hips, it's like heaven. This is the kind of "time stands still" pleasure that stops the aging process. Our bodies, minds, and spirits are hardwired to seek this kind of sensual or even sexual experience, which can be available to every one of us.

Your brain and hips are not supposed to be experienced separately from each other. In fact, your pelvis has wisdom just as your brain does. Awakening to your sexual pleasure doesn't mean being indiscriminate and mindless about your partners or sexual behaviors. The aim is not to be like the lost young women on the HBO series *Girls,* who have sex often but are disassociated from their own pleasure and wisdom. Nor should you aim to use sex to manipulate other people, because your Aphrodite power is not a commodity to be exchanged. Using sex that way wouldn't be wise or ethical. It's like the power of fire: you can cook with it or you can burn down your village, so use it responsibly. Jungian analyst and psychic Llorraine Neithardt, host of *Venus Unplugged* on Blog Talk Radio, points out that the aura of our sexual partners remains in our own energetic field for quite some time. When a woman is penetrated by a man, his energy stays with her for a year, while a woman's energy stays with a man for a month. Hence, you want to be very discerning about whom you allow into your body—because that person is also entering you emotionally and spiritually.

To trust in the wisdom of your pelvis is to trust your own connection to Source, to the energy that creates worlds. Ageless goddesses own their sexuality and sensuality—shamelessly but also with great discernment. You draw in what you desire. Then you use it to bring forth something new and delightful. Nature doesn't "use up" resources; she recycles them. You take in life force, enjoy it, and send it back out again in a different form. This is what women's sexuality researcher Gina Ogden is referring to when she says that a woman's pleasure reverberates out into the world, healing all of us.

YOUR SEXUAL BIRTHRIGHT

A fulfilling sex life, however you define it, is possible at any age. Your perception of yourself is what has the biggest impact on your experience of sexuality, and this has little to do with your age. If you believe you're sexy and sensual, you will be, no matter what your age or physical condition.

Most women have been brainwashed into thinking that after the age of 50 or so, they're no longer sexually attractive or desirable. Others have been faking orgasms and putting up with less-than-fulfilling sex for years—all because they simply don't know there is no ceiling on sexual satisfaction and delight. Nor do they know that experiencing sexual pleasure is a skill that can be learned and enhanced at any age. Sheri Winston, author of *Women's Anatomy of Arousal: Secret Maps to Buried Pleasure* (Mango Garden Press, 2009), explains that anyone can learn to play a few notes on the piano, but to become a virtuoso takes years of practice. It's the same with sexuality. There's always room for more skill and more pleasure.

Women have been hoodwinked into believing that the desire for sex naturally wanes after menopause. The truth is that there are times when the sex drive is expressed by going deep into the body's root system to reinvent yourself rather than just "putting out" for others. It's not waning, it's finding a new direction for a time. Women have big sexual appetites if given half a chance to know and express their desires with individuals who love and respect them. Not realizing this, many women are "hexed" by mainstream medical research that pathologizes women's sexuality. When research suggests that almost half of women have FSD (female sexual dysfunction), you know that it isn't women who have the problem. It's the culture that is adversely affecting them. A 2008 study showed that while 42 percent of women had FSD by this definition, only 12 percent of those women were upset about it.[1]

Mainstream sex research narrowly defines normal sex as intercourse twice a week—an incredibly limited definition. Women's sexuality is a whole-body experience that is not limited to our vaginas and clitorises. By the way, the word *vagina* is Latin for "sheath," as in the sheath for a sword, so this major part of our female anatomy is referred to by its relationship to a man's penis. Regena Thomashauer, leader of Mama Gena's School of Womanly Arts in New York City, where women learn to reconnect with their sexuality and graduate as "sister goddesses," refers to a woman's vulva and vagina as a "pussy." Now, I'm not totally comfortable with that word in casual conversation, but I have to say it has some better origins than "vagina" does. "Pussy" is said to come from Old Norse and Old English words for "pocket" and "bag" (for holding money or possessions—in other words, for holding your power!). And the P-word may also come from an old Germanic word used to call a cat—and what's more seductive and powerful than a cat who answers to no one and luxuriates in her own skin? "When a woman owns her pussy, she owns her life," says Mama Gena.[2]

Mama Gena teaches that every time a woman discovers her pleasure—on all levels, including sexual—she sets another woman free somewhere else. It's kind of like in the movie *It's a Wonderful Life* when the angel Clarence tells George that every time he hears a bell ring, another angel has earned his wings through saving a life or doing another good deed. This makes perfect sense to me. Quantum physics has proven beyond a doubt that all of us are interconnected energetically. So when one woman awakens to her birthright of pleasure, she makes it that much easier for the next one to do the same. Awakening to our pleasure and sexual power is an act of power in a culture that is sexually repressed or shaming. As a woman awakens sexually, she connects her intellect and her spirituality with her erotic anatomy, becoming a fully integrated force for good on the planet. So ring your bell and invite other women to ring theirs!

We can reinvent ourselves from the inside out at any age or stage, and there's something especially potent about the rebirth that occurs for so many around menopause. One aspect of rebirth is the reclamation of our sexuality, as we take it back from a dominator culture that says it has no value after it's no longer needed for baby making. Our sexuality is far more than a vehicle for bringing sperm together with an egg.

Research has shown that the number-one predictor of good sex after menopause is a new partner, but there's no need to take that literally. Research has failed to show a consistent link between a woman's hormone levels and her sexual satisfaction. It also hasn't shown a link between her age and her sexual satisfaction. So why is a new partner so potent? Because with a new partner, you become awash in DMT, the hormone produced by the pineal gland that makes you feel blissful. It's also the hormone produced in so-called "enlightened states." The good news is it's entirely possible to generate DMT on your own! When you cultivate a new relationship with your sexuality and sensuality, you're actually connecting with what Sheila Kelley, the founder of S Factor pole dancing workout classes, calls "your inner erotic creature." You connect with the archetype of Aphrodite as she comes through you. Her expression is unique to you.

No matter what your relationship status, you can use your sexual power to source your life and activities. If you're currently single and not in a sexual relationship, you can express your sexual drive in a virtually unlimited number of healthy, positive, and uplifting ways. You start by acknowledging that your body was created by sexual energy and is still fueled by that same energy. You are an expression of Source—pure and simple. And Source is flirtatious, sexy, and full of pleasure!

As an ageless goddess, you can enjoy your sexuality well into your 60s, 70s, and beyond. Although it may fly in the face of everything you've been told, research shows that older women have far better sex lives than many younger women. Gina Ogden, Ph.D., author of the ISIS (Integrating Sexuality and Spirituality) study and a researcher of women's sexuality, says that women in their 60s and 70s are having the best sex of their lives.[3]

A fulfilling sex life begins first with your thoughts and beliefs. As you start to feel sexier, you soon become more attractive on the outside. Both men and women know that women who are turned on and in touch with their own desire for pleasure are sexy. *There is no more powerful aphrodisiac than a woman who feels irresistible and relishes it!*

Like many baby boomer women, when I was younger, I didn't know how to express my power without turning off men or feeling asexual or unattractive. Many women were taught that to be desirable, we had to be weak and submissive so that a man would feel strong and, well, manly. Or we were told that the feminine arts—donning lingerie, makeup, and beautiful clothing, for example—were not worthy of our time or attention. And we also learned to focus on our partner's pleasure at the expense of our own. Talk about a double bind! Be a strong woman who acts like a man—where's the fun in that?

In many ways, women of all generations are still in that struggle to own their power in a way that's aligned with the inner erotic self. Women wrestle with how to be sensual, strong, feminine, and confident in their bodies and self-expression. We judge ourselves relentlessly about our weight, our breast size, our thighs, our hair—the list goes on and on. Our self-judgments and shame turn off the life force within us. To turn it back on—and have great sex at the same time—you just have to know, and practice, four things:

1. Align with the goddess energy of Venus/Aphrodite and allow her to come through your body in a way that is unique to *you.*

2. Awaken and cultivate your female erotic anatomy as a regular health practice.

3. Become a student of your own pleasure (when you do, you not only turn yourself on, you turn on your partner too, if you have one).

4. Understand the powerful connection between your spirituality and your sexuality.

RECLAIMING APHRODITE

Many ancient cultures had goddesses of love, sex, and pleasure—there was Freya in Scandinavia, Oshun in West Africa, and Rati in India, just to name a few. It's interesting to note that the Greek goddess Aphrodite, whose Roman name was Venus, was not just the goddess of beauty, sexuality, and seduction but also of prosperity and victory. She was also all about relating deeply and profoundly to life. The archetype of the sacred sexual goddess lived in our collective psyches for eons until the rise of agriculture, when the collaborative societies that worshipped the goddess were replaced by societies that worshipped the male god. Afterward, for thousands of years, cultures around the world tried to deny, suppress, control, and demonize the power of women's sexuality, severing the connection between women's bodies and the creative, divine life force. These dominator societies were focused more on individual triumph than on collaboration, and the power of people at the top of the hierarchy headed up by a king or emperor. While this may *seem* like ancient history, we can see the same ideas playing out today, even in the U.S., where some states actually have laws to force vaginal ultrasounds on women who choose abortion. There are legislators who believe women can't be trusted to know their own hearts and bodies well enough to make the choice without this invasive procedure. You think you're living in the modern world and then someone proposes a law that makes you wonder what century you're in!

After millennia of influence from dominator culture, it's no wonder we're so disconnected from our bodies and the creative life force associated with the earth. But deep down, we know we're meant to be sexual, sensual, life-giving, ageless goddesses. And deep down we know that sex and Spirit go hand in hand. In a survey of 4,000 women, Gina Ogden found that 47 percent reported that during orgasm they had experienced God, while 67 percent said that they needed sexuality to be infused with spirituality to be satisfying.[4] Likewise, neurotheologian Andrew Newberg, M.D., who studies the relationship between the brain and spiritual belief, has suggested in his book *Why God Won't Go Away: Brain Science and the Biology of Belief* (Ballantine Books, 2001) that sexuality influenced our ability to experience religious ecstasy.[5] That's not something you are apt to learn about while sitting in a church pew!

Sexuality is power. It's our connection to the creative life force. When you connect with your Aphrodite energy, you remember that you're worthy of receiving what you desire. You surrender to sexual and other pleasures without fear of displeasing anyone, and you enjoy a bounty of sexual delight that can include multiple orgasms. To embody Aphrodite is to be a diva in the original sense of the word, unapologetic about your longings and cravings and unchecked in your pleasurable pursuits. That's hard for many of us to imagine, because we've been taught not to take too much, not to laugh too loudly, and not to be too aggressive in getting what we want. We've been taught to question our yearnings and make sure we're not being selfish.

To become ageless, we must learn to distinguish selfishness from self-nurturing, because self-nurturing is the replenishing act of reconnecting to the energy of Aphrodite, the creative and sensual force of life itself. To be self-nurturing *is* to serve the world. As Judy Harrow wrote in *Gnosis* magazine, "Aphrodite's rituals of love and pleasure are the acts which connect the inner and outer planes . . . we must actually dance, sing, feast, make music, and love in Her honor. It is with our bodies that we worship Her, and through our bodies that She blesses us. By these earthy rituals the false divisions between body and spirit, between mind and nature, are healed. We find the Sacred within us and all things, within our beautiful, living Mother Earth."[6]

You offer your own joy and irresistible deliciousness for others to savor even as you're recharging your own batteries. The Breathing In Aphrodite exercise, inspired by Laura Bushnell's book *Life Magic*, is a great practice for connecting to your pleasure.[7]

Exercise: Breathing In Aphrodite

Take a walk, whether in nature, by yourself, or on a crowded city sidewalk. As you're walking, imagine that a very sexy woman is pressed up against your left side—the side of your body that represents receiving and femininity. (Your right side represents giving and masculinity.) When I do this, I imagine that Sophia Loren or Salma Hayek is on my left, but you can use any woman you find sexy and powerful.

Now, breathe in that woman and her energy. Imagine drawing in her sensuality and sexuality, and increasing your life force with each breath as it is channeled directly from the Divine through her into you.

Do this exercise for two to five minutes a day for 21 days and watch what happens. You can combine it with affirmations about your sensuality, such as "I am Aphrodite. I make love with wild, unleashed abandon. I am an irresistible force of nature."

Libido is the life force coursing through our bodies. It's the natural yearning for more pleasure, and for more of what pleasure creates.

The life force is creative and abundant. Trees generate a far greater number of seeds than will ever sprout and grow into new trees. This past year, the yellow pollen from the pine trees in my yard was released all spring in huge amounts whenever the wind blew. The pollen covered everything on the ground and fed the other plants with its rich nutrients. I recently learned that it is this same pine pollen that awakens the forest floor and signals the growth of plants and mushrooms. Talk about fecundity! Fish lay far more eggs than will ever hatch. And women are wired to experience multiple orgasms because that moment of ecstasy is an expression of the life force accompanied by a burst of nitric oxide. Our bodies are not designed to limit or contain our pleasure. They are meant to experience it as the medicine it truly is. Orgasm is a gift that, quite literally, resets our personal energy fields and radiates out from there.

If you want to live healthfully and as a goddess, you need to know how to work with your innate sex drive and spiritual life force, bringing it down into your pelvic organs and your female erotic anatomy. Spirituality and sexuality are two aspects of exactly the same thing, despite the fact that they have been separated by many cultures and many religions for millennia. If you expect to shut down sexually as you grow older because that's the accepted cultural norm, you're likely to do just that, but it isn't necessary and it won't lead to agelessness. You can become a sex goddess right in the privacy of your own mind, your own body, and your own bedroom.

REPRESSION BEGINS—AND ENDS—AT HOME

Part of my own journey to sexual wholeness involved teaching others to use pleasure to fuel their lives, which I did at Mama Gena's School of Womanly Arts (www.mamagenas.com). As I watched the women I was helping to teach break open into healthier and happier versions of themselves, I realized that I needed to learn the womanly arts as much as any woman there did—and my daughters decided to take the "Mastery" course with me.

At one of the after-parties, a woman invited me to get up on a bar and dance. I don't drink alcohol and have never been drunk or high on drugs. But cheered on by the love, support, and urging of all the other sister goddesses, I figured I'd give it a try. Up until then I had never ever experienced myself as a sensual, sexy anything. I saw myself as a serious doctor who had worked hard my whole life to have my point of view accepted. But there was something about dancing sensually on top of a bar in New York City while being encouraged by dozens of joyful women that felt really good.

But I noticed that my daughters were not exactly thrilled with my performance, even though I wanted their approval. My youngest said, "Really, Mom. I don't like seeing you like that."

Wham! Instantly, I'd been smacked down from ecstasy and fun to shame and constriction. Not wanting to embarrass my daughters further, I considered shutting back down into my maternal, asexual Mom self. But then I spoke with Anne Davin, Ph.D., a cultural anthropologist who, at that time, was part of the Mastery staff. She's an expert on addiction, psychology, and anthropology. Anne told me that in indigenous cultures that have coming-of-age rituals, girls are initiated into the rites of womanhood by mothers who have been initiated separately, years earlier. In Western culture, which has few cultural coming-of-age rituals for girls, both adult mothers and their daughters are, in essence, uninitiated girls. Consequently, it feels uncomfortable for both mothers and their daughters to be undergoing the same "rites" at the same time. She suggested that I shouldn't let my daughters' reaction stop me. It was too important to claim my right to sexual pleasure.

Months later, while still in the Mastery program, I had run out of the room to get something, and when I came back, I realized everyone had paired up for an exercise and the only person who didn't have a partner was my daughter Ann. Neither of us knew what the exercise was about, but then we were told we each had to do a sensual move and have our partner comment on it. I laughed. Of *course* my daughter and I would end up being partners in this exercise! I went first and did the move with all my heart. Ann responded, "Mom—you moved like a snake. That was so beautiful it almost made me cry." Breakthrough! And when she did her beautiful, sensual move, I complimented her. Since then, both my daughters and I have come a very long way in supporting each other in being fully alive and fully embodied.

In freeing ourselves, we free our daughters. They will get to see and experience a woman past her childbearing years feeling powerful, sensual, and beautiful and know that they, too, can continue to be sexual and alluring, ageless goddesses.

Women are rising at warp speed! Back when my father was growing up, the sight of a woman's bare ankle as she stepped into a carriage was considered risqué. At the height of the American feminist movement in the late 1960s and 1970s, women were wearing miniskirts one day, maxi dresses the next, going bra-less, or wearing high-collared, puffy-shouldered prairie-inspired wedding gowns and cosmetics with "baby" in the name, completely confused about how we "should" present ourselves! In the 1980s, we learned to "dress for success," which meant wearing suits with big shoulder pads to make us look like men and little floppy silk bowties that suggested we were authoritative, like men, but soft. These fashions reflected the cultural ambivalence about looking feminine that was part of that time. The old staples of Hollywood glamour, from bold lipstick to draped satin, were discarded, but now we're reclaiming them. Finally, we're realizing that the glamour queens were no pushovers, and like them, we can be sexy, powerful, and smart. You have to love the fact that 1940s movie star Hedy Lamarr, known for her classic glamour-girl looks, had an onscreen orgasm in a European film back in the early 1930s—and also invented a key piece of technology that she incorporated into a torpedo tracking system designed to help the Allies in World War II and that became integral to the cell phones we use today. Soak that in!

The fact is that you can enjoy lipstick and draped satin even if you're a breadwinner and mother. You can dress in a uniform during the workday and sweatpants at night, and then become a divine, erotic goddess in bed. You can be the hot librarian or rock a pair of yoga pants. It's not what you wear but how you carry yourself. Clothing and makeup just serve as accessories. I love the women's bathroom scene in the movie *The Heat* where Melissa McCarthy tries to explain to Sandra Bullock why she needs some serious wardrobe help to express her sexuality. McCarthy's character can do it simply through movement because she owns her womanly power. She doesn't need to be thin or traditionally beautiful. The challenge is to let go of the virgin/whore archetype that disempowers and disrespects women. Find your own unique blending of the earthy woman who knows how to shake her stuff and the bold and brainy woman in hot pants who is selective in choosing her partners.

As Dolly Parton has said, "Find out who you are and do it on purpose." You don't have to justify your personal expression of your Aphrodite nature. Don't apologize to anyone for what makes you comfortable. All humans have feminine aspects. Don't deny yours out of a misguided notion that to be feminine, or womanly, is to be weak or inconsequential. Then you'll be able to own your womanliness and express it in your own unique way.

Male Sexual Health

Just like women, as men reach their 40s and 50s, they typically undergo a transition into a new stage of life. Though this is medically called andropause, I really dislike the term because it can be a form of the same "hexing" of men's sexuality as menopause is of women's. (By hexing, I mean that as soon as you set up the cultural expectation that people will face challenges at a particular time in life, people will respond by having crises they might not have had otherwise.) Yes, at this stage of life, testosterone levels in a man may drop, but this is not inevitable. It depends on a man's health and well-being. (It also depends on how big his gut is. That "beer gut" that so many men develop creates all kinds of hormonal havoc because it produces inflammatory chemicals and excess estrogen, which shuts down testosterone.) And just as in women, men's old buried emotions may come to the surface in the form of physical problems. For men, it tends to be erectile dysfunction and circulation problems. Erectile dysfunction drugs, such as Cialis and Viagra, may resolve men's difficulty with attaining an erection but mask deeper problems of unresolved anger, fear, and grief that may stem from sexual abuse. I once heard Dr. Oz call the penis the "dipstick of men's health." By this, he meant that erection problems may be the first thing that signals the beginning of heart disease. And as we have already discussed, heart problems are often associated with old, unresolved resentment and grief.

If a man in your life is having health or sexual issues, his main issue may actually be his fear of mortality, which is showing up as a loss of potency. Share with him what you know about cultural portals and biology. Suggest to him that he hasn't even begun to reach his peak of effectiveness! (And yes, erectile dysfunction is far more common in men who sit all day long, so if you have a male partner, tell your partner to get up off the chair and join you in pleasurable movement!)

Because a man's sexual prowess is so deeply connected to his sense of power in the world, he may act out by having an affair or develop a sudden obsession with pornography to prove to himself that he's still "got it." Remember the movie *Moonstruck* when Loretta's (Cher's) mother, Rose, played by Olympia Dukakis, asks the character Johnny why a man would need more than one woman? He replies, "Maybe because he fears death." Men may have sex with a new woman to feel alive again. As his partner, you can be that new woman yourself by reconnecting with your own vitality. Several years ago, I met a man who was in his 70s who told me that he no longer needed Viagra for sex since

his wife started the Mama Gena Mastery program and connected with her own sexuality and sensuality. Unfortunately,
some men are so overwhelmed by the challenge of opening
their own hearts that they can't maintain their commitments
to their partners.

As a woman partnered with a man who is having a so-
called midlife crisis, you can best support him by being your
most joyous, flourishing self. He may not like this at first.
He may feel as though he is losing control of you—because
he is! But that will most likely save both of you from discon-
necting from each other.

You need to take the lead in being a role model for pleasure and joy in life. Women set the tone for men. Don't allow
his anger or sadness to drag you back down, which would
be a disservice to you and to him. Do *not* make the mistake
of waiting to have fun until your man agrees to accompany
you on the pleasure train. Board it yourself, and then invite
him to come along!

EROTIC ANATOMY

For years, I've been teaching women about their erotic anatomy, something that even ob/gyns are not taught in our formal
training! Trust me, most don't ever address it. Few women have
been shown how to use a hand mirror to examine and explore
the external part of this erotic anatomy, which is part of the reason they're unfamiliar with it. How often do you hear women
talk about their vaginas when they really mean the clitoris, inner
lips, and outer labia, all of which make up the vulva? How ridiculous is it that most of us weren't even taught what the terms
are for our organs "down there"?

And it's not enough to simply know the map, although that's
very useful. In fact, Figure 1 shows what your erotic anatomy
looks like, minus the part that is located in your brain, which is
very much involved in your experience of your sexuality. When
you can name something and simultaneously feel deep in your
body the sensations associated with it, you have access to your
personal power. You no longer think of your pelvis as an unknown

area that only some outside expert can negotiate. Becoming familiar with your female erotic anatomy also helps you own and operate it sensually. Energy follows thought. Even just seeing this illustration and thinking about and putting your attention on your erotic anatomy will begin to bring blood and pleasure to that area of your body. This is how you light your own pilot light—and ignite your own engine of power and pleasure!

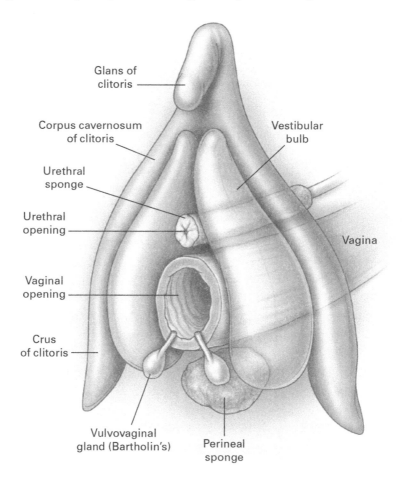

Figure 1. The erotic female anatomy

Were you shown an illustration of the erotic female anatomy back in your school days? Probably not—or if you did, the class discussion did not work its way around how to own and operate this part of your anatomy. I want you to start exploring and learning about your erotic anatomy by yourself, through self-pleasuring. Get a hand mirror, or stand over a large mirror, and start looking at yourself between your legs—spread them so you can get a really good look. Describe what you see. Is it a beautiful pearl, nestled in folds of rich purple satin? How does it feel and look when you massage the lips surrounding it? Observe how your genitals look in both aroused and non-aroused states.

Practice stimulating yourself around your own clitoris. Use plenty of lubrication. For most women, the most sensitive hot spot is slightly to your left and to the top of the clitoris. The G-spot is a quarter-shaped, slightly raised spot inside your vagina at 12 o'clock, two to three inches in, on the top of your vaginal canal (toward your front, not your back). You will feel it only when you're in a sexually aroused state—and you have to squat down and insert into your vagina your second or third (or both) fingers, fingernail toward your tailbone. If you rub yourself in that area, you will feel its sensitivity because the G-spot is abundant in nerve endings. Try up and down strokes and circles. Work it with your fingers—stroke it, as if you were kneading out the knots in a sore muscle. At first, you may experience pain or numbness. Over time, you can make this area wake up to bliss—and a loving partner can assist with that. If you have vaginal dryness, use plenty of lubricant.

A Word about Vibrators

I am not a fan of vibrators for self-pleasuring because they emit a constant strong sensation that, over time, can deaden sensation, not enhance it. Yes, they might jump-start an orgasm. But I prefer you learn how to feel more and more with less and less stimulation, not become desensitized so that you require increased clitoral stimulation over time to have the same feeling. As with everything related to sexuality, this is a very personal choice.

In addition to self-pleasuring, you can also have your partner massage your vulva and around your clitoris. But even if you have a partner, don't deny yourself the delight of self-pleasuring, or, as the ancient Taoists called it, "self-cultivation." This practice is also known as masturbation (an awful word believed to have derived from word roots meaning "to defile with the hand"). Self-cultivation is a healthy way to experience sexual pleasure, orgasm, and the release of rejuvenating nitric oxide into the bloodstream. Consider making self-pleasuring a ceremony in which you offer your pleasure and your time to your inner Aphrodite. Feeling good emotionally and physically is the sacrament.

SHAME-FREE SELF-PLEASURING

Think back to the first time you self-pleasured. Did you feel uncomfortable? Secretly ashamed? Or elated? As one woman put it, "I felt as though I had just happened on the best thing my body ever did—available for free . . . at my convenience." Self-pleasuring might at first bring up a feeling of shame because you've internalized the dominator culture's messages about women's sexuality. Take a moment to illuminate the shame so it dissolves and you can embrace your inner erotic creature fully and joyfully.

Self-pleasuring is the ultimate safe sex, which may be why then U.S. Surgeon General Joycelyn Elders was asked in a UN forum on AIDS prevention back in 1994 if masturbation should be taught as an outlet for healthy, safe sexual expression. She agreed it might be a good idea and was almost immediately forced to resign because of the backlash. That's how powerful the self-pleasuring taboo in America was back then. But even today, there are still some states that try to control or ban self-pleasuring, as well as the sale of vibrators because they're often used for this purpose.

Taboos against self-pleasuring can be found in most major religions, and they have affected policy and practice in the medical community over the years. Circumcision of boys and men became popular in the U.S. in the 19th century because it was thought to prevent them from self-pleasuring, which was blamed for a host of ailments from tuberculosis to blindness to insanity.

Victorians sometimes tied the hands of boys and girls when they went to sleep so they wouldn't touch themselves, a practice advocated by Dr. John Harvey Kellogg (who also created corn flakes as part of a bland diet designed to reduce sexual desire). In fact, Kellogg once said, "A remedy [for masturbation] which is almost always successful in small boys is circumcision . . . The operation should be performed by a surgeon without administering an anesthetic, as the brief pain attending the operation will have a salutary effect upon the mind . . ."[8] I've done hundreds of circumcisions on infant boys as part of my job as an ob/gyn, so I've seen how traumatic these operations are—and how unconscious about this trauma our culture is. Circumcision is a practice rooted in fear and it needs to end.

Why are we so afraid and ashamed to talk about self-pleasuring? Let's look at what it does that some might find scary or threatening. For both men and women, it bestows the power of sexual expression without sanction from a church or another authority. It provides pleasure for the self, not others—unless it's incorporated into sexual activity between two people, with one watching the other, which apparently the anti-self-pleasuring folks are unaware of. Self-pleasuring by men prevents them from impregnating women because they "spill their seed," as it says in the Bible. That means the self-pleasuring person isn't following the Christian and Jewish teaching to "be fruitful and multiply"—the purpose of sex, according to these religious traditions.

What's more, self-pleasuring bestows power on women who practice it because once you know how to trigger your own orgasm, you don't need a partner to do it for you. A 22-year-old lesbian who had just discovered self-pleasuring said to me, "Now I don't need to go out to bars anymore, because I don't need a partner to get me off." As far as the old dominator culture is concerned, women having sexual pleasure without men threatens the status quo. So what are we going to do with all these women pleasuring themselves? I say, encourage them! You can start by checking out Betty Dodson, a pioneer in encouraging women's self-pleasuring who is now in her 80s. She has a marvelous website devoted to this topic: www.dodsonandross.com. She can teach you just about anything you'd want to know about how to pleasure yourself with your erotic female anatomy, and she is wonderfully frank. I also enjoy the work of Layla Martin, who teaches an online course in female sexuality and pleasure at www.layla-martin.com. She makes the important point that a woman's relationship to and comfort with her erotic anatomy are key to her overall happiness. All manner of depression, anger, and sadness can be eliminated when a women honors this area of her body and takes the steps necessary to work through the shame and judgment that can reside there.

Self-pleasuring is a positive practice that will help you understand your own sexual response and needs while making you feel good. And if you think about it, how is a partner supposed to know how to touch you to make you feel good if you don't know yourself?

UNLIMITED PLEASURE IS YOUR RIGHT

Your ability to experience orgasm is infinite because of how you are wired as a woman. Now that is a right to celebrate! The clitoris has more than 8,000 nerve endings and is the only organ in the human body designed solely for pleasure. I think we ought to respect evolution on this one and use the clitoris as it was intended. As part of your erotic anatomy, the clitoris is connected to the G-spot and through glial cells to the pineal gland in the brain. That's the gland responsible for the release of DMT, the brain's endogenous hallucinatory neurotransmitter, and melatonin, the neurotransmitter that causes us to dream.

You are sitting on a throne of gold, the fountain of youth, and it is your erotic anatomy. Explore it and get to know it. Turn back to Figure 1 if you want to. Don't be squeamish about inserting your fingers into your own vagina. We should be teaching our daughters and granddaughters to familiarize themselves with their anatomy and let them know that many girls and women explore and touch their genitals for the sake of pleasure.

We want the real deal and so do our partners. Faking it is never a good idea. You're robbing yourself of pleasure and your partner of the pleasure of learning how to make you lose yourself in sexual ecstasy. Don't do it! Your partner wants to be invited into that delicious expression of your inner Aphrodite. Healthy, strong men are not afraid of our Aphrodite power. They enjoy it. In fact, the reason men are so turned on by the sight of two women sexually pleasuring each other is because their bodies respond powerfully to the creative, erotic, female energy in those women. It awakens their own inner desire to be a part of that powerful, ecstatic experience.

Most women don't experience orgasm through intercourse alone, which only indirectly stimulates the clitoris and much of the erotic anatomy. By combining intercourse with other forms of stimulation—or skipping the intercourse, for that matter—you can experience orgasm more easily. In their personal teaching and writings, Drs. Vera and Steve Bodansky call the first contraction of the PC (pubococcygeus) muscle with sexual stimulation the beginning of the orgasm. The minute you begin to think of your first sensation as an "orgasm," the performance anxiety about struggling to "achieve" something goes away. You just sink into the sensation of every stroke. And that changes everything. It removes performance anxiety from the entire discussion. The minute you begin to feel pleasure is the beginning of the orgasm. There. Doesn't that definition feel better?

If you have a sexual partner, offer feedback to guide him or her. When you're engaging in pleasure, teach yourself how to vocalize and use positive reinforcement—"wow," "that feels fantastic," "you have great hands," "you're the best," and so on—to give directions and encouragement. Release sounds of pleasure, which will turn you on as well as your partner. There's a very strong connection between the throat and the genitals: a relaxed, open throat enhances energy flow and pleasure. Make a list of positive words: *yes, ahh, more pleasure, thank you, wow.* If you're intimidated, play some music. Don't hold back because you're afraid of what the neighbors, or your kids, will hear or think. Invest in some soundproofing if you want to. Find a way to be sure you're comfortable letting yourself vocalize the energy that's coming straight from your lower chakras. The sounds of lovemaking and the sounds of birth are remarkably similar. This is what pleasurable creation sounds like.

In Sanskrit, the penis is referred to as a wand of light imbued with the sacred masculine life force, so when it penetrates a woman's vagina, it brings healing power. That is very different from what many women have experienced in intercourse! But whether you are having intercourse with a male partner or you are stimulating your erotic anatomy in some other way, imagine your vagina as a sacred portal, bringing divine, loving energy into your body. Imagine each loving stroke removing sadness, anger, trauma, and pain that's embedded in your tissues.

You probably know that our major organ systems are represented by reflexology points elsewhere on the body—on the soles of our feet, the palms of our hands, and our ears. The vagina also has reflexology points that correspond to the major organ systems (see Figure 2). Note that the innermost part of the vagina—near the cervix—is energetically connected with the heart. And that is why having intercourse or stimulating yourself vaginally can be a healing practice, stimulating and awakening the entire body. It's also the basis of what is known as "sex magic," in which you dedicate a session of raising sexual energy to attracting more abundance (which is nothing more than creative energy). Remember—the health of the pelvic organs is related to money, sex, and power. So sexual energy and abundance are highly correlated. You are, quite literally, ramping up the energy that created the world in your own body! However, this same creative energy is one of the key reasons why a woman can become addicted to a man after having sex with him. The very act of having intercourse turns on her heart and causes the release of bonding hormones. In a loving, committed relationship, this kind of physical/energetic bonding is glue that helps keep the couple together. But in a noncommitted relationship, a woman can be left with longing and an addiction to the man that feels as intense as a crack cocaine addiction. Hence, it's very important to be selective of whom you "let in." And remember, you can always stimulate these reflex centers on your own until the right partner arrives.

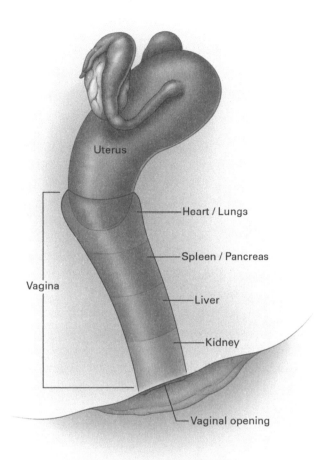

Figure 2. Vaginal reflexology

If you'd like to learn more about how couples can use clitoral stimulation with the hands as a most enjoyable form of intimacy and pleasure, I highly recommend the husband-and-wife team Steve and Vera Bodansky's book *Extended Massive Orgasm: How You Can Give and Receive Intense Sexual Pleasure* (Hunter House, 2013). I also highly recommend a DVD called *A Guide to Your Orgasm*, produced by The Welcomed Consensus (www.welcomed.com).

Making your sexual and sensual pleasure a priority will change your life and fill your cells with life-giving nitric oxide, the molecule of life force. Let your inner Aphrodite and your emotions be your guide, have fun with your erotic anatomy—and remember that there's no more powerful aphrodisiac than a woman who feels irresistible. Be a goddess of sensual pleasure!

SEXUAL HEALING FOR TRAUMA AND BLOCKAGES IN THE LOWER CHAKRAS

If you've suffered sexual trauma, or are holding on to the energy of fear and loss in your pelvic area due to surgical procedures there, such as a hysterectomy or removal of a cancerous tumor, you can use sexual energy to heal the blockages in your pelvic center. There are many ways to reawaken this area of your body and begin its energetic healing.

The psoas muscles are part of your core muscle groups and run from your lower spine through your groin to your upper legs. These muscles support range of motion, balance, and proper functioning of organs in the pelvic region. They get stretched and worked in Pilates and in some other types of exercise, such as erotic dance.

The psoas muscles have a close relationship with the emotional centers in the primitive, limbic brain, so emotional stress, particularly fear and anger, can affect the health and flexibility of the psoas. These muscles are located near the first chakra, the seat of the kundalini life force—the female energy located in the base of the spine, connecting the body's energy to that of the earth. The kundalini life force is often depicted as a coiled serpent that holds the potential to rise up, bringing chi into the rest of the body. The first chakra is associated with survival instincts, while the second chakra is the seat of sexuality, power, and creativity. Moving your hips, relaxing your psoas, and letting go of your fear that you'll be shamed for being a sexual, sensual, creatively expressive goddess is vital to your health.

It's crucial to have a physical practice that addresses these chakras—and every other muscle in the body. It could be yoga or Pilates. It could be dancing. Horseback riding is another way to reconnect to your hips and reclaim your relationship with the force of your inner Aphrodite. To have a huge, strong animal attune to the movements you make with your pelvis and the area between your legs, and respond to them, is empowering and deeply sensual.

Erotic dancing, such as pole dancing, belly dancing, and close-embrace Argentine tango, also reconnects you to your pleasurable core. I once took a private pole dancing class to learn some of these fluid and beautiful movements. In a dimly lit room, my instructor encouraged me to truly surrender to some slow, sensual hip circles with erotic music. As I began to move my hips in circles that grew ever wider and more sensual, I thought, *I have waited my entire life to be given permission to move my hips this way!* Taking a private or women-only class taught by a woman can help you get past any shyness or embarrassment to discover that you were born to move sensually. Belly dancing was originally taught by grandmothers to their granddaughters as a way to help with birth—not to seduce men. Whatever you want to give birth to, believe me, it will help if you reconnect with the power in your pelvic bowl.

OVERCOMING THE OBSTACLES TO BLISS

What gets between women and their pleasure? For one thing, many women are exhausted. An uninterrupted night of sleep is the most desirable activity they can imagine. Most blame it on hormones, and those can certainly play a role. But hormones aren't really the issue. The fatigue comes after several decades of putting your own needs last and caring for others instead. Your body just says, "Stop it." If sex is just another item on the To Do list to attend to because you "should" have a sex life to please your partner, of course you're going to have trouble feeling sexual desire!

As adults, we don't talk about how overwhelmed we are by what we have to do because we don't want to be seen as whiny or angry. The striving for perfectionism, for never letting them see us sweat, for not giving anyone reason to shame us, sucks the life out of us. Our desire for sex naturally suffers. This has nothing to do with age or hormonal changes. Women are presented with unattainable, conflicting expectations topped off with a huge serving of shame, and *that* is what kills sex drive.

Recently, it was announced that a pharmaceutical company is working on a drug to boost the libido of women who are on antidepressants, because those medications have the side effect of killing sexual desire. Hello, we don't need more drugs to address the side effects of drugs! Women need to grieve and rage, let their feelings out, and nurture themselves so that they feel pleasure. Then their sexual desire will increase automatically.

Some women have fear surrounding sex because they've been sexually abused and exploited, or they have looked around and seen how other women have been sexually violated or simply shamed. Secrecy, silence, and judgment make matters worse. Many women don't even remember traumatic events until somewhere around menopause, probably because survival depended on forgetting. Given that most abuse takes place in the home, we really can't allow ourselves to get in touch with what we know and feel because there's no safe place to retreat to—even as adults, women who have been traumatized may associate "home" with abuse and a lack of safety. It's hard to be open and trusting when you know you're vulnerable to being hurt again.

Brené Brown says, "Vulnerability is not weakness and that myth is profoundly dangerous. Vulnerability is the birthplace of innovation, creativity, and change."[9] *Vulnerability* comes from a Latin word for wound. When you're vulnerable, you're more easily wounded, but that doesn't mean you're weak. It takes a lot of strength to open your heart again and trust another person enough to be physically intimate. If you've been hurt in sexual relationships, or hurt sexually, of course it's going to be difficult to reclaim your sexuality and your vulnerability, but it is definitely worth the effort!

Another obstacle to experiencing our "inner erotic creature" is the shame that comes from having an "imperfect" appearance. Brené Brown wrote a book on rejecting shame and delivered a magnificent TED talk on the topic. Afterward, many people shamed and judged her in the comments section of the TED website for her clothing, weight, and hairstyle, making catty and cruel remarks. Apparently, those viewers didn't get what she was saying at all! She admits she cried her eyes out and then, over time, realized that if someone wasn't out in the public arena like she was, "daring greatly," as she calls it, she wasn't interested in what they had to say. Bravo! Better to feel sorry for someone who is so unhappy that he has to resort to shaming a brave woman to feel better about himself. When a well-known male film critic used rude terms to shame actress and comedian Melissa McCarthy for being overweight (and what does being overweight have to do with her performance in movies?), her response was, "Why would someone be O.K. with that? I felt really bad for someone who is swimming in so much hate. . . . That's someone who's in a really bad spot, and I am in such a happy spot. I laugh my head off every day with my husband and my kids who are mooning me and singing me songs."[10]

To experience earthly pleasures and nourish the life force within you, you've got to release the shame—and anger, guilt, grief, and fear—that kill the libido by constricting blood flow. The truth is that you'll never get it all done and you'll never be perfect. You're a goddess just as you are. Stop worrying and put pleasure and play *first*. And then, believe it or not, you'll find that you are so energized, you'll be able to get far more done and you'll be far more relaxed.

Exercise: Body Love

Many women have been shamed for not measuring up to some elusive ideal of beauty, or simply for being sexual. Many have been sexually violated. Unhealed wounds from sexual abuse or shaming can cause a woman to become out of touch with her body. This exercise will help you reconnect to your body and its natural beauty. To do it, you will need a full-length mirror and a candle. Find a time when you will be alone and uninterrupted in a dark room. You'll need at least ten minutes to receive its full effects.

Light a candle, place it on a table nearby, and look at yourself in the mirror. As you do, relax your face and jaw. Allow your shoulders to drop. Notice any thoughts that arise, such as *This is really a stupid exercise.* Or *I'm so fat.* Or *Look at all those wrinkles.* When these thoughts arise, just smile. Relax your face and jaw, and breathe—slowly and mindfully. Observe how the candlelight casts a flattering, soft light on your skin, making it glow.

Remove all your clothing and stand before the mirror. Breathe consciously and slowly as you gaze at your reflection. Slowly move your eyes around your reflection so that you look at every part of yourself.

Notice when your breathing changes, your muscles tense, or you feel the desire to look away. Just relax your face, your jaw, and your shoulders. Don't judge your reaction or yourself. Simply make note of what you're experiencing. Focus on your breathing for a few moments, and say aloud, "Divine Beloved, change me into someone who sees the incredible beauty in my body." Then, look at yourself in the mirror again—at the part of your body that caused you to have a defensive emotional or physical reaction when you gazed at it. Affirm your beauty, or say the Divine Beloved prayer, several times.

When you have gazed at your entire body in the mirror, using affirmations and prayer whenever you feel resistance to the exercise, end by affirming, "I am a beautiful, valuable, sexy, and sensual woman. I appreciate my body."

Get dressed before turning on the light and blowing out the candle.

Repeat the Body Love exercise at least twice a week for a full month or until you find you're no longer experiencing resistance and it's easy to send your body love and appreciation. The shift in your feelings toward your body can be dramatic.

ADDRESSING PHYSICAL OBSTACLES TO ENJOYING SEX

Of course, there can be physiological reasons for sexual desire waning, one of which is pain during sex. If sex is painful, it may simply be because of vaginal dryness—which is easily addressed with lubricants. But it can also be due to repressed anger or trauma manifesting as scarring or vaginal adhesions. These can form after inflammation, infection, and surgery. In the late 1980s, it finally dawned on gynecologists that women with chronic pelvic pain very often had experienced rape or other sexual abuse. Given that every year one in three women on this planet is raped or abused, it's not surprising that so many women experience pelvic pain and painful sex.

One of the most effective modalities for women with pelvic pain, urinary problems, and sexual pain is the subspecialty of physical therapy known as Women's Health Physical Therapy. Therapists trained in this modality know exactly how to retrain the muscles of the pelvic floor and help reestablish normal function. You can learn more at www.thebathroomkey.com or www.obgyn-physicaltherapy.com.

Sometimes, manual therapy, a type of massage, is required to break up fascial scarring in the pelvis. My colleagues who do manual therapy work have reported many cases of women who've had painful sex being cured in a very short time with this type of therapy. Women's health physical therapist Tami Lynn Kent (www.wildfeminine.com) reports some incredible results with using manual therapy on women who find sex painful due to fascial scarring and lesions. So do Larry and Belinda Wurn (www.clearpassage.com), who developed the Wurn Technique and have trained many other physical therapists. Jennifer Mercier, M.D. (www.drjennifermercier.com), is also an expert in this area and has trained other practitioners in manual therapy for pelvic scarring.

To avoid pain during intercourse, you need adequate lubrication. Lack of lubrication does not mean a lack of sexual interest or response. Some women naturally generate a lot of fluid when aroused—others, not so much. If you have difficulty with lubrication, go ahead and use lubricant liberally. There are many types available over the counter. Low estrogen can also cause a decrease in lubrication. My favorite approach to this problem is to use *Pueraria mirifica* either orally or topically. It is very effective for restoring vaginal moisture.

Birth control pills, patches, or shots, while highly effective, may alter your natural testosterone levels in such a way as to quell libido. Continue using some kind of birth control scrupulously if you're still *physically* fertile—and you have to consider yourself fertile for a full year after your last period ends. Consider using a type other than those made with synthetic hormones. IUDs and tubal ligation are good choices as well.

Cholesterol, too, can affect your sex drive: The lower your cholesterol, the lower your libido. Statin drugs to lower cholesterol also lower the libido. If you're on a very low-fat diet, it's time to get off that and start adding healthy fats back into your diet.

Usually, it's stuck emotions, not hormones, that are the main issue when it comes to low sexual desire or sexual discomfort. If so, you might work with a physical therapist or do self-massage of your vagina to release any emotions that are energetically stuck in your pelvis, destroying your libido and sexual enjoyment. Signs that emotions are stuck in your pelvis include any and all gynecological problems, such as pelvic pain, large fibroids, recurrent urinary tract infections, and inability to experience sexual pleasure. Consider talk therapy for bringing to the surface your thoughts and feelings about your sexuality and past sexual trauma. I have to warn you that while a great sex therapist or sexological body worker may be able to help you quite a lot, it's important to choose someone who will respect your sexual boundaries. I've known far too many women who've been traumatized trying to get help. If you don't get a good feeling working with someone, and you sense it's not the healing work but the person who is the problem, walk away and find a different healer.

WHEN YOU CRAVE TOUCH

Humans are designed to give and receive touch in many different ways. In orphanages where babies don't experience regular, loving touch, the children end up with serious developmental problems. Experiments have even shown that baby monkeys will choose the touch of a mother over food—it's that important to have pleasurable touch. Whether or not you're having sex with a partner, you need to make sure you get plenty of touch.

Fertility, Childbirth, and Becoming a Mother in Midlife

I consider fertility a lifelong blessing even when you can no longer get pregnant. After a certain point, a woman's body is not meant to experience pregnancy and giving birth.

When you look at the statistics on abortion, the majority of women ending their pregnancies are younger women, but the next largest group is women in their early 40s who thought they were no longer fertile and were inconsistent about using contraception. Don't kid yourself—you still need birth control in your 40s and sometimes even in your 50s, unless you've gone through perimenopause and are definitely postmenopausal. Of course, for many women, sex gets better simply because they are no longer worried about pregnancy after menopause. Sometimes, switching off of a hormonal method of birth control makes a big difference. Getting off the pill and rid of the fear of pregnancy may not return a woman's sex drive to normal instantly, but it should come back fairly quickly. If you've written off sex as a thing of the past, and you are using hormonal contraception, I urge you to look at your other options until you've crossed the threshold of menopause.

If you feel drawn to become a mother in some way during this new stage of life, and you're thinking of adopting, or taking in a foster child, or working with a fertility specialist to have a baby despite being in perimenopause, think hard about what it is you want to create. There are many ways to express your mother energy. Becoming a mother to a child at this point in your life may be right for you, but it's not the only way to express yourself creatively. Be honest with yourself about your fertility and the ways your body is changing. That way, you're more likely to make the best decision for yourself. Don't make the decision unconsciously by not being scrupulous about birth control. Start envisioning what you want to give birth to—and give yourself permission to be "fertile" in a new way.

Unrequited, the desire for touch can lead you to make sexual choices that aren't right for you. Acknowledge your need for tactile input as well as your longings for companionship and affection, and it will be easier to make sexual choices that support you as an ageless, pleasure-seeking goddess.

Touch is a basic human need, so meet it shamelessly. I hug men and women in my tango community all the time—and, of course, tango offers a marvelous opportunity for touching another person. I remember that soon after my divorce, I began to miss being hugged by a man. I loved that Dave, my favorite waiter at a restaurant near my home, would give me a big, loving hug every time he saw me. My body soaked up his embraces like a desert after a rain.

Research shows human beings need not just touch but affectionate touch into adulthood. When you experience affectionate touch, your body releases the bonding hormone oxytocin. That not only makes you feel good, it may reduce inflammation in your body.[11] Be sure to bring into your life people who are comfortable with the kind of touch you like, whether you're someone who craves hugs and neck massages or you like kisses on the cheek. It's important that two people agree on how to touch each other. If your partner is emotionally affectionate but not big on touch, find someone you can touch nonsexually to get your hugs, back rubs, and cuddles. And get massages if you can; that's another way to bring touch into your life.

A massage therapist will typically work on your arms and hands, legs and feet, neck, and scalp, but not your pelvis or breasts. I prefer that a massage therapist focus on the sacrum and pectoral muscles around the breasts because so much needs massaging there! Trust yourself. A good massage therapist will respect that a lot of trauma may be stuck in this area and will help you release it. But if you don't feel comfortable when you walk into the room, or during the massage, speak up or leave.

Choose a massage therapist carefully to be sure it's someone whom you can trust to drape you carefully and respectfully during the body work, and who will respond to your requests for altering his or her touch. Keep in mind that it's common for emotions to come up and out during massage—even if the massage therapist isn't working directly on the parts of your body that are holding the emotions—so don't feel embarrassed if the touch brings up some tears or laughter.

Listen to your instincts about what feels nurturing and pleasurable and what feels uncomfortable. Don't be afraid to speak up for yourself and your needs. You may find that the ritual of a massage, in which you're just in underpants and kept covered by a sheet that is carefully adjusted as the masseuse moves on to work on another part of your body, is a marvelous way to experience respect for your body and your boundaries.

If you have never had a massage, start with one that involves lighter touch (for example, Swedish massage) and avoid any that involve deeper pressure. Sports medicine clinics often focus on the kind of massage that is uncomfortable, even painful, and can leave you sore afterward. You're looking for a massage in a quiet, dimly lit room with spa music, and a massage therapist who almost whispers when she has to give you an instruction and who keeps chatter to a minimum as she gives you a relaxation massage. The other types of massage have their value, but when it comes to reconnecting to your body in a pleasurable way and releasing any stuck emotions or energy, go for the softer, gentler massage rather than the kind that will have you yelping in discomfort. Drink plenty of water after a massage to help release toxins.

Massage increases your circulation and lowers your levels of cortisol, the hormones associated with stress. It also boosts your immunity and is a wonderful way to nurture your whole body. In fact, I think massage should be a cornerstone of your self-care and wellness program. If you have trouble affording regular massages, go with a friend to take a course on how to do them, and once you've gotten the training, give each other massages. Sign up for coupon deals, buy massages in bulk, or get them at a spa school to save money.

Another way to experience sensual, tactile pleasure is foot massage. In the somatosensory cortex of the brain where we experience sensations, the area where we experience clitoral sensations is right below where we experience sensations on our feet. No wonder a foot massage can be a turn-on!

Ageless Sex: Eleven Tips

Regardless of your age, you can experience the best sex ever if you follow these 11 tips.

1. *Put the focus on your pleasure.* Whether you're having sex with a partner or alone, connecting with your vital life force and enjoying the experience are paramount.

2. *Ask for what you want.* Recognize that your pleasure matters, and don't settle for a partner who doesn't value your needs.

3. *Take the time you need.* Stop looking at your watch and surrender to pleasure! Enjoy every moment and don't worry about how long it is taking you to get warmed up or to reach a pinnacle of excitement. Remember that the orgasm begins with the first contraction of your PC muscle. Don't try to "achieve" anything.

4. *Use plenty of lubrication.* When you get enough stimulation and your blood is circulating well, the mucosa tends to thicken on its own, but you can get a little help with over-the-counter lubricants. I highly recommend ones made with *Pueraria mirifica.* Prescription estrogen creams can also make your vaginal lining thicker and slicker.

5. *Build a flexible, functional pelvic floor.* Instead of using the old Kegel muscle squeeze techniques, work out the entire pelvic floor muscle group so that you can better enjoy intercourse and be free of stress and urgency incontinence. Check out the book *The Bathroom Key* by Kim Perelli and Kathryn Kassai, P.T., C.E.S., for a program for working out and building up your pelvic floor, and see the quick hints in Chapter 4 on page 110. Also check out *"Down There" for Women,* a DVD by Katy Bowman.

6. *Know, treasure, and express love to your erotic female anatomy.* Your erotic anatomy is a marvelous gift! Be familiar with your erotic anatomy and how to stimulate this area pleasurably.

7. *Keep vitamin D levels optimal.* Between 40 and 80 nanograms/ml is ideal. Sufficient levels of vitamin D can help prevent anxiety and depression, which are common libido killers. You can get vitamin D from exposure to the sun and from vitamin D3 supplements.

8. *Get adequate sleep.* Most women need eight to ten hours for optimal functioning. Sleep is restorative at a cellular level. It allows you to clear accumulated stress hormones that cause inflammatory processes that lead to disease.

9. *Awaken your pelvic energy centers.* Your first chakra is the center of kundalini energy, where you experience your life force. The second chakra is your second energy center, and it can become sluggish and blocked if you have unresolved emotional issues about sex, money, and power. Let go of anger, hurt, and fear, and recharge your lower chakras with activities that get your hips moving.

10. *Get a new partner—or become a new partner.* When you experience your delicious sexuality and indulge in self-pleasure, you become even more desirable. Better sex starts with you.

11. *Consciously bring the Sacred into your sex life.* Light candles, burn incense, play beautiful music, and be a goddess whose bodily pleasure is a channel for healing the world.

EROTICA VERSUS PORN

One powerful way to reconnect to your sexuality is through the written word. Men tend to become sexually turned on by images, while women often become turned on by words. That's why a man will log on to an Internet porn site rather than read an erotic novel, and a woman will go for *Fifty Shades of Grey.* Whether you read and enjoyed that bestseller or not, its huge success is a reminder of what women are looking for sexually but are often denied. The woman in the story is able to experience sex guilt-free because she can't protest when she's tied up, so any shame about pleasure goes out the window. The man is dedicated to giving her pleasure and has an entire room devoted to sexual enjoyment—that's a turn-on to women who are unlikely to make room for pleasure in their own lives. The male lover pampers the woman, showering her with gifts and taking her out to the most delicious and romantic dinners—again, something women fantasize about. And all of this is described in detail so that the reader can create her own image of what her pleasure room and devoted lover look like.

Erotic writing connects us with our earthy desires. I appreciate a spicy romance novel and the erotic writings of authors such as Anaïs Nin. My all-time favorite erotic scenes in literature feature the characters Jamie and Claire in Diana Gabaldon's Outlander series. I encourage you to awaken your erotic anatomy by reading erotica and erotic passages. The world is a little short on really good erotic movies at the moment, but I expect that will change with more women becoming empowered sexually.

Frankly, the porn industry has done more to warp the erotic imagination of men than just about anything else has. The standard "formula" porn movie is cheap to produce and features a vacuous woman with breast implants and no pubic hair who is mounted by a guy with a big penis, who penetrates her for a very short time before "finishing" with his own climax. The woman doesn't appear to experience much pleasure at all. It's because of porn, after all, that Brazilian pubic hair waxing has now become standard for so many women. Removing pubic hair was first done in porn flicks simply because a hairless vulva makes it easier to see the "penetration shots." It's now considered "personal care," as though pubic hair in and of itself were somehow dirty! Shaving this area of the body can make a woman more vulnerable to infections when bacteria enter tiny cuts in the skin caused by shaving, and it can cause ingrown hairs.

Now, if you want to trim or remove your pubic hair, that's your choice. I just want you to know it's a choice—not another "should." Many men and women are turned on by the body's natural state of hairiness, so don't feel pressured to do something that makes you uncomfortable because of some mistaken idea that it's "hygienic." Don't let pornographic images dictate how you feel about your body or what you think is sexy.

In general, porn perpetuates a very substandard sexual experience for both men and women. However, unlike pornography, which has no heart or soul, erotica is enlivening. If, like many women, you aren't turned on by sexual video and photographs, you might want to try reading an erotic novel or story collection. And if neither makes you feel sexy, don't worry about it. There are many other ways to reconnect with your sexual self.

ROOM FOR PLEASURE!

Every woman should make room in her life for pleasure, so let's talk about the two rooms in the home most associated with a woman's body—and most likely to be uninviting, cold, and/or cluttered: the bathroom and bedroom.

Women so often settle for whatever their surroundings are. If they're renters, they convince themselves it's a "waste of money" to decorate—even if they've been in the same apartment for ten years. Is your bedroom a love nest or a storage space you plop down in after you're exhausted by the demands of your day? A bedroom should be a boudoir—inviting, sensual, visually reminding you to reconnect with your body and its capacity for endless pleasure. Get rid of the electronics, such as the TV and computer. Clear any clutter; use beautiful fabrics on the bed, pillows, and windows; and have plenty of soft spots to sink into, whether it's a bed or a chair. Give the walls a fresh coat of paint and choose a color that turns you on—according to feng shui, flesh tones are best because they'll remind you of your connection to your body.

Install new lighting that enhances your skin tone. Candles are great, but it's dangerous to fall asleep with them still burning, so you might use Himalayan salt lamps instead. Have fresh flowers or at least fresh plants around, as well as natural objects. Make sure that your windows are open to the starry, moonlit sky and to sunlight, if possible, to make nature a part of your bedroom experience. Set up the room as if for a visiting queen.

And make room for a partner if you desire one—or want to keep one. An expert in feng shui told me that having two night-stands, one on either side of the bed, is one way to change your bedroom's energy from being perfect for a solo sleeper to being just right for a couple. On that note, take down any photos or paintings you have of single women if being alone in your bed-room isn't the message you want to send to the universe.

And now, on to the bathroom! Don't you just love those com-fort stations in the ladies' lounges of finer hotels and restaurants? They set out a perfect little display of lotions and sundries, in-cluding perfume, to make a woman feel beautiful and connected to the pleasure of her body in a space that, let's face it, often involves some not-so-romantic activities. Make your bathroom a space where you feel inspired to nurture yourself and get in touch with your sensuality and sexuality. Stock up on big, fluffy, soft, and absorbent towels that feel heavenly against your skin. Keep some in the bathroom to dampen harsh sounds and echoes. If you don't have windows in the bathroom, use natural, full-spectrum lighting.

I book hotel rooms based on whether or not they have a tub and even bring my own rubber drain stopper in case the tub doesn't work properly! And in my home, I built my ultimate fan-tasy bathroom, with a shower that has two showerheads and a large sunken oval bathtub facing a window with a view of the river near my house. It's surrounded by green marble that forms a shelf that's the perfect area for flowers, candles, and incense. I also built a bookcase right behind the tub because it's my favor-ite reading spot. And I have a great sound system, with Pandora radio stations playing sensual or relaxing music. Yes—it's an amazing room. And I describe it only to inspire you. It took me years to come to this. Don't wait. You can create a wonderfully sensual space even in the smallest bathroom.

When I bathe, I make it a ritual with bath salts, aromatherapy or incense, candles, music, and a good book. I crave a bath before I go to sleep—maybe because my moon is in Pisces, a water sign. Immersion in water is always soothing. Doing affirmations, massaging your breasts, journaling, and singing while soaking in the bath will all awaken your sensuality and pleasure.

In the language of dream interpretation, water represents abundance and the flow of life and emotions. Maybe that's why we're so often drawn to it. All life starts in amniotic fluid, which has roughly the same chemical composition as the ocean. If you have a chance to swim in clean, natural bodies of water—lakes, an ocean or sea, or even a pool cleaned not with chlorine but an ionization process—you can experience the sensual pleasure of water against your skin and a sense of oneness that comes from immersing your body in the caress of water. Let yourself be infused with the spirit of the river goddess who teaches you to go with the flow and the goddess of the ocean who is teeming with abundant life.

We can all become deliciously seductive pleasure goddesses— not predatory cougars but golden tigresses luxuriating in the delight of our own sexual power. My late cat, Francine, who still appears in my dreams regularly, taught me more about being a woman than anyone else has! When she sashayed over to me and deemed me worthy of having her place her soft, silky, warm body on my lap, I'd feel as if I was the chosen one. And *that* is how the world will respond to you when you truly own and operate your inner erotic creature.

CHAPTER SEVEN

GODDESSES LOVE WITHOUT LOSING THEMSELVES

Run my dear,
From anything
That may not strengthen
Your precious budding wings.
Run like hell my dear,
From anyone likely
To put a sharp knife
Into the sacred, tender vision
Of your beautiful heart.

— HAFIZ (TR. DANIEL LADINSKY)

In the 1970s, Gloria Steinem used to say, "We have become the men we wanted to marry." I have my own twist on this: become the kind of woman to whom the kind of person you are looking for would be attracted. This is the path I decided to follow. In the year or two following my divorce, as I thought about getting involved with a man again, I resolved to become the kind of woman that the kind of man I wanted would desire.

How do you feel about yourself? Here's the truth: *the number-one relationship that determines the quality of all the others in your life, and sets the tone for them, is the one you have with yourself.* Are you willing to learn to love yourself enough to discover your depth, own your beauty, and articulate your deepest desires? Or are you going to neglect the work of mining your inner treasures while waiting for someone else to sweep into your life and rescue you from your loneliness, your yearning, and your despair? Each of us is confronted with this choice every day. Only when we have the courage to love ourselves as the divine, ageless goddesses we are do we have a real shot at creating heaven on earth with someone else.

Post-divorce, I believed that finding Mr. Right would completely solve all my problems and make me feel happy and whole again. That was a worthy goal, but at the time I had no idea that my soul had a much bigger plan for me. I was driven by longing for a relationship that would complete me. Now, I knew intellectually that this awful feeling of yearning was about far more than the lack of Mr. Right in my life. Still, I wanted that "perfect" man and "perfect" relationship.

Though I met a lot of men, the few I desired weren't available—but all of them *were* soul mates for me at some level. They were meant to be in my life to wake me up—to show me my need to reconnect to Spirit and find happiness inside me instead of looking for it somewhere out there.

In the process of becoming the woman the right kind of man would want, I transformed into a woman more whole, happy, and confident than I've ever been in my entire life. Now, instead of feeling like a woman who has been neglected and left behind, I am happy and whole and know that my presence is an asset. Why? Because I finally mated with my soul and became my own soul mate.

I know many of you are seeking a flesh-and-blood life partner. We are mammals and herd creatures, after all. But I can assure you that the only way you're ever going to be fully ready to step into true partnership with the person of your dreams is to release the constant craving to be completed by another. You must learn how to complete yourself. You have to see yourself as irresistible and set a high price on your head. And you have to believe that your ideal partner has already been picked. He (or she) will show up at exactly the right time and in the right way. In the meantime, your job is to live happily ever after, starting right now!

The truth is that when you feel whole, complete, and lacking in nothing, that aching abyss you think only a mate can fill will finally go away. And you will stop choosing mates or even friends who ultimately disappoint you. Trust me on this one. No one expresses this better than writer Tosha Silver in her poem "The Kiss," which you can read on the next page.

BEING LOVE

To have a better relationship with yourself, begin to think of yourself as love itself. Imagine you are both a transmitter and receiver of an infinite amount of life-giving energy. Share this love with others. You can do that with just a smile.

A man and his wife and daughter sat down at a table near me at one of my favorite local restaurants. He radiated life force and joy, even though he spent most of the lunch absorbed by his smartphone. When I finished lunch, I stopped by his table and told him how strikingly happy he appeared. He beamed from ear to ear, and in a German accent said, "Even though I was spending too much time looking at my phone?" We all laughed and I left, both of our days lightened with love and joy. You can do the same thing wherever you are and whatever you are doing. Before you post something on a social media board, saturate it with Divine Love first, and don't make the mistake of expecting a particular response—a validation from someone else. Freely send your love outward and trust that love will always come to you.

Find your inner voice and sing as an offering to the Divine and to love itself, whether you do it literally or figuratively. As Wayne Dyer says, "Don't die with your music still in you." It doesn't matter whether your song is an offering of love to yourself

The Kiss

Since the Divine
will never be closer
than
She is this moment
Her kiss
never waits
'til you meet your soulmate
have a baby
or adopt that stray dog
No need to nab
the perfect handstand
or hope that Venus
might finally submit one day to Mars
No need to grow more worthy
burn extra sage
or light
one more flame
Her kiss descends
when the torrid lust
for future and past
expires in a fit of pure exhaustion
And you bless
This Very Moment
As It Is
turning your full-on gaze
to the One
long waiting
and just say
Now

—Tosha Silver, from *Make Me Your Own: Poems to the Divine Beloved* (Alameda, CA: Urban Kali Productions, 2013)

or to someone else. When you love yourself, you contribute to the abundance of love, and we all benefit.

A few years ago, my mother won an award from the state of New York for being a "distinguished woman." At the awards ceremony, I noticed that the other women who had won the award had all been recognized for something they had done for others in their communities—everyone had performed unselfish, charitable acts. My mother was the only woman being recognized for having simply followed her passion, climbing mountain peaks, hiking the Appalachian Trail, and continuing to lead a physically active, adventurous life in her 80s. It's not as if she had never served her community directly: she had been mayor of her town for five years. But then, even though both the Republicans and Democrats in town wanted her to run for reelection, she decided not to because she had other interests that were important to her. Many in the audience came up to my mother after she received the award and were buzzing with a sense of excitement about her. It was as if they could feel the joy of my mother's life flowing into theirs. They wanted what she had—the willingness to put herself first, enjoy life, and follow her passions. Her relationship to herself was inspiring to women and men alike.

But how many of us buy into the idea that following our heart's desires is selfish? Anita Moorjani, author of *Dying to Be Me,* says, "Selfishness comes from too little self-love, not too much." And she explains, "When I'm *being love,* I don't get drained, and I don't need people to behave a certain way in order to feel cared for or to share my magnificence with them. They're automatically getting love as a result of me being my true self. And when I am nonjudgmental of myself, I feel that way toward others."[1] By having a great relationship with yourself, by loving yourself fully, you *are* serving the world. You're inspiring others to truly appreciate themselves by modeling what it looks like to appreciate yourself without conceit.

To truly love yourself, you have to get to know who you are instead of repressing all the parts of yourself that you might have been shamed for in the past. For years, I wanted to learn how to dance. But whenever my husband and I took dancing classes, I simply ended up being criticized by him for what I was doing wrong. Unbeknownst to me, in many ways I was shut down emotionally because I was always trying to make myself into someone I wasn't.

Often, we go along with other people's plans for us and expectations of us because underneath it all, we're terrified that if we really go for all of what we want, we'll be abandoned. Better to get crumbs than risk being left alone, we tell ourselves. We leave ourselves undeveloped and emotionally malnourished. Then we yearn for someone to rescue us and provide what we think we can't provide for ourselves. That makes us needy, not alluring. It's not the beauty of youth that we lose when we're constantly compromising ourselves but the beauty of youthful courage. You're never too old to take risks and do what makes you feel alive.

Whether you love horses, dance, gardening, fitness, making jewelry, or travel, it's clear that they all contribute to agelessness and make others feel attracted to you. As Julia Child, who discovered her joy of cooking late in life, said, "Find something you are passionate about and keep tremendously interested in it." That's what makes you ageless.

In relationships, your job is to fill yourself up until you're overflowing with love and enthusiasm for life, and then allow a relationship to unfold. The point is *not* to find your missing part so that you can be rescued from your problems—and it is *not* to be someone else's missing part and rescue him or her. In the movie *Jerry Maguire,* there's a famous scene that demonstrates what a fine line this can be. In the movie, Jerry (played delightfully by Tom Cruise) realizes that he misses his wife (Renée Zellweger), having put his career far ahead of his need for connection. He's left her, but he rushes to her after one of the biggest career successes of his life because he realizes how empty it is to feel that he has no one to share that success with. He stands in front of her with his heart in his hands, pouring out his desire for a partner to be by his side. Through teary eyes, he says, "You complete me." And every woman in the audience sighs and wishes a man (or woman) would say the same thing to her. But make no mistake. He's not really saying that he is incomplete without her. Instead, he's acknowledging that she brings out the best in him, and that he's a better person when he is with her. *This* is what a relationship is supposed to be: a partnership between two people who enhance each other, and who become more than each could be alone because of the power of the partnership. A relationship should not be the result of two half people trying to complete each other. In a great co-creative partnership that keeps us ageless, one plus one makes more than two.

Whether you're heterosexual or a woman looking for a romantic relationship with another woman, you can find a romantic partner who is exciting and dependable in the important ways. Many women now have much more freedom to create a relationship that's going to meet their needs—and realize they don't even need a partner to meet them anyway. A romantic partner is just icing on the cake.

WHAT DO I DO WITH RALPH?

When women and men get into their 50s and 60s, their experiences and interests often start to diverge. Women become free of old obligations and want to start a business, travel, or learn something new. Men finally stop focusing solely on the competitive world of work, or even retire, just as their testosterone levels may drop and their energy moves up from their lower chakras to the heart chakra. In other words, their energy becomes less concentrated in the energy centers associated with survival, self-expression, sexuality, and power, and stronger in the energy center associated with feelings and relationships. This change is good for men—in fact, all of us should be living from a heart-centered place. The electromagnetic field of the heart affects our hormonal balance, so it's beneficial for our health to have a well-functioning heart chakra. But this shift to a more heart-centered energy in middle-aged men causes them to start to feel more domestic, and they may become homebodies, which some women see as a problem. Ralph starts a garden, putters in the garage, and tries out new recipes. Meanwhile, his wife complains, "I can't seem to get Ralph out of the house and *doing* something!"

A woman who retires from a full-time, high-pressure job may enjoy taking the time to read novels, empty out the basement at last, and redecorate her bedroom, but more often than not, restlessness soon sets in. She is hormonally and spiritually driven to get out into the world and launch into deeper self-discovery and new adventures. As one woman who retired at 65 said, "I was going to go on the vacation of a lifetime to celebrate my thirtieth wedding anniversary, and then I remembered how boring my husband is. He complains all the time and he's just no fun. So I called my girlfriend and said, 'We should do this together.' And she said, 'Oh yeah. Absolutely. I'm there!'" Clearly, the woman who is itching to spread her wings and the mate who wants to nest can drive each other crazy unless both are willing to grow and change.

Divorce is certainly not the only answer. As long as the two of them recognize that they have different desires and interests, they can rediscover each other and fashion a new relationship.

Many of us began our adult lives thinking it was a man's job to take care of a woman financially and a woman's job to take care of a man emotionally. We rid ourselves of that stifling idea, but accepting the new paradigm of a supportive partner back at the nest as we stretch our wings for the first time in ages can be challenging but very rewarding. Women who aren't coupled may find they are ready for an entirely different kind of lover and partner, whether it's a man or a woman.

THE GOOD GUYS

If you're heterosexual and have no partner, know that the "good guys" who don't bore you to death are out there—they always have been. Men are closeted romantics who are dying to please women—unless they're narcissists, in which case all bets are off. And even if you're not interested in a romantic partnership with men, know that there are plenty of great men in the world. They just have difficulty making themselves known when they're shamed for being in touch with their romantic side—and the screwed-up men who use violence and posturing to hide their vulnerability grab all the headlines. Those men attract women who have unresolved issues about their own feminine sides.

Embrace your womanliness in your own way and the sexy good guys will show up.

As women, we absolutely must acknowledge how scared men are, and how much they are criticized by the women in their lives. They look to women to make them feel competent and strong. When I have invited men to men's night at Mama Gena's School of Womanly Arts, the first response from many of them is, "Oh, great. A whole room full of women. Are they going to rip me a new one?" I've always been stunned by this response, but I'm starting to realize it's common for men to fear women's disapproval. And I'm equally stunned by the few men who, when surrounded by a roomful of beautiful, wholehearted women, feel so threatened that they leave. But this experience of feeling vulnerable and hurt by rejection, which is familiar to both men and women, speaks volumes about the fact that we're all in this together.

Because we live in a dominator culture, the soft, feminine, feeling side of men is as wounded as it is in so many women. Playwright Eve Ensler travels a lot and tells me that more and more, she's seeing men on planes watching romantic comedies and "chick flicks" on their personal viewing devices (maybe because watching it on a phone screen or tablet is more discreet than watching it on a larger screen). The Hilton Hotel chain started offering rooms decorated with softer colors and lighting to appeal to female travelers—and found male travelers eager to book those rooms. It's good to see men acknowledging their softer side and indulging it. We need more of that! And we need to let go of the old dominator culture's attitude that men in touch with their female aspects are weak and unattractive.

We women have to lead the way toward healthier male/female relationships by healing ourselves, reclaiming our womanliness, embracing our own desires, and tapping into Spirit. We have to bring love into ourselves, through ourselves, and out into the world in a way that benefits the men around us as well as the women. Men are desperate to feel connection through the feminine life force—and not just in the most literal way, by penetrating us sexually. They want touch and emotional connection. They want to come into our circle of healing. Holistic healer Tami Lynn Kent, whose books include *Mothering from Your Center: Tapping Your Body's Natural Energy for Pregnancy, Birth, and Parenting* (Atria Books/Beyond Words, 2013), has pointed out that we can see this in our sons. Even into their teens, boys are drawn to their mothers, and hug them and try to sit on their laps, because they're hungry to get in touch with Mom's feminine life force. She calls this behavior "returning to the mother ship."

As women, we aren't as emotionally vulnerable as men can be because we aren't socialized out of our feelings. We also take better care of our bodies than men do. We know how important it is to get support from our girlfriends and to have strong relationships with people who love us and look out for us. Men are slowly coming to realize that they, too, need to have a "tribe" to support them. Without women in their lives urging them toward wellness and giving them love and support, men often fall apart. That's why married men experience greater longevity and better health than unmarried men do. It's also why so many men remarry so quickly following divorce or the death of a spouse. Men sense they'll age quickly without a woman to keep them young—and the woman doesn't actually have to be younger than the man for him to feel she is helping him remain vibrant. Ageless goddesses are alluring to partners of every age. Who doesn't want to be around a woman who lives with gusto?

When it comes to our culture's damaging messages about the feminine force, I firmly believe that men won't heal until women do their own healing work and express their strength and womanliness in the world. It's going to have to start with us. We're the stronger ones, unafraid to look at what needs to be healed. But we have to make the first move so that men aren't shamed for wanting contact with the feminine force—whether it's through touching and being physically near women or being in contact with the feminine force within them.

Men could have healthier relationships with women *and* other men if they were allowed to own their emotions and need for connection. Recently, a very manly, accomplished sailor was visiting our tango class and I had him dance around the floor with my good friend Leftari, a young Greek man who dances right from his heart. Leftari knows how to make other men feel comfortable with the connection. Afterward, the sailor texted me to say, "The connection I felt in such a short period of time dancing is kind of funny. Your head is trying to fathom—does it feel this good dancing with a man while my heart and energy know without a doubt it is exactly what I need and yearn for, connection. Interesting that you had had me watch that Brené Brown TED talk beforehand. Very clever of you!"

The good news is that more and more, men are letting go of their shaming, owning their need for connection to the feminine life force wherever they can access it, and not apologizing for it. Men who are in touch with their need for connection and who are not shamed for it will stop trying to control women. In fact, they'll begin to appreciate competent and strong women even more. Once they have a better balance of masculine and feminine within themselves, they'll become capable of healthier relationships resulting from a healthier relationship with the vulnerable aspects of themselves.

In ancient cultures where people interacted collaboratively instead of giving one leader, or a small group of leaders, power over everyone else, men were warriors and hunters who served the life force. They protected and served the mothers and children literally and figuratively. The men didn't bring down a mammoth to serve themselves or to gain power over the tribe. They did it so everyone would have enough to eat. A man's ability to provide something of value for his loved ones is key to his well-being and sense of self. Men require respect. When they don't get it, they don't function very well.

Today, what do men really want? To protect and to serve. They want to be seen as useful and worthy of admiration. They also love giving pleasure to women. In her book *Swoon,* about the great lovers of the world, feminist historian Betsy Prioleau, Ph.D., writes that Casanova reported that two-thirds of his pleasure arose from giving pleasure to his lovers. Countless men agree with this and say that the biggest turn-on in their lives is providing pleasure to the women in their lives. Most men want to be heroes. I have seen this over and over again. All you have to do is acknowledge them for stepping up. It's so simple and powerful.

As women, we must allow them to serve us as the goddesses we are. It's good for men's souls and psyches to be connected to women who are full of the life force and to serve them in a loving and balanced way. We don't want men becoming perfectionists who give too much and deplete themselves as women have. Together, we can create new relationships with men that support well-being, health, and agelessness.

I was clueless about men's needs in my younger years, but fortunately, I'm a quick study. I think my willingness to learn about this aspect of men is part of the reason my two daughters have partnered with wonderful, strong, wholehearted men whom I adore. I have learned how to treasure the men in my life and all they do for me, including all the men who dance with me and do their best to provide me with pleasure. I also treasure my male plumber and male electrician! I feel so blessed to have such wonderful men in my life.

If as women we do everything by ourselves all the time and leave no room for men to serve us, we prevent men from doing what they're meant to do as powerful, sensual, masculine beings. We have to stop exhausting ourselves and end our endless quest for perfection. Let men serve us, even if they don't always do it perfectly. We need to set the bar higher and expect more of them when it comes to their attentiveness. If they put real effort into serving us, we need to appreciate that rather than become hypercritical and micromanage them.

If you want men's support, become attractive and kind to the men who can serve you. Send the message that you appreciate a strong man willing to give you what you need but that you also don't need to be rescued from utter helplessness.

SEX, MONEY, AND POWER

One thing that stands in the way of healthy male/female partnerships is women's discomfort with their own power, both sexual and financial. Money, sex, and power are all second-chakra issues. If we have good relationships with these things, then our second chakra, which is also our creative center, will be energized and strong. If we don't, we'll have a diminished sex drive, trouble attracting and holding on to money—and a boatload of gynecological issues!

It's important to look at money and sex as energy forces: Money represents power and security while sex represents the creative life force that balances receiving and giving. You've probably heard the myth that if a woman makes more than her husband does, their sex life will suffer. This doesn't have to be the case, but a man needs to be honored for his role, whether he's a breadwinner or a mate and father serving his family. Forty percent of families with dependent children are supported by a female, not male, breadwinner. If we don't let go of the myth that men need to make more money to feel virile, women will feel ambivalent about their financial power and start to feel that they'll be too strong for men to handle. A strong, healthy man is attracted to a woman who has power and uses it confidently.

It's the fear and shame we feel when we defy the old ideas about how men and women are "supposed" to act that age us. Creating relationships based on what fills our hearts and the hearts of our partners is far better for our health and well-being than trying to conform to old notions about gender roles. Men need to learn how to get their sense of power and success from living wholeheartedly, not just from their second chakra where they experience sexual and financial power (or powerlessness!). And women need to learn to be soft and receptive without giving up their own sexual and financial power. Achieving balance is much easier when both partners give up their fear of not having enough power and resist having a "ledger" relationship in which they keep track of what each other has contributed.

My daughter Kate was 16 when her father and I divorced. After that, I experienced the biggest financial success of my life. Seeing this, Kate developed a fearful belief that she could either have money or love but not both. She worked through that during her 20s and is now married to a wonderful guy with whom she shares both a life and a business. Her book, *Money: A Love Story* (Hay House, 2013), chronicles her healing of money and love issues and provides a blueprint for others to do the same. To get to a place of balance and healing, she had to recognize how her mother's experiences had colored her beliefs about power, sex, and money. You, too, may be holding on to beliefs about your own limitations. If you're having physical issues that correlate with your second chakra, such as fibroids, uterine cancer, abnormal Pap smears, ovarian cysts, or other pelvic health problems, you need to start looking at those beliefs and the fear that's wrapped up with them. (I had a fibroid the size of a soccer ball that developed several years before my divorce. It was all about funneling my creative energy into a dead-end relationship—but being afraid to strike out on my own.)

Work through your fears, and your issues about men, sex, power, and money will start to resolve. This is a process, not an event. And it can take a while. But you don't have to pass on those issues to your daughters and sons. In fact, the work you do to resolve these issues will change your entire family legacy. Kate's wedding to the man of her dreams marked this transformation for both of us. After the ceremony she gave me a card with the following message: "I also want to acknowledge you for all the work you've done around your own heart to allow you to be present during this time. To be able to enjoy this time free of worry about any tension between you and Dad or around the blending of families is the biggest gift. THANK YOU!!"

MOTHER-DAUGHTER RELATIONSHIPS

Let's talk about a different type of relationship that's affected by your beliefs regarding growing older, shared power, and emotional security: mother-daughter relationships. It's sad that women often have toxic relationships with their mothers or their daughters. If you haven't come to acceptance of your own mother and her limitations, you probably haven't come to peace with your daughters. Your ageless years are the time to work on healing these relationships at last if you haven't already.

We each have to own our part in the toxicity. Now is the time to release all the old anger, resentment, grief, and guilt and remake these relationships. And if your mother is no longer living, you may still have work to do—reread Chapter 5 and start releasing those stale feelings you have been holding on to in your energy field and your body.

I have a friend who decided one day that she was done with the dysfunctional relationship she had with her mother. She called up her sister and discovered that her sister, too, was more than ready to stop the pattern of their mother being "the ultimate squelcher of joy." Don't we all know someone like that? Mom was constantly saying to her daughters, "Who do you think you are to try that?" or "You're never going to make that happen!" Whatever the parade, Mom was there to rain on it.

My friend called me for advice, knowing I had done mother-daughter healing myself. I told her that the reason it's so very uncomfortable to have a conflict with our mothers is that our bodies were created in their bodies. When we were in the womb and our organs were forming, our mothers' moods and behaviors directly and powerfully affected the amount of blood and nourishment our bodies experienced. If Mother was upset or depressed, just as if she smoked a cigarette, the blood supply through the umbilical cord decreased, and we felt it. There was no escape from her happiness or grief, and that biological imprint remains with us throughout our lives until we bring it to consciousness and transform it. We've all heard the saying "When Mama ain't happy, ain't nobody happy." As young children, most of us do what is necessary to keep Mama happy. But when you're an adult with a mother who hasn't figured out how to make herself happy, it's counterproductive to allow yourself to get drained by her and keep her happy at your own expense. The same goes for a daughter who isn't happy by the time she reaches adulthood. It's not a mother's job to sacrifice herself for the good of her children, either.

The fact is that in freeing themselves from the weight of their mother's negativity, guilt mongering, and control, my friend and her sister were freeing their mother too. There's no reason for everyone to suffer because of a pattern set years ago. Even so, a complaining adult mother may be extremely resistant to changing a pattern that has allowed her to get her needs met (although in an unhealthy way) for years. The trick is to invite your mother—or your daughters—into turning the relationship around. But be prepared for the fact that the "problem" person who is sucking energy will resist this. Do it anyway. Notice the weight of the guilt. Celebrate yourself for noticing. This alone begins to change the pattern because you are honoring yourself.

Mothers can become very controlling and martyr-like if they haven't had the opportunity to express themselves and explore their passions. This often happens when they feel that to be good mothers and wives, they have to constantly sacrifice to serve their families. There's a great depiction of this phenomenon in the movie *Moonstruck* with Cher. Her character's fiancé, Johnny Cammareri (Danny Aiello), can't get married because his mother back in Italy is dying and won't approve. He can't live without Mama's love, so his entire life is on hold until the old broad kicks off, which she's been on the verge of doing for years. Because most men access feminine life force through women, and because their bodies were literally created in their mothers' bodies, some men never become untangled from Mom—and some mothers aid and abet them in this behavior. A son can become so enmeshed with Mom that she rules over him for life, casting a spell over him that isn't lifted until she dies. There's an old saying that a man is twice born: once from his mother's womb and once again when his mother dies. A daughter may end up in the same position if she doesn't learn how to tap into Source energy for herself and stop looking to Mom to be her Source.

Is your aging mother becoming even more dictatorial because of dementia? I've come to the conclusion that the reason so many old women get really cranky when they develop dementia is because of all the unspoken resentment and self-sacrifice they succumbed to in their early years. The first part of the brain to go in dementia is what's known as the "frontal lobe inhibitory circuits," the area of the brain that, when healthy, inhibits you from saying what you really feel. These circuits are important if you want to fit into the group because they allow you to conform to others' expectations and avoid conflicts. When this area of the brain starts to go, hang on to your hat. You're going to hear what your mother (or whoever) really thinks now that the inhibitory circuits aren't working as they had for so many years. It's payback time. She is going to demand her due, and often in the most unpleasant way. What an awful way to get all the attention and devotion that the person has denied herself for years because she was afraid of being seen as selfish. Dealing with a mother who has dementia is very, very difficult, and it brings up everything—generally a potent mixture of shame, guilt, anger, and exhaustion, but mostly guilt. Know this: there is no way that you, as a daughter, can possibly be responsible for your mother's happiness or expect yourself to be the medicine she needs to heal the pain of her own lifetime. Daughters and mothers have been lugging around a chain of pain for too long. It's time to break it—starting with yourself.

If you're dealing with a mother or mother-in-law who seems determined to suck the life out of you, there's a way to pull the plug and give her a chance to breathe on her own. You do it by no longer participating in the power struggle. (Believe me, if it's a power struggle, she's going to win, because for her it's a life-or-death struggle.) If you can, get your siblings involved. Mothers will often pit one sibling against the other to retain their power. You start to break the spell by getting your sisters and brothers on board with your plan to reconnect Mom to her own life force.

Most women think they have to confront their mother directly about her behavior. That rarely works with a controlling mother. Instead, you just change your reaction to her. When you do that, the game is over.

Carol noticed that her very able-bodied mother had started to be overly dependent on her—always calling when she was taking her kids to school or in the middle of dinner. Carol's siblings noticed that their mother was starting to act feeble and a bit confused and helpless, especially around their oldest brother, though less so around her daughters. She had depended upon her husband for support and cheerleading for years. But he had died ten years before, leaving her widowed at the age of 60. When Carol noticed her mother's increased dependence on her and her brother, she gathered her siblings around and told them what she had observed. Because every child has a unique relationship with a parent, Carol knew that her other siblings might be surprised to hear about what was going on between her and her mother. She told them all the ways in which their mother was driving her nuts so they could see what she was seeing. And she warned her oldest brother that if he continued to coddle their mother

either physically or emotionally, he would actually be contributing to her decline. After she broke the silence about what
was going on with Mom, the first thing they did as a family
was to create a game plan to deal with their mother before she
developed health or other problems as a result of her cling-
ing behavior. Forearmed with information, they all agreed to
stop enabling her by dropping everything to solve her minor
problems whenever she called them or visited them to complain about some aspect of her life. Their mother resisted the
changes at first, but soon learned to get her needs met in a different, healthier way.

You have to be willing to endure the discomfort of setting
a limit with a controlling mother or father. Dr. Mario Martinez calls this becoming a "guardian of your heart." Notice
that visits with your mother may follow a pattern of starting
out well and then deteriorating into negativity. She may have
that "upper limit" problem and be able to stand only so much
joy and fun before taking the visit south into complaining and
fault finding. Instead of enduring the negativity, simply guard
your own heart, and when the dynamic between you and your
mother begins to sour, know that it's okay to take your leave.
End the visit. Say, "Thanks, Mom. Nice to talk. Gotta go," and
hang up the phone. If she's angry at your withdrawal, you have
to take on the challenge of not being upset by this. Your inner
child will be scared, but be gentle with yourself. Stifling your
need to escape, only to lose your temper with your mother, isn't
the way to go.

At first, like a baby in the womb who is not getting enough
oxygen, you may find that establishing a boundary with your
mother feels awful, as if you'll lose her forever and be disconnected from her love. This won't happen. A mother's love is too
strong for that—at least, in most cases. If she's one of the 20
percent or so of women who have a personality disorder, you've
got to make the break with her for your own mental, emotional,
physical, and spiritual health because she won't be able to change
without self-awareness and a lot of therapy.

One of my friends got caller ID just so that she could identify
her mother's calls beforehand and not get sucked into an overly

long conversation—a "donating bone marrow" call—with her mother. She had trouble getting her mother off the phone, and eventually learned when to call and when to hang up: while it was still enjoyable for both of them. Another friend, who had been in the habit of calling her mother every morning after her father's death, began to string out the calls to every other day, then every third day, and finally, once per week. Her mother was healthy and independent, but simply not interested in living life fully or joyfully despite many opportunities to do so.

What a gift it would be if her daughter freed her from her cultural beliefs about growing older and becoming irrelevant to the people she loves. Too often, the overbearing or needy mother is an unwitting victim of ageist cultural messages. By helping her to see that she doesn't need her daughter rescuing her from this problem or that one, a daughter can free up her mother to become an ageless goddess.

AGELESS GODDESSES AREN'T HELICOPTER PARENTS

If you're a mother, you also have to look at the relationship you have with your own children. By now, they're probably teenagers or adults. They need their independence. Are you having a hard time letting them go? I remember the first time I went to New York City to visit my oldest daughter, who was sharing her first apartment with friends. I stayed in a hotel. At midnight that first night, she walked away from our meeting to catch a subway back to her apartment, waving good-bye. I hated to see her go. I worried. I fretted. After all, I'm from a small town in Maine, and for me, the fast pace of New York still takes some getting used to. But then I realized that because she had visited the city with her friends all during college, she knew her way around. I hadn't been with her even once when she was exploring the city. It was time for me to let her take flight, and I did.

Today's parents have more opportunities to be overly involved with their kids than ever before. Though I applaud close family ties, I don't think this trend is ideal. A friend whose daughter has just gone off to college on a sports scholarship tells me that the college has a very strong parents' association for this sport. My friend has been warned by other parents in the association that if she is not present for all of her daughter's games, her child is likely to feel depressed and left out. The problem is that the daughter's college is a 20-hour drive or a plane ride away. I was shocked! My friend, who has three younger children who are also involved in sports and other activities, is feeling enormous pressure to go to all the games—mostly from the other parents, not her daughter.

The cultural pressure to be a "good mother" by staying actively engaged in your children's lives really should start to lessen when they go off to college. Otherwise, when are they going to develop the skills necessary to live independently and happily without you? When are you going to develop the skills to live without them? I am extremely close to my daughters and to my siblings. But each of us has a separate, large circle of friends and activities of our own. When you're together with your children, bring your fullness, not your neediness. If you love sports and it's easy for you to spend every weekend away during that sport's season, flying to your son's or daughter's college games, then good for you. But it's distinctly unhealthy for you to expect your children to fill holes in your life, or for your children to expect you to fill holes in theirs.

Recently, my oldest daughter, Ann, moved back home from New York, with my blessing. She was at a crossroads in her career and there were problems with her apartment, so she asked to come home for a bit. Ann had been self-supporting for nearly ten years, so I knew she wouldn't get stuck in dependency. Plus, a move back home for a while would give us a chance to bond again. She had left for college the year of my divorce, and we hadn't spent much time together since then.

As I mentioned earlier, she soon became interested in participating with me in the local tango social life. There she met and befriended Paul, a good friend of mine. Eventually, a romantic relationship between the two of them blossomed.

Quite suddenly and unexpectedly, I began to feel like a fifth wheel. On one level, I was thrilled for both of them. They seemed like a great match, and I knew both of them intimately. But I couldn't help thinking, *Ouch. What about me?* Luckily, my good friend Deb called me while this was happening and I was trying to talk myself out of how I was really feeling. Deb encouraged me to get my feelings off my chest on my own so that Ann, Paul, and I could all move forward into the future freely. I invited Deb over to be my supportive witness as I lit incense and waved it around to clear the air while I ranted and raved. I let all of my feelings of loneliness and abandonment and jealousy out. After about 45 minutes, I told Deb I felt ten pounds lighter from having released the feelings. She said, "Okay, good. Now turn around and walk into your new life." I never had another moment of pain about the situation. Only after I processed the feelings did I mention to Ann and Paul how I had felt. They didn't need to start feeling guilty about what I was going through. And after doing my healing work, I found that other people and opportunities came rushing into my life. My social life flourished with a slew of new friends and experiences because I had created space for something new to come in.

Like most of us, I had been trying to cover up my grief and loss by painting a happy face on it instead of releasing my emotions so that they wouldn't get stuck in my tissues and age me. Always let go of shame and accept your emotions so you can move through them. Create a safe way to get your feelings up and out of your body, with a friend to witness and emotionally support your process if possible. Being embarrassed about how you really feel and trying to be the perfect mom who doesn't have human needs and feelings leads to illness.

My relationship do-over with my oldest daughter has been one of the biggest gifts ever. Living together with your adult children offers an opportunity to redefine the dynamic and make it a healing one instead of an unhealthy one marked by power struggles and hurt. The heavy lifting involved in the growth of the soul happens with family. You will have to negotiate with each other to ensure both of you have your needs for independence and togetherness fulfilled. With Ann and me, there was a lot of texting that went on around dinner plans, movies, and other things. We were mindful of including each other but not burdened with unreasonable expectations.

So whether you're living in a two-generation household, or you're thinking about it, or you realize you're stuck in the same old dynamic with your mother or daughter, start the healing process today. Let your new relationship unfold. It's tempting to revert to your original nurturing role of caring for your child if you're a nurturing type. And it's tempting for a child to let herself be pampered and mothered as if she were still seven years old. But if you and your daughter live together and you do your daughter's laundry and put it away in her drawers, and remind her to fill up the gas tank, you're both going to drive each other crazy. Cook as a love offering, not a duty. Don't keep score or keep track of who does what. That's the only way to make a mother-daughter relationship—or any relationship—work over the long haul.

A do-over can happen at any time. I have a former patient named Eva who is 87 and has just begun family therapy with her daughter. After becoming widowed, Eva moved in with her daughter. Soon her daughter told her she couldn't deal with the fact that her mom was going to die someday and leave her motherless. Eva recognized her daughter's pre-grieving of her death as a sign that the two of them ought to work out their relationship. When issues are unresolved, we hold on to the people we love energetically even after they've passed. And nine times out of ten, those who "hang on" are mothers.

And if you're a mother holding on to resentment about the way your daughter treated you when she was a teenager, or you're a daughter still steaming about the way your mother raised you, you have to let it go. You need to release the emotions and choose to forgive her—and yourself—for what happened in the past. There's nothing more pathetic than two older women still having the same argument they had 30 years ago. Aren't you both sick of the old story? Have the courage to write a new one. Otherwise, as I delight in telling people, in your next life, you will come back as identical twins!

THE CHOICE OF FORGIVENESS

No matter who hurt us or what they did, we played a role in getting hurt. That can be hard to admit. But freedom and joy begin when we acknowledge that on an energetic level, we invite everything that comes into our lives. On a soul level, we pick our parents. Of course, this intellectual knowledge doesn't help the hurt child within us.

If you're still holding on to resentment or blame toward someone, you not only have to release the feelings—you have to make the choice to tell the story differently so you don't get stuck in emotional responses, such as resentment, that will age you. Blame is defined as a way to discharge pain or discomfort. Forgiveness means being willing to remember the past differently instead of trying to force the facts to be different. The facts will remain the same. How you frame them is what changes.

Forgiveness has to include not just the other person but yourself too. Here's what you can forgive yourself for: Not being perfect. Not knowing better. Lacking the courage to stand up for yourself and speak your truth. Needing a loving mom and wishing your mother were able to be the mother you needed at that moment.

Many women hold on to feelings about their former spouses but feel guilty for failing at marriage. Our culture is relentless in driving home the screwed-up message that divorce is devastating to children and that women who divorce are selfish. This myth doesn't seem to go away even though there's no evidence for it. Every article on how divorce devastates children cites the same old study by Judith Wallerstein that's based on substandard social science. That bad nickel of a study simply will *not* disappear! And its message is just plain wrong. What's devastating for any of us is chronic unresolved stress and conflict, which you're all too likely to find in a family where the parents are still married despite their anger, resentment, and unhappiness. I am certain that neither my daughters nor I would have the level of health and happiness we now enjoy if their father and I hadn't divorced. I consider my 24-year marriage a huge success. It supported me during the formative years of my career and produced two beautiful daughters who are loved by both their father and me.

Let's rethink the idea of a "broken home." Why is it "broken" just because the parents are divorced or separated? A split is better than chronic depression, anger, and conflict. By addressing the unhappiness instead of just deciding to stay in the marriage "for the sake of the kids," parents can transform the family and make it healthy and whole. Then, if they do stay together, it will be a better situation for all—and if they don't stay together, the family won't be "broken." It will just be shaped differently. Chronically being unhappy ages you and leads to health problems. Make a conscious decision to live happily—with or without your partner.

And get over the idea that because a relationship has reached its conclusion, it is somehow a "failure." At this time in history, marriage is no longer the economic arrangement that it was for centuries. Now both men and women want more from their relationships than ever before. We want true partnerships in which both of us can grow and thrive, not everyday familiar misery nailed in place by the outmoded belief that divorce is the worst thing that can possibly happen to us.

After we got divorced, both my husband and I flourished. (Not instantly, of course. But in time. And with a tremendous amount of effort and healing on my part.) He's happily remarried, and my daughters love their stepmother and little half-sister—the daughter my former husband had with his second wife. My daughters also have an excellent relationship with me. They don't have a broken family; they have two families who love them unconditionally. If my husband and I had stayed together, they wouldn't have the loving relationships with their father's second wife or their half-sister. While we don't all spend holidays together as one big happy family, we get along well, without conflicts. You can have that too.

You and your kids and your former husband get to choose how to frame the experience of divorce. By being willing to see what everyone gained from it, you can forgive each other for causing each other pain and commit to enjoying what you have to offer each other now. Forgive your ex and yourself, and let go of any residual emotions from the divorce. And if you're thinking of divorce but figure there's no one out there for you and you might as well end your days in the marriage, you need to stop thinking that way. You are *not* too old to start over. Choosing to stay in a bad relationship will quickly age you because of the stress you'll create for yourself.

PERFECTIONISM AND RELATIONSHIPS

Beating yourself up or stressing yourself out for not being the perfect wife, mother, sister, daughter, friend, or neighbor is a sure route to premature aging. In *Working Ourselves to Death: The High Cost of Workaholism and the Rewards of Recovery* (HarperSanFrancisco, 1990), Diane Fassel, Ph.D., writes that most women do too much and develop what's known as the "disease of doer-ship." Workaholism, she explains, is the addiction of choice for those who feel unworthy.[2]

Goddesses who never age give up the insanity of trying to make everyone love and approve of them at all times. The belief that you must be active all the time, working to please everybody, leads to worry, overwork, and obsession. It also results in an increased amount of inflammatory chemicals in the body that set the stage for chronic degenerative disease.

I'm inspired by the words "You are my beloved child, in whom I am well pleased." God knows us completely, with all our failings and faults, and loves us fully and unconditionally—and wants us to love ourselves the same way. God is not looking to get us to iron the sheets, iron over everyone's hurt feelings, and be Little Mary Sunshine every minute of the day.

When you try too hard to make everyone happy or get them to conform to what you think is the perfect way to live, you end up being too controlling and smothering—and you drive people away. Perfection in relationships doesn't come from being perfect people but from allowing ourselves and others to be who we are. Do this and you *will* achieve perfection—the perfection of harmony.

Timeless Time

In his book *The Big Leap* (HarperCollins, 2009), Gay Hendricks has a chapter called "Living in Einstein Time," in which he explores the idea that since time is relative, we can change our relationship to it and experience "timeless time." For many overworked people, time has become a commodity as precious as gold. But every one of us is given exactly the same amount of time. I wrote this poem as a way to help me remember to slow it down and truly experience the expansiveness of time in a delightful way.

Say the following out loud—slowly—while breathing deeply.

I brag that time is on my side.
That time is standing lusciously still for me.
That I am creating timeless time.
That I have enough time.
That I am having the time of my life!!!
That I am where time comes from, in slow, sexy, sensual rhythms of joy and pleasure that stretch out into eternity. Ahhhhhhhhhh . . .

CARETAKING AND TAKING CARE OF OURSELVES

Though sickness and infirmity are not inevitable as you get older, you may find yourself in the role of caretaker of a sick or ill parent—or needing care yourself. The flow of offering and receiving is a part of life, but it's easy to become cranky and difficult instead of submitting to it gracefully.

Caretaking for others can be so stressful that it zaps your energy, makes you depressed and anxious, and even causes you to develop stress-related illnesses. It's no accident that women often develop autoimmune diseases after the stress of caretaking for their parents. An autoimmune disease is characterized by the immune system not recognizing the body's tissues as its own. In caretaking for those you love, you can lose yourself and start to wonder, *Who am I? What's my role? Am I daughter or nurse?* If at all possible, even if you *are* a nurse, get professional caretakers to help you with your parents should their health start to fail. Becoming all things to Mom and Dad is a surefire way to age yourself. As daughters, we have to learn to express our love to our parents without losing or exhausting ourselves.

Years ago, the dying process was very different. We didn't have the medical interventions we have now that can prolong a fairly poor quality of life at great cost for an average of five years, causing enormous stress on the person dying and on the family caring for her. In her book *Passages in Caregiving* (William Morrow, 2010), Gail Sheehy writes, "Today's average family caregiver in the United States is a forty-eight-year-old woman who holds down a paid job (more than half work full-time) and spends twenty hours a week providing unpaid care for an adult who used to be independent. One-third of family caretakers are actually on duty forty or more hours a week. One-third also still have children or grandchildren under the age of eighteen living with them and take care of two or more people, usually parents. Not surprisingly, one-half report a high level of burden and nearly one-half say their own health is fair or poor."[3] When perfectionism enters the picture, the burden on the caretaker becomes even greater.

Sheehy has written that caretaking should be approached as a marathon, not a sprint. We all want to believe that once Mom gets the surgery and the post-surgery physical therapy, she'll get right back to her active life again. We all want to believe that Dad's mild confusion and forgetfulness will be checked by some medication. Unfortunately, often, one small loss of health or independence leads to another and another and we're unprepared for how quickly the situation snowballs.

The typical scenario is that the daughter—and if there's more than one daughter, it's usually the oldest daughter or the unmarried one—steps in to do the caretaking while the other siblings check in here and there, and maybe offer some money to the caretaking daughter (or son). The other siblings don't understand how much of a burden Mom and Dad are on the caretaker. If you see this beginning to happen in your family, call a family meeting and set a plan. Expect some denial all around. No one wants to admit that Mom and Dad aren't able to be totally independent anymore. Push for everyone to come to an agreement on what to do so that you don't end up doing all the caretaking.

If your parents are still independent and in good health, talk to them and your siblings now and set up a plan for what to do should Mom or Dad become frail or ill. Urge your parents to do estate planning and end-of-life planning. Have them set up and sign a health care POA (power of attorney) so someone can deal with their finances if they become incapacitated. Also, have them set up a living will so you have a legal document spelling out their wishes when it comes to end-of-life medical interventions, and a MOST (medical orders for scope of treatment) form. The MOST form, which must be reviewed yearly, is far more explicit and detailed than the living will. For example, a MOST form includes an option to choose a do-not-resuscitate (DNR) order, which means that if your parent goes into cardiac arrest, she does not want cardiopulmonary resuscitation administered. The harsh truth is that CPR often breaks the person's ribs and rarely even works, or if it does work, it often leads to diminished quality of life. It's important to know whether your parent wants to spend his last minutes of life on a floor or hospital bed having someone pound on his chest—or to risk surviving and becoming an invalid. You can get the forms I've mentioned on the Internet; they can vary from state to state and country to country, so you want to read them carefully to make sure they cover what you need covered. The MOST form should be printed out on bright-colored paper and posted visibly on your loved one's bed so that every person can see it and follow the instructions clearly.

If your parent is open to it, you can plan even further ahead. I recently took a walk with my mother and asked her what she wanted for her funeral. Given her relationship with organized religion, she was most clear on the fact that she didn't want a minister anywhere near when it came time for the funeral. She's fine with a Vedanta monk, however, who is a friend of the family. And she wants to be cremated and have her ashes strewn from a small airplane over the back hill on the farm where we all grew up. I asked her if she wanted to have one of us make a video of some "parting comments" in the next year or two that we could play at a memorial service after her death; Mom said she'd think about it. She also wants her service within a couple of days after her death—that matters to her, and I want to honor that.

While we're on the subject of making end-of-life wishes clear, start thinking about your own plan for leaving this world for the next. I don't care if you're 30—there's no time like the present to create a vision for your transition. Remember, healthy centenarians usually die in their sleep, not in a hospital bed. Don't set up your loved ones to try to guess at your wishes and wrestle with the doctors and the state and your other relatives to try get everyone on the same page. Develop a loving relationship with yourself, with the people in your life, and with the Divine. I don't think it's death we fear so much as the possibility that we won't get to truly complete the unfinished emotional business that is part of our soul school in the first place. Consider what we can all learn from the many who have had near-death experiences and now teach us that when we pass over, we will find that we are loved and cherished beyond anything we can imagine. Anita Moorjani says that having died and come back, she no longer works so hard at being "spiritual." Instead, her near-death experience taught her that truly loving and taking care of herself in daily life were most important. Live fully now, trust the process of life, and plan for how you want to make your exit. No one wants to be a burden on the people they love. Avoiding the conversation about planning for the end pretty much ensures that will happen!

Ira Byock, M.D., former director of palliative medicine at Dartmouth-Hitchcock Medical Center, has said, "When people die well, their families grieve lighter." He explains that what matters most as your relationship with your loved ones in this life draws to an end is saying four things: "please forgive me," "I forgive you," "thank you," and "I love you."[4] Truly, the deathbed can be a place of amazing healing. My sister and brother-in-law lived with his mother, Thelma, for the last six months of her life until she finally passed at age 94. Thelma had been a successful research chemist and a natural leader in her community. She wanted to die in her own home, and was a fighter until almost the very end of her life. One day, toward the end, she could no longer stand up, and she laid her head on her son's shoulder. Then she told him, "You've done a good job." These were words he'd never heard her say before—and they healed not only him, but his children as well.

After that, his mother slipped into a coma and didn't eat or drink for five days. Meanwhile, her entire extended family gathered around her. On what would be the final day of her life, her great-grandson, who was just a toddler, said, "When is she going to die?" The child's mother was embarrassed because Thelma had always been a most proper individual, with a strong personality. But immediately after the boy asked his question, Thelma suddenly had a moment of lucidity and said with great compassion, "He can't help it, dear." And with that, she took her final breath. She had a good death.

If all this talk of death is making you want to get on with life, good! To quote Rebecca Authement, "Thoughts of death are best used to get on with life. Death will come in its own time. Get your affairs in order should be a daily mantra, not something said to a person with a terminal diagnosis."

THE ERA OF COMMUNITY

It's hard not to be scared in times of uncertainty, whether it's a transitional time in your life or a transitional period that everyone is facing. As I write this, there are astrologic events happening that we haven't experienced since 1966—perhaps before you were born. The last time the celestial bodies were in a similar position was a very chaotic time when the women's movement, civil rights, gay rights, and the very unpopular Vietnam War were all in the news. It was also the beginning of waves of women and nonwhite individuals entering professional schools in significant numbers for the first time in history. Today, we're entering a new era and experiencing what shamanic astrologer Daniel Giamario calls "the turning of the ages." You won't find security in money, power, or doing things the way you've always done them. Give up the fear habit and replace it with faith, love, and community connections. You *will* find support and sustenance in your relationships with those around you. We need to be thinking about community support as a primary way to help us release fear, anger, and grief and develop a greater sense of safety, happiness, and optimism—and to keep us healthy and ageless. Social isolation and loneliness are a major health risk, right up there with smoking cigarettes, high blood pressure, obesity, and a sedentary lifestyle.[5]

The happiest people are those who have a tribe. In the documentary *Happy,* the elderly women of Okinawa, Japan, one of the famous Blue Zones where people enjoy an unusually long healthspan and lifespan, talk about being sisters to each other and interacting and playing with the children on the island; a single mother in Denmark explains why communal living with a dozen or so families was key to overcoming her loneliness and fear. We aren't meant to live alone and disconnected. In his study of healthy centenarians, Dr. Mario Martinez finds that they all live in "subcultures" of like-minded individuals who support their joyful and healthy outlook.

Many people feel close to their family and close friends who serve as their tribe, but we can also receive support from the larger tribe of the human race. Social media has helped us recognize our interconnectedness. I'm a regular over at Tosha Silver's Facebook page, where a tribe of us follow Tosha's wonderful writing and example of turning our lives over to the Divine Beloved. On my birthday, I was on a family cruise of the Greek islands and Turkey—a dream-come-true vacation for all of us—and I checked Tosha's page, where she'd posted about my birthday. A woman named Yesim had posted "Happy Birthday all the way from Istanbul." I loved her picture—she looked so vibrant! I took a chance and asked if she wanted to meet my family when we arrived in her city. Not only did Yesim meet us, she became our family tour guide for the weekend, getting us into places we would never have been able to visit without her. She also became my friend. The moment I met her, I knew that I had met a true kindred spirit. My entire family felt the same!

This is how we're designed to interact with each other: remembering that we're all sisters and brothers, and letting go of our social anxiety, fear, and shame to reach out to say hey, let's enjoy this experience together. When we do that, we share cardiac coherence. Our hearts actually synchronize with each other and change the energy field we share. We also begin to attract persons, places, and things that reflect our celebration of life. The universe reaches out and gives us a high five, and the Goddess herself smiles. So move into the new era of community by building a sustainable tribe of support.

And when it comes to your tribe, be judicious about who is in it. The people around you can help you reconnect to the life force and flourish or they can drain you and depress you. When we first started the Women to Women health center years ago, at a time when women doctors and nurse practitioners treating only women was a radical shift, some colleagues I respected responded with resistance and sarcasm, the way most people do when confronted with new ideas. I learned to be careful about choosing the people I shared my ideas with. I didn't need colleagues who were highly critical and unsupportive of the changes I was making in my practice and my perspective, especially when my ideas were new and tender. Some of these colleagues were people I had known for years; we had shared a long and rich history in the trenches of medical training. I loved and respected them. But just as plants outgrow their pots, I was outgrowing them.

You may have to turn the volume down on some relationships, or even let go of them, and commit to bringing new people into your life who will be more supportive of you. The good news is that the universe will provide you with new members of your "tribe," sometimes in the most extraordinary ways. Once you make the change inside of you, your energy will shift; those who resonate with you energetically will gravitate your way and those who don't will start to fall away. Years after transforming the way I practiced and thought about medicine, I find that I'm a magnet for people who believe in inspiring women to experience wellness through feeling connected with their joy and their life force. I regularly meet people I want to add to my tribe.

There are people who truly want to vibrate at a higher frequency and be happier and lighter in mood and attitude. But some people who will be attracted to your lightness of being will bring to the table their old, negative emotional patterns. They will love what they get from you, but they will drain you because they're not committed to becoming lighter themselves. They are emotional vampires. You might not realize that they are sucking you dry because they seem to be so nice and supportive at first. They may not realize what they're doing to you. But in time, you'll see that whenever you interact with them, you come away feeling as if someone just took a pint of blood out of you. I have felt as though I had to get down on the floor and go to sleep after interacting with certain individuals. In fact, sometimes I feel this way just from reading an e-mail from one of them! Those people are mostly gone from my life at this point, but it sure took a while to figure out this pattern.

As you begin to tap into your own vitality, you have to be cautious about letting people drain it out of you as quickly as you fill yourself up. Encourage family and friends who want what you've got to get it for themselves and stop seeing you as their Source.

In fact, people can energetically hook into you so strongly that if you stop, focus, and tune in, you can actually sense the cord of energy that goes from you to them. I like to use the following exercise to cut them loose so they can find another source of energy.

Exercise: Cutting Energetic Cords

Use this exercise whenever you suspect you have an energetic connection to someone who is draining you of life force. Cutting the energetic cord is good for you *and* for that person. You can do this when the cord is between you and a living person or when it's between you and someone who has crossed over into the spiritual realm.

There are many ways to remove an energetic cord, but I learned the basic technique from the late shaman Peter Calhoun—and it is explained more fully in Peter and his wife Astrid Ganz's book *Last Hope on Earth* (World Service Institute, 2013). To remove dark energies' connection to your energetic field, you will call upon Archangel Michael, an angel of protection and love who wields a cobalt-blue sword of light. You'll also use the energy of what's called the Violet Flame, a living spiritual energy that's an aspect of Divine Love. Before beginning, take a moment to clear your mind and take a few deep breaths so that you can tune in to your energy field.

1. Take a minute or two to become quiet and relaxed as you focus on your breathing.

2. Start by asking any dark or wandering energies to leave. Say, "If there are any dark or wandering energies, I now send you to the light. If there are any dark ones, I encapsulate you in black light and bar you from ever returning."

3. Draw your attention to your lower chakras, from your solar plexus down. Do you sense, feel, or see a cord or a hook extending outward toward someone else, or do you see one coming into you? If so, you need to cut it so it stops draining your energy. Then visualize and feel yourself cutting the cords while saying aloud, "With Archangel Michael's cobalt-blue sword of light, I now cut all attachments and cords." You can make sweeping movements around your body with your hands.

4. Identify where you feel an uncomfortable sensation in your body. For most people, it's in the belly, where the third chakra is located, or in the heart area, where the fourth chakra is located. Next, identify the person who is connected with this feeling who requires your forgiveness and release.

5. Now say the following out loud: "(Name of the person), I forgive you for (fill in the blank; for example, for sexually abusing me, betraying me, abandoning me, for not stepping up, or whatever it is—name everything you need to forgive that person for)." Allow yourself to feel the full power of your emotions as they come up. Don't hold back out of guilt or shame!

6. When you're ready, say, "I send you on your path of healing."

7. Repeat steps 3 through 6 until you feel finished with the work, that is, until you have no more emotions to release or words to say.

8. Now see yourself standing within the Violet Flame (a brightly burning violet flame) and say, "I now transmute this pattern with the Violet Flame." If you prefer, you can say, "I now transmute this pattern with Divine Love" (or use any other wording that is in sync with your beliefs about the Divine).

9. Draw your attention to the area of your body where you'd felt discomfort. Chances are very good that the discomfort will have resolved. If not, repeat the steps until it's gone.

10. You've just removed an energetic imprint, and it leaves an energetic hole. For your protection, visualize "packing" the area where the imprint was with healing midnight-blue and golden light.

11. Make sure to drink plenty of water and get rest following this exercise. You may find yourself very sleepy. If so, don't fight it. Removing an energetic imprint is like doing surgery on your energy field, so it's very important to rest afterward.

The imprint removal process is like peeling an onion. You may find that once you've cut a cord and released one energetic imprint, others arise or the cord reforms. Take it slowly—don't expect to heal all your grief or emotional pain in one sitting. Do imprint removals as the need arises—by yourself, or with another person leading you in the process.

Cords can easily reattach if you don't change your daily relationship patterns, so you can take precautions. Before you interact with someone you've had a draining energetic connection to in the past, imagine zipping up a bag over yourself, starting at your feet and zipping right up over your head. This imaginary bag will protect you energetically.

AGELESS RELATIONSHIPS

Being around people who depress and frustrate you will age you quickly. Do you want to spend your most creative years surrounded by the people you're currently spending most of your time with? Agelessness means discerning which relationships are worth keeping, starting, and nurturing, and which need to end— and then withdrawing from those. You can do this simply by allowing them to wither on the vine. It's not that you have to stop speaking to an old friend for good or write her off forever. It's just that you no longer donate your precious energy to trying to save her from her choices. Your ageless years are also a time for making new friends with youthful energy who don't dwell on the past or talk about illnesses and doctors. Healthy centenarians are focused on their future, not their past.

I've often said "community is immunity," and research has shown this to be true. People who have varied community connections live longer and enjoy a longer healthspan than people who are loners or in unhealthy relationships (bad marriages, for example) that cause them stress.

Unhealthy community fosters poor health. Healthy communities foster true flourishing. If you want to remain ageless, you need to create a subculture of individuals who are living healthfully and joyfully. Affirm and imagine your supportive tribe and be patient as the universe works to bring it to you. Then make a point of getting together with others. Maybe your group of girlfriends, whom you used to meet at the bar in your 20s and then at the playground when you had young children, is ready to meet at the yoga studio or the cooking demonstration at the food co-op. As I've always told my daughters, "Everyone is looking for a good gig." Attend classes or events you find interesting and go to places you like to visit, and see who shows up.

There's a new science called sociogenomics, which is the study of the relationship between people's social connections and their health and gene expression. The truth is that your health will pretty much be the same as that of the people you hang around with (just as your income tends to be the average of that of your five closest friends). *The Social Network Diet* by Miriam Nelson, Ph.D., a nutritionist at Tufts University, and Jennifer Ackerman, explains that it really isn't willpower that makes us stick to our goals for eating and exercising so much as whether we have a social network of people who support us in those goals. If your family brings junk food into your home daily, and complains when you want to turn off the television in the family room and work out in that space, it's going to be hard to stick to better habits. Healthy centenarians all have subcultures that support maximizing their ability to live agelessly, so start looking for individuals to hang out with who make it easy to be happy and healthy.

There's nothing like a group of girlfriends to enhance each other's life force. I like to say that women can be a placenta for each other. However, what you want is a relationship that is nourishing for all, not a sisterhood based on one-upping each other on who has more trouble keeping weight off or who has more aches and pains. When I pass a restaurant table of women all having an "organ recital"—talking about their doctor visits and so on—I get out of there quickly.

To create positive sisterhood, you have to be an uplifting, ageless goddess who knows how to have fun. Bond over funny online videos, a healthy recipe you invented, or a hilarious movie you saw. Design an evening or weekend around doing something none of you have done before that sounds daring and fun. Get everyone together to go surfing, sailing, or hot air ballooning, or to enjoy karaoke or dancing. Go birding or kayaking or to an indoor climbing wall. Have a spa weekend or attend a spiritual retreat or music festival. Clothing swaps are also great fun, and you can score a new wardrobe!

And if you want to have fun with girlfriends, don't forget to invite women you've recently met who clearly have great energy. Loyalty is wonderful, but we do tend to hang on to female friendships after they've become stale and depressing.

FURRY FRIENDS

For more and more women, pets are a part of a loving community. I'm not exaggerating: the amount of money people spend on their pets has increased exponentially in my lifetime, and we've seen a huge shift in how people relate to animals. When I was growing up on a farm, cats belonged in the barn and dogs in the yard, never on the couch. You had pets but didn't necessarily think of them as furry friends or members of the family. Now, people are connecting to the animals in their lives to a degree that's unprecedented.

Our relationships with our pets aren't just emotionally nourishing. They're spiritually nourishing and good for our health. Having a pet lowers your stress, your cortisol levels, and your blood pressure. Cats and dogs keep our heart chakras open and clear. They love us unconditionally, which humans aren't truly capable of without Divine intervention. No wonder the amount of money we've spent on our pets has exploded. The image of the woman surrounded by cats being someone lonely and pathetic has to go. More often, the woman who has cats—or dogs, or birds, or some other type of pet she's connected to—is happy and less lonely because she's surrounded by unconditional love and affection.

Let's own this: Our pets are more than just friends. They're creatures who come here to share love with us. And they can be extraordinary healers. Both of the cats I got after my divorce died from cancer within 12 years, even though they ate quality organic food and there was nothing in the environment of our home to cause cancer in any of the humans. Those cats came here as souls to serve me, and I believe they took on my post-divorce grief. I've talked to other women who have had similar experiences. Although my cat Francine has been dead for several years, I still feel her around me even now, and I dream about her regularly. Her spirit visits my house. Sometimes, a very intuitive person will come to my house and pick up on Francine's energy too. She's still looking out for me.

As for relationships with people, your intuition will never steer you wrong. You know when a relationship is serving you, and when it isn't. You're no longer willing to spend your precious time and energy trying to fix people or get them to change. You want to be around whole people who take responsibility for their side of the street. What a relief! As you begin to reclaim your goddess nature, you also reclaim your intuition and your inner knowing. You stop trying to justify yourself to other people because you know your worth regardless of what they think of you. You're more secure and sure of yourself—and your identity as an ageless goddess.

CHAPTER EIGHT

GODDESSES
SAVOR THE
PLEASURE OF FOOD

*We all eat. And it would be a sad waste
of opportunity to eat badly.*

— ANNA THOMAS

Recently I enjoyed dinner with some family and friends.
We sat down before a bounty of delicious, gorgeous food:
baked organic chicken breasts seasoned with garlic, her-
bes de Provence, and sea salt mixed with rosemary; baked sweet
potatoes with some coconut oil; and onions, carrots, and kale
sautéed in coconut oil with a bit of balsamic vinegar added at the
end. Dessert was slices of organic honeycrisp apples sprinkled
with cinnamon. Before we feasted, I lit some candles, we joined
hands, and I performed my usual ritual of saying an impromptu
blessing. I thanked everyone and everything who had contributed

to this meal, and threw in some humor and choice details from the day. After grace, all of us dug in. The meal had taken my sister and me 45 minutes to prepare rather than my usual 15. We ended up lingering around the table, savoring the meal and the company, for a good hour. When you eat like this, you automatically feel satisfied and "fed." You don't spend the rest of the evening "grazing" in an attempt to bring into your body the sweetness, love, and belonging that are missing.

Study after study shows that the age-old ceremony of "breaking bread" together is an effective way to combat stress, build solid relationships, keep your family together, and bring joy and pleasure into your daily life. The longer I live, the more aware I am of just how important this ritual truly is. As my Greek friend Leftari always says, "Food brings people together." It's simple and so true. We were not designed to eat alone watching bad news on television. We are creatures who seek connection, and when we sit down to enjoy a meal together, our differences melt away. The emotional bonding allows us to rebuild our tissues and organs with a sense of love and belonging. Enjoying a home-cooked meal prepared with love and pleasure always feels good. And the energetic imprint of love and caring in those who prepare the food can even override the adverse effect of some less-than-ideal ingredients that you might find yourself being served from time to time.

If you read over the menu for the dinner I described, you will note the following: no dairy, no grains, no soy, no sugar, and no sweeteners of any kind. At the time, I was following a one-month nutritional reset program called Whole30, with meals that included meat, fish, vegetables, nuts, seeds, and fruit, with some healthy oils and herbs for flavoring. The only thing I missed was having a little stevia in my coffee or iced tea, but now that I have a sweet life, I don't need to import as much sweetness via my food as I used to. I'm back to using stevia now, but much less than before. I see I was mindlessly consuming it more than I really felt the need to.

Enjoying life makes it easier to enjoy food that nourishes your body. You don't have to look to food to be your friend or therapist. If you have a love/hate relationship with food, this chapter will help you learn to make peace with it. It can be done! If you want to live agelessly, break the old habit of mindlessly tossing processed convenience foods into your grocery cart. By knowing what healthy and delicious foods to enjoy (think creamy avocados, fresh nuts or blueberries, and so on), you'll find it easier to make changes in your diet. Eating well is never about deprivation or being "bad." And it's simple to eat for your heart, your brain, your hormones, and your overall health because the right food takes care of the entire body. What's more, you'll find that healthy food is delicious and satisfying, not boring, repetitious, or lacking in taste and texture.

I want you to notice something. I purposely started this chapter with a description of a pleasurable dining experience complete with candlelight and good company. It sounded good, right? Though I was describing a meal created within dietary "restrictions," I wasn't telling you what I was depriving myself of and what I was "allowed" to eat. I was describing a meal that tasted wonderful and was rich in delightful textures, colors, and smells. It was a meal I shared with others who weren't following the program but who also enjoyed it and had a wonderful evening. When it comes to food, you must learn to eat like a goddess who loves the bounty before her and deserves to enjoy every bite. The language and thought forms of restriction, deprivation, and shame when it comes to food will hold you back from flourishing. They have to go!

TAKING THE "DIE" OUT OF "DIET"

There are hundreds of "miracle diets" out there. You read about them in every magazine. All of them work for a while, but none of them is sustainable. I know you've probably tried many of them only to go back to unhealthy eating, bouncing between deprivation and plenty, frustration and indulgence, pride and guilt. Food has become too much of a drama for too many of us.

I've personally been on dozens of diets, fasts, and juice fasts since the age of 13. Back in my 30s, I was a macrobiotic vegan until I noticed that my hair and nails were brittle and I was gaining weight on all that grain. I've done Atkins, HCG,

Fuhrman—the list goes on and on. And because of my large bone structure and ease at building muscle, I've always weighed more than the "ideal" that my five-foot-four self is supposed to weigh. I happen to know that if given the choice between being fabulously healthy but 20 pounds heavier or being glamorously slim, most women would choose slim. That's why women continue to smoke and take diet pills.

My weight is now stable—and all my clothes fit. I ditched my daily weighing habit about a year ago because I realized that I was treating my body like an enemy who would betray me with weight gain if I didn't keep her on a really tight leash. Talk about a setup for shame and failure! Yes, I'm probably five to ten pounds heavier than I'd like to be, the same five to ten pounds I've battled with for the past 30 years. I would "lose" them, but they would inevitably "find" me again. I had a cold war going on with my weight for decades! But today, those pounds and I are coexisting in peace. And after a year of "recovery," I can now step on the scale without a surge of adrenaline or self-recrimination.

I have said again and again that women need to think and talk about health differently. Constantly expecting that something will go wrong, and watching for it warily, is a sign of not trusting your ability to remain healthy. The same thing can happen with weight. You have to trust that your body is capable of reaching and maintaining a healthy weight. Otherwise, what you resist, in the form of "forbidden" foods and excess weight, will persist. You'll feel deprived and eat the brownies and chips, or stress yourself out over your weight, which will end up causing soaring stress hormone levels that, all by themselves, result in weight gain and inflammation—no matter what you eat. I now realize that by resisting that "last five to ten pounds," I was cementing them into place.

For some women, weighing themselves daily keeps them feeling in control of their weight. They see the number on the scale go up toward the top end of that five to ten pounds and they become a little more mindful of what they eat, how much they exercise and sleep, and how well they're handling stress (since stress and weight gain are often related). The number goes down a little after some minor adjustments to their choices for a few days or weeks. Other women rarely weigh themselves and rely on how their pants fit as an indicator of whether they need to be a bit more mindful about making healthy choices. However, for many women, stepping on a scale every day just adds to their stress over their weight. As you develop a healthier attitude toward food and your body, you'll know whether you want to get rid of the scale or not. Trust yourself. Trust your body to do what it needs to do with the food you eat. And take pleasure in preparing and eating good food fit for a goddess.

WHAT'S EATING YOU?

Sometimes callers on my radio show will tell me that they're eating beautifully—meals and snacks that any nutritionist would rate an A-plus—yet they're having health problems. It's not what they're eating but what's eating them. In their quest to be the perfect woman who takes care of everyone and never breaks a sweat, they dutifully fill their plates with wild-caught salmon, pomegranate seeds, and organic broccoli—but they're moody, bloated, and losing their hair. The real problem for them isn't the occasional piece of chocolate they might have. The real problem is forgoing the sweetness of life in an attempt to achieve "perfection" and beat their true appetites into submission. This is what raises stress hormones to levels as toxic as the most highly processed foods do!

Shame about what you're eating creates tremendous anxiety, so just take a moment right now and pay attention to your stomach. Is it relaxed? Happy? Content? Or is it tense? Worried? Bring awareness to your stomach. That's all you have to do. Awareness itself begins to heal the problem. No one eats perfectly all the time. You can enjoy food. You can recover from food fundamentalism. But first, you have to become aware of it.

Doesn't it seem that no matter what you want to eat, there's somebody who thinks you should feel guilty for putting it on your plate? The food police are everywhere, and most of us have internalized their scolding voices. I remember years ago when I was newly macrobiotic and went to the local macrobiotic restaurants, people who knew me from my work would come over and say hello, and their eyes would quickly run over my plate. I could tell they wanted to be sure I was following the rules of macrobiotic eating. Was there a forbidden food there? Was I a "good" macrobiotic eater? As I got to know them and hear them talk obsessively about what you should or shouldn't have in your diet, I learned most of them smoked and drank. Their attitudes toward food and their bodies were as dysfunctional and destructive as the attitudes of people who brag about eating the quadruple bypass burger with extra bacon. (And the pride those people take in that is reflective of an outmoded way of thinking anyway, because, as you'll learn shortly, fat—even saturated animal fat—is not the problem we've been led to believe it is.) Extremes in eating aren't the way to go, but it's hard to resist those judgmental voices about "good foods" and "bad foods" when they're everywhere.

Often, food represents "mother" and what we did and didn't get from Mom. How an infant is fed trains that baby's gut and brain to internalize what is good, loving food and what isn't. Taste is learned at our mother's breasts. In fact, breast-fed infants of smokers actually learn to prefer the taste of milk laced with the taste of cigarettes. As adults, we often try to nurture ourselves through food when what we really want is affection, love, and attention. Now is the time to stop meeting your emotional needs with unhealthy foods. As an ageless goddess, you deserve better.

Often, as you enter your ageless years, your body does you a big favor by sending you clear signals that it is no longer okay for you to nourish everyone but yourself—to eat whatever's available, whatever's left over, whatever no one else wants, whatever feels good in the moment but not so good in the long term. "Good enough" food is no longer good enough. You have to start taking care of yourself in a sustainable way. Over the years, after a few decades of the wrong foods, the digestive system changes and the body produces fewer digestive enzymes, which means the sugary treats or deep-fried foods that contain gluten, trans fats, monosodium glutamate (MSG), and refined sugar start talking to you very quickly in the form of bloating, gas, cramps, and other stomach distress. You can walk around with a baggie of enzymes and probiotics to use in a pinch, but it's better to listen to the wisdom of your body when it says, "Enough. I deserve real food. I love you too much to let this continue!"

The question is, do you know what you can be eating instead to fill you up, satisfy you, nourish you, and keep your body humming?

WHAT TO EAT

In recent years we've learned so much more about food and nutrition that it can be hard to keep up with just what constitutes healthy eating, so let me start by keeping it simple. I love what author and food activist Michael Pollan says: "Eat food. Not too much. Mostly plants." He also says if your grandmother wouldn't recognize it, you probably shouldn't eat it.

While it's important to eat whole foods—mostly plants—you do need to be moderate when it comes to eating grain because our bodies rapidly turn grain into sugar, which causes all sorts of problems, including weight gain. Believe it or not, there's evidence that even the ancient Egyptians got overly fat on grain. We eat far too much sugar to burn it off quickly, and too often our meals center on bread, pasta, cereal, muffins—you name it. Even whole grains are problematic and too easily become a substitute for vegetables and healthy proteins.

Because of addictive and ubiquitous fast foods, along with the combined effects of high insulin, blood sugar, stress hormones, and our current culture, eating well takes more planning than it used to. My father, who was a holistic dentist, used to give his patients who were on antibiotics natural yogurt that my mom made at home. He understood that the probiotics in yogurt would counteract the negative effects of antibiotics, which kill bacteria that cause infections (a good thing) along with bacteria that are beneficial for digestion (not so good—and you'll learn why in a bit). Nowadays when you go to a typical grocery store to buy yogurt, if you read the labels, you find that what's in those little plastic cartons is very different from what yogurt used to be. You can even get yogurt that's neon pink and green and comes in a plastic tube with a cartoon character on it—and they sell that at health food stores!

You have to read labels and understand them, or prepare foods yourself with ingredients you trust that are whole and fresh. The more processed a food is—the further removed it is from nature—the more likely it is to spike your blood sugar or contain toxins. You may already know that if the label for a simple food has 12 ingredients, most of which you can't pronounce, it's best to put it back on the shelf. It's likely to sit there unspoiled for many months, because bacteria can't break down something that really isn't food. It's also important to avoid food dyes and artificial flavors (which sometimes are called "natural flavorings" because some lawyer for a large company got the food labeling laws changed). All of these ingredients are better off remaining in the chemist's lab where they were created! And too much refined sugar, artificial sugars, and processed sugars from corn (think high fructose corn syrup) aren't good for you either. Now add to that the adverse effects of MSG, which is added to huge numbers of foods, and you have a perfect setup for weight and health problems.

ENJOYING EARTH'S BOUNTY

As I was preparing a lecture for a large group of nutrition students recently, I was going through some of my very striking before-and-after photos of individuals who had radically improved their health by switching to a whole-food, organically grown diet. Their faces and bodies had transformed within a matter of a couple of months. Indeed, improving your diet is one of the most powerful reset buttons available. Thinking about the power of organically grown food to improve appearance and health, I realized that eating organic food is like breast-feeding from the earth herself. Improving the quality of what you eat is like a rebirth because the earth produces the very foods you need to flourish.

Begin with rich greens and reds and oranges and yellows that burst forth in the garden at harvest time. There's nothing more delicious than taking the time to prepare a marvelous meal with fresh ingredients and enjoying it thoroughly—especially if you do it with people you're close to, as I've mentioned. It turns out that most of the members of my Argentine tango community

A Word about MSG

MSG, or monosodium glutamate, is a highly addictive flavor-enhancing chemical found in many processed foods. To avoid it, look on the label for any of these terms for MSG, compiled by Mark Hyman, M.D., in his book *The Blood Sugar Solution 10-Day Detox Diet* (Little, Brown, 2014).[1]

- Anything with the word *glutamate* in it
- Gelatin
- Hydrolyzed vegetable protein
- Yeast extract
- Glutamic acid
- Autolyzed yeast
- Vegetable protein extract
- Protease
- Anything "enzyme modified"
- Carrageenan
- Bouillon or broth
- Any flavors or flavoring
- Barley malt
- Malt extract
- Natural seasonings
- Yeast food or nutrients
- Anything containing "enzymes"
- Maltodextrin

are foodies. That makes sense. Those who savor the pleasures of close-embrace dancing also savor the pleasures of eating. Our potlucks are legendary feasts. My friend Leftari says, "I love to cook so much that honey drips from my fingers into the food."

Believe me, when you eat his food, you can *taste* the love. Here's a prayer to reinforce healthy, pleasurable eating: "Divine Beloved, please change me into someone who is surrounded by beautiful healthy food and those who love to prepare, serve, and eat it."

Not every meal is going to taste divine or be divine for you. Sometimes you may get stuck having to order something off the menu of a fast food restaurant known for its high-salt, high-sugar, highly processed food that has been factory designed to be addictive. This is the food responsible for the obesity and sickness epidemic all over the world, so do your best to avoid it. However, if you are going to eat food that isn't of the highest quality because you're stuck with nothing else to eat, take a moment and imbue the food with Divine Love. When you sit down to unwrap your meal, say to yourself, "Thank you for this food. May it nourish my body." Then eat it without guilt. Take your time as you chew. Let your body recognize that you're slowing down and providing it with the nourishment to keep it going. Feel gratitude for the fact that you have a healthy body and food available to you. Give yourself a moment to breathe and feel relaxed. For one thing, if you engage in this ritual, you'll realize you really don't want to make a habit of eating lifeless food! Real food filled with life force feels so much better in your body. And a little goes a long way because your body feels satisfied with far less than you might imagine.

If it feels easier to get takeout than to cook for one, start thinking about how cooking simple foods that nourish you might be possible. The key is planning ahead as though you were planning what to serve to guests. You can assemble a meal of protein and vegetables in as little as 15 minutes, and make soup to last you a few days—and swap a few portions with someone else for variety. Prepare and eat meals with others when it's easy and fun.

THE FAT-SUGAR RELATIONSHIP

We're born to enjoy fats, and the body and brain need them, but they've gotten a bad rap in recent years. Some experts have even recommended consuming as little as 10 percent of calories from fats when we probably need more like 50 to 70 percent.[2] Here's the truth: *you don't become fat from eating fat.* A 2010 meta-analysis of the research on fats showed *no* significant evidence that eating saturated fats (the kind associated with meat and dairy foods) increases your risk of stroke or heart disease.[3] Unfortunately, many women have taken saturated fat out of their diets and reduced their overall fat intake under the impression that this is the way to health. But when you take out the fats, the food isn't as tasty or satisfying, and you end up eating more sugars and simple carbohydrates like bread and pasta. As low-fat, high-carbohydrate diets have become popular in the U.S., obesity rates have skyrocketed.

Not all fats are alike, so it's important to understand that fats per se don't make you fat. It's the trans fats (hydrogenated and partially hydrogenated oils), highly processed vegetable oils, sugars, starches, and MSG (in many different forms) that pack on the pounds and lead to all sorts of health hazards. There's no reason to fear *healthy* dietary fats.

In fact, fats are brain food.[4] Your brain is made up of mostly fat, specifically fat called DHA. And your brain, like those of humans who lived hundreds of thousands of years ago, will fuel itself on fat unless glucose—sugar—is available. If the brain has sugar to keep its engines running, it will switch to that for energy. Because we have a lot of sugar in our diets, our brains are running on glucose and storing a lot of fat as fat, even as we're also storing a lot of sugar as fat. We're also storing toxins within the fat, so our bodies are holding on to pesticides and heavy metals that affect us at a cellular level. Now, this system of storing fuel for lean times worked out beautifully when humans were living in caves and had to live off stored fat when food was scarce. It's not such a great system now that we lead more sedentary lives and can get low-quality, highly processed carbohydrates everywhere. We can even buy candy and chips in the vending machines at health clubs and hospitals, and get free cookies in bank lobbies. And fast food advertising supports the mainstream media. The commercials are for chips, not carrots.

With all those cheap carbs staring you in the face, you have to pay much more attention to the amount, quality, and types of fat and glucose you eat. Otherwise, you just end up consuming what's easily available—typically foods that are very bad for your body and your brain. You have to be vigilant so you don't snack constantly on cheap carbs when you're distracted or upset. The more stressed out you are, the more your body will cause you to crave fats laced with sugars, because the primitive part of your brain thinks that what you need are sources of energy to outrun whatever is chasing you! What you really need is to rebalance your brain and body chemistry. When the levels of hormones and neurotransmitters in your body are what they're supposed to be, you won't crave the high-carbohydrate comfort foods such as mashed potatoes, French fries with ketchup, cookies, pasta, breads, and sugary cereals. These highly addictive foods boost your mood and energy temporarily but then cause an inevitable crash in energy later, along with a host of other problems I'll talk about shortly.

Are you surprised by the news about fats and sugars? There's been an incredible amount of confusion about the pros and cons of low-fat/high-carb diets and moderate-fat/low-carb diets. Let me explain why you don't need to worry about healthy fats and why it's best to consume healthy sugars and whole grains only in moderation, if that. I'll talk about fats first, and then sugars and grains.

HEALTHY FATS

Fats from plants, such as avocados and raw seeds and nuts, aren't a problem. And minimally processed oils from organic plant sources—extra virgin olive oil, coconut oil, almond oil, sesame oil, flaxseed oil, hemp oil, and so on—aren't a problem either. Be aware that heating some oils changes their chemistry and makes them less healthy, so cook with olive or coconut oil. You can also use clarified butter, known as ghee, a staple food in India, for cooking or flavoring food. Don't use canola oil, which is highly processed and derived from seeds likely to be genetically modified. Avoid any oils or spreads that contain trans fats, which contribute to type 2 diabetes. If you are of the generation that gave up butter for margarine, let go of that old habit and go back to healthier, more natural fats.

Animal protein is fine, even though meat, fish, and poultry have saturated fats. If you're not a vegetarian or vegan, go ahead and eat wild fish—not farmed—and beef, chicken, pork, or other meats from animals who moved freely in a natural environment and ate their natural food (grass-fed beef from cows raised on a small farm, for example). If you eat dairy foods such as yogurts and cheeses, the ones made from raw milk are the best, but know your sources and the laws in your area; raw milk products are illegal in many places because of fears of foodborne illnesses. If you can't find or aren't comfortable with raw milk products, choose milk from cows raised by organic farmers who don't add hormones such as rBGH (recombinant bovine growth hormone) to the animals' feed. Usually, it's the processing involved with dairy foods that makes them hard to digest, although you might be intolerant of lactose (the sugar in milk) or casein (a milk protein). Listen to your body. If you feel good eating clean, organic meat or cheese in small quantities, use those as protein sources.

You've probably been told for years to cut out saturated fat, but that advice could not be more wrong! Avoiding fish, meats, healthy dairy foods and oils, and nuts and seeds is likely to lower your so-called "bad" cholesterol (your LDL) on a standard, obsolete lipid profile, but as I explained in Chapter 4, you have to think about cholesterol very differently. LDL is *not* inherently bad. It's not even cholesterol. LDL transports much-needed cholesterol to cells, while HDL, so-called "good cholesterol," transports unneeded extra cholesterol away from cells to where it can be processed and recycled by the body. Think of your LDL as your delivery trucks and your HDL as your garbage trucks. When you avoid healthy fats, such as fats from fish and coconut oil and nuts, all you do is reduce the *good* LDL—the less-dense particles that do a great job of getting much-needed cholesterol into the cells and are not easily oxidized. When you cut sugars and include healthy fats in your diet, you won't have as much *bad* LDL, the delivery trucks that have been battered by too much sugar in your system. The bad LDL particles are indicators of progression toward insulin resistance. Your good HDL can transport away extra cholesterol, but not if you don't have enough of it (and you can increase HDL through meditation and regular exercise). Please don't worry so much about HDL and LDL and cholesterol. I'll fill you in a bit later on accurate tests for cholesterol and HDL and LDL levels, but for now, just remember that the old advice is obsolete.

Having healthy fats in your diet means you'll be more likely to fuel your brain on fat—the superior brain food. Plus, you won't get into the habit of experiencing low blood sugar and cravings and reaching for a sugary food to spike your blood sugar. Remember, when I say healthy fats, I'm talking about the natural, saturated fats in foods such as coconut oil, grass-fed beef, wild-caught salmon, and eggs from free-range chickens that eat organic foods. "Free-range" chickens can walk around and eat plants, their natural foods, which makes their eggs higher in omega-3 fatty acids. "Cage-free" chickens typically have little room to move around and don't eat foods high in omega-3 fatty acids, which means their eggs are lower in this essential fatty acid that is very important for optimal brain health. Remember, what animals eat affects their flesh, milk, and eggs![5]

What you really have to think about eliminating from your diet for health reasons isn't meat and dairy but sugar and grains. Again, commit this to memory: fat, including saturated fat, is *not* a problem. It's crucial for health!

SWEET TREATS AND BLOOD SUGAR

From an evolutionary standpoint, a sweet tooth was a good adaptation we humans made to our environment. We are born preferring sweet tastes, and fruits and vegetables at the height of their ripeness and sweetness are packed with the highest amount of nutrients. Mother Nature puts plenty of sweetness in pumpkins and strawberries. Foods like these that are naturally high in sugar also have fiber, which slows your body's absorption of their sugars. They're not going to spike your blood sugar levels the way refined sugars will—and by refined, I mean any sugars that have been extracted from the fibrous fruit or vegetable. And chances are you're probably not overeating pumpkins. You can have small amounts of real maple syrup and honey, but don't go overboard on those.

If you do want a little bit of sweetener in your food, at least take the processed sugars off the table. You can use a bit of stevia, which is natural and very sweet so a little goes a long way. Avoid the sweeteners you can find in little packets at a diner: refined sugar (white packet), aspartame (blue packet), saccharin (pink packet), and sucralose (yellow packet). And absolutely avoid high fructose corn syrup, which manufacturers have put into all sorts of foods. Read all labels, and look for the sugar content. You'll be appalled at how much sugar is added to just about everything processed. I read the label of some organic squash soup sold at a health food store recently and the amount of sugar in it shocked me. Sugar is as addictive as crack cocaine, so the compulsion to overeat it in any form is almost impossible to resist—and that includes so-called "healthy" foods like granola and trail mix.

The meal I described at the beginning of the chapter had plenty of sweetness—the honeycrisp apples (an especially sweet variety) and sweet potatoes—without added sugars. Even that amount of sugar, though, will cause unhealthy blood sugar fluctuations in those who are no longer sensitive to their own insulin from years of unhealthy eating. If that's the case for you, remove *all* sugars and sugar-producing foods from your diet for seven to ten days. One day every week or two, you can eat them. Reducing your consumption of these foods to this degree generally resets the insulin receptors, preventing type 2 diabetes and sometimes even reversing it. If you have an exhausted pancreas from the overproduction of insulin, you will probably find that getting rid of the sugars, breads, and pastas—and getting enough protein—will support your pancreas in keeping your blood sugars more stable. Maintaining stable blood sugar levels also prevents complications of diabetes such as neuropathy. And believe it or not, if you already have complications, it's never too late to start improving your health with dietary change.

Even if you show no signs of diabetes, one of the most important things you can do to remain ageless is to keep your blood sugar levels from going haywire all day long. That requires avoiding sugars unless they're in whole fruits or vegetables. If your levels are fluctuating wildly during the day, you'll have high energy at some points and very low energy, and difficulty concentrating, at other points. You'll also tend to crave cookies and candy, and if you make a habit of giving in and eating them, you'll only worsen the situation. Over time, uneven blood sugar levels and high sugar consumption cause cellular inflammation and insulin resistance, and those lead to diabetes, cancer, dementia, and heart disease. In fact, sugar is more strongly associated with the development of type 2 diabetes than any other type of food—and it's even more strongly associated with it than a sedentary lifestyle is. Eating lower glycemic foods is associated with lower rates of diabetes whether or not you're sedentary or obese.[6]

If you're experiencing strong dips and peaks in your levels of energy and focus most days, or if you already know you have a prediabetic condition, you must start paying attention to your blood sugar and what you're eating. Ideally, you want a fasting blood sugar of about 70 to 85 mg/dl and it shouldn't spike more than 40 points after you eat. In other words, it should stay at 120 mg/dl or below in the two hours after eating. For years, 100 mg/dl after fasting has been considered the high end of normal, but that's too high given that the PATH Through Life project study (PATH stands for Personality and Total Health), released in 2011, showed that the higher your fasting blood sugar, the greater the damage to the hippocampus in your brain (hippocampal damage is associated with dementia).[7] Research shows a very strong connection between diabetes and dementia. In fact, Alzheimer's disease may be thought of as type 3 diabetes.

To measure and monitor your fasting blood sugar, buy an inexpensive glucometer at the drugstore. Even if you're not worried about your blood sugar levels, try it anyway for a few days in a row just to see where you are with your levels. Take the test before breakfast, and don't snack during the night. (If you're experiencing insomnia and middle-of-the-night cravings, or if you have bowel or stomach problems after eating sugar, you probably have unstable blood sugar levels.) You can also ask your doctor to do a hemoglobin A1C test to determine your blood sugar levels over the past several months, which is an even more accurate measure. If your blood sugar has not been stable, look at what you're eating. Also, listen to your body. If around 3:00 in the afternoon you're cranky and ready to eat the wallpaper, you've probably got uneven blood sugar levels.

The food you eat early in the day sets the stage for your blood sugar level for the next 24 hours, so make sure you get some protein and fat first thing in the morning. Think eggs with avocado and maybe some berries. For sweetness, use stevia, as I've said. You have to have some pleasures in eating. If you make a ritual of enjoying small amounts of chocolate, sweetened tea or coffee, and the like, you're less likely to eat so much of it that you develop inflammation and unstable blood sugar. But know yourself—and remember what I said in Chapter 2 about "moderators" and "abstainers." *Many* people cannot stop after even one bite of chocolate.

Even if you think blood sugar isn't a problem for you, it's important to recognize that sugars affect your body at a cellular level. If you're eating a lot of sugars and grains, even whole grains, your gastrointestinal system is probably leaking some food particles into your bloodstream in a condition known as leaky gut syndrome. Remember, the genetically altered grains of today are very different from those our grandparents enjoyed. They have much higher gluten content. That causes cellular inflammation, because the cells don't know what these particles are and they want to neutralize them by surrounding them with fluid. Your hormonal system responds to all the sugars by having your pancreas pump out more insulin to get the extra sugar in your blood to go into cells, where it can be used. Some of that sugar is stored as fat, but much of it just travels around your bloodstream, looking for a cell that will take it in. Meanwhile, the inflammation in your body and blood vessels causes oxidative stress, which means you've got cells that are missing electrons scavenging electrons from other cells, destabilizing and injuring them.

As oxidative stress and inflammation get out of control, everything goes haywire and your body begins to break down and turn on itself. The next step is a prediabetic condition known as glycemic stress. This condition is reversible if you change your diet and release repressed emotions such as resentment and grief. Glycemic stress causes cellular inflammation, which first

Basic Recommended Lab Tests

There are several lab tests I recommend for every woman to assess how her eating habits are impacting her health. The first two measure blood sugar levels directly; the third is related and was discussed earlier in relation to heart health. I recommend that you ask your health care practitioner to work with you to get these tests and interpret the results.

1. *Insulin response test.* Also known as a glucose tolerance test, this measures both your fasting blood sugar and your insulin levels one and two hours after consuming a 75-gram glucose drink. Since fasting insulin levels will be the first thing to become abnormal with a high-sugar inflammatory diet—long before your blood sugar starts to change and long before diabetes can be diagnosed—this test is really valuable as an early warning that you can do something about! An alternative is to purchase a glucometer yourself and test your own blood sugar. Fasting blood sugar should be 70 to 85 mg/dl. And two hours after eating, you don't want your sugar to go any higher than 120 mg/dl.

2. *Hemoglobin A1C.* This test measures your average blood sugar over the prior six-week period. Anything over 5.5 percent is considered elevated. Over 6.0 percent is diabetes.

3. *NMR lipid profile.* This is the most up-to-date way to test your cholesterol. Unlike the standard but obsolete lipid profile, this test identifies the particle number and particle size of each type of cholesterol, LDL and HDL, as well as giving you a triglyceride count. See the section in Chapter 4 for a full explanation. The NMR lipid profile can be obtained only through LabCorp or LipoScience. You can order the other tests yourself through SaveOnLabs at www.saveonlabs.com. Ideally you'll want to work with a health care practitioner who understands nutritional and functional medicine (www.functional medicine.org) to help you interpret and act on your results.

shows up as physical discomfort, such as aching muscles, bloating, headache, insomnia, and weight gain. Over time, chronic degenerative diseases such as heart disease, arthritis, high blood pressure, Alzheimer's, diabetes, and cancer are the result. Fortunately, this domino effect of sugar/inflammation/disease can be counteracted and reversed if you just lower your sugar intake and pay attention to the types and form of sugars you eat.

HOW TO AVOID FOOD ADDICTION

Are you a sugar addict? A sugar-fat-and-white-flour craver? Or are you addicted to a different type of treat? Notice the foods that "sing" to you—the ones you're tempted to overeat. One of my friends recently posted on Facebook that she was finally facing up to her chocolate addiction. She's realizing that when it comes to chocolate, she can't eat it in moderation, whether it's organic cocoa nibs or a chocolate bar. She knows that the only answer is to go cold turkey and never eat it again. Announcing it publicly is helping her gain the support she needs to stick to her decision.

For others, the addictive food might be mashed potatoes, or brown rice, or anything salty. If you're tempted to overeat a food, it's probably addictive for you. Don't battle yourself and your cravings—just avoid the food completely. If it's hard for you to commit to that, decide to avoid the food for at least a month and then see what happens. Getting it out of your system and breaking the habit might make you realize that you'd rather be free of the addiction than continue to fight it. If you've been addicted to sugar, you're likely to find that fruits and vegetables taste much sweeter than they did before because you've down-regulated your sweet taste receptors. And by eating more natural foods and ensuring you get enough blood sugar–stabilizing protein, you will retrain your taste buds to appreciate real foods and your cravings will be reduced too.

Author Anne Wilson Schaef has said, "Addictions serve to numb us so we're out of touch with what we know and what we feel." If I tell you to take out of your diet refined sugar, alcohol, or high-glycemic foods—all of which increase beta-endorphin and make you feel better temporarily—you may be able to do it. But if you don't deal with the feelings that drive you to look to foods for life's sweetness, to caffeinated beverages to get energy, and to a bottle of spirits to find Spirit, your underlying issues will make you crave these substances again.

It's well established that food manufacturers tinker with the chemistry of foods to make them more addictive. Knowing this, be conscientious about choosing which foods to eat—and be honest with yourself about whether you really can handle them in moderation or if you have to let them go altogether. The only long-term, sustainable cure for food addiction is to generate natural feel-good chemicals in your body and at the same time work on your emotional body and the issues of your soul. Then you can align with the goddess within you.

If you have very powerful cravings for sweets, there are two reasons. The first is that you ate something for breakfast that spiked your blood sugar temporarily. After that breakfast bagel sends your blood sugar up, it inevitably comes down in a blood sugar crash. The second reason is that your taste buds have become used to all the highly processed foods out there that have thrown off your gut flora balance and your brain chemistry. As you eat healthier foods, you'll crave sugar less. Then a handful of berries really will satisfy you in a way that a cupcake or ice cream won't. And if what you're really craving is the sweetness of life, go outside, sit in the sun under a tree, and have a conversation with someone who makes you laugh. By now you know there are plenty of ways to experience pleasure without reaching for a substance that will spike your mood artificially.

And if you love your soda pop, you'll have to cut that out. It's liquid candy and it's common to be addicted to it. Don't drink the diet versions, either; they use artificial sweeteners and trick your brain into craving real sugars. Diet soda with aspartame has been linked to obesity, probably because that no-calorie drink tends to make you crave something like a high-calorie piece of bread with a sugary spread on it, or a cookie. But aspartame is also an excitotoxin that kills brain cells and is associated with everything from seizures to multiple sclerosis.[8]

Many women become addicted to caffeinated diet colas and mistakenly believe that because these beverages have no calories and less caffeine than coffee, they are no problem. Wrong! Drink water as your main beverage. If you want a little variety or fizz, try some natural mineral water, or put a slice of lime or lemon in your water, or drink a little seltzer with juice flavoring or fresh mint and stevia (which is low calorie) or herbal tea. You have plenty of choices. Don't make regular soda or diet soda one of them.

As for alcohol—and yes, alcohol is a sugar—it's not going to kill you to have wine once in a while, but are you having it once in a while? Be honest. You don't need it, and it has a greater downside than upside. If you're telling yourself that research shows moderate drinkers live longer and enjoy better health, remember there are plenty of things those healthy, long-living wine drinkers could be doing that simply correlate with drinking a little alcohol. It's probably the relaxation time on the porch, or the time spent with friends, that makes their drinking health-protective. The fact is that even moderate alcohol use significantly increases the risk of breast cancer. Thousands of women "run for the cure" and wear pink wristbands, yet they drink enough wine to double their risk! And recent studies have indicated that most women are not interested in hearing about the alcohol–breast cancer connection.

Alcohol, which can be highly addictive, is also a depressant. What's more, when your estrogen levels are low during perimenopause or after menopause—or during the few days before your period—alcohol is especially effective at lowering your mood by depressing your brain chemistry. What is your mood before, during, and after drinking? Do you need the drink to find the courage to be charming and witty, to dance on the bar or flirt with a stranger, or to say no to someone else's idea of what should give you pleasure? Ageless goddesses don't need an excuse to have fun!

If you're a recovering alcoholic, avoid sugar. It will trigger cravings for alcohol and depress your brain chemistry. Don't substitute one for the other. And keep in mind that alcohol, like other sugars, also worsens and even causes hot flashes.

A Word about Balancing Your Hormones

You've heard that hormones naturally get out of balance in midlife. Want to balance your hormones quickly? Eliminate sugar, gluten, and alcohol from your diet. Journal about it and see how quickly you experience changes in your mood, energy level, mental clarity, and cravings for unhealthy foods. Taking phytoestrogens such as *Pueraria mirifica* and maca can also help since these contain what are known as adaptogens. Adaptogens sit on the hormone receptors in your cells. And if your hormone levels are too low, they safely act like low-dose estrogens. If your levels are too high, they block any adverse effects from the excess. (See Resources for Chapters 3 and 4 for more information.)

GRAIN BRAIN AND WHEAT BELLY

If you've heard of menopause belly, or wondered why it's so common to misplace your cell phone and keys when you hit midlife, let go of the idea that the problem is your hormones or "early old-timer's disease." Don't think that way or talk that way. It isn't your hormones, or early dementia, or a "natural" part of midlife that's got your belly sticking out and your brain muddled. It's what you're eating. The culprit is probably grain, as two terrific books—*Grain Brain* by neurologist David Perlmutter, M.D. (Little, Brown, 2013), and *Wheat Belly* by William Davis, M.D. (Rodale, 2011)—explain in detail.

For most of human history, people ate very few grains—perhaps a little wheat, barley, rye, kamut, spelt, and other grains that grew here and there. People weren't planting and harvesting crops, so these grains weren't a major part of their diet. When the agricultural age came in thousands of years ago, we started eating considerably more grains and our bodies adjusted to them—to some degree. But as Dr. Perlmutter explains in *Grain Brain,* using glucose from grains as our brain's primary energy source, and using grains as our primary food source, is not ideal. As I said earlier in the chapter, fats are brain food: it's better to fuel our brain cells and the mitochondria, or power stations, within them by using dietary fats, mostly from plants. All that grain in our diets—even when it's eaten in whole form, with the hull mostly intact—turns to glucose and acts like sugar in the body and brain. The extra sugar from grains is also stored as excess fat in the body. Cattle are fed grain to fatten them for market; our bodies grow fat on grain too.

There's increasing evidence that most of the diseases we're experiencing in the West lately, from cancer to autoimmune disorders, Alzheimer's, and autism, are caused by inflammation related to our diets. Think about how you eat grain. Are you eating a whole-grain slice of bread smothered in honey or concentrated fruit spread for breakfast or a snack? Cereal with dried fruit? Do you have grains at most meals in place of vegetables? You've probably taught your brain to run on regular, not premium, fuel.

Another reason we're not doing well with grain in our diets is because we changed the grain after World War II. Most of us are eating what's called dwarf wheat, which was introduced to alleviate starvation around the world because it's very high yield. It's also very high in gluten—and we all know someone with celiac disease or gluten intolerance. Many people are now gluten intolerant to some degree. Eating so much of this new wheat that's highly processed and loaded with gluten, in addition to all the refined sugar and toxins we're consuming, has tipped the scales. These aren't Grandma's grains. And you'll have plenty to eat without bread, cereal, and pasta made from wheat in your diet. You won't miss bread and pasta if you're getting a little sugar from fruits and natural sweeteners and eating plenty of healthy fats and fresh foods, because your food will taste good and you'll enjoy it. You really don't need grains at all as long as you're eating plenty of vegetables and getting healthy fats to feed your brain.

A LITTLE HEALTHY PROTEIN GOES A LONG WAY

Healthy protein keeps blood sugar stable, and protein sources that contain fat provide essential fuel for the brain. And you don't need a lot of protein—about 45 grams a day. A serving of meat, which is three ounces and the size of your palm, has about 21 grams of protein, so you don't need to go overboard with fish, poultry, or grass-fed beef on your dinner plate.

There's no "clock" inside our bodies that suggests we limit ourselves to three meals a day. Some people do fine with two while others need five. It all depends upon your metabolism. Between meals, eat some protein-rich snacks and add a little fat. A handful of nuts, a hard-boiled egg, a spoonful of coconut oil, some blueberries, an apple with peanut butter, or a slice of cheese will keep you from feeling light-headed or ravenous between meals. It is the refined sugars—especially when mixed with fat— that do the most damage. So avoid those foods. (You know the ones—they're from the vending machines!)

A Word about Beans and Legumes

So now you know you can enjoy the bounty of the earth in the form of vegetables, fruits, meats, and dairy products from animals that live close to the land as they did back in your grandmother's day. What about beans and legumes? These plant foods quickly boost blood sugar for some people but not others. They're not a part of what's called a Paleo diet, which has been highly touted lately, but let's get real. Pinto beans and navy beans are not exactly cupcakes or white bread, and they're a cheap, readily available form of protein. A bean or split pea soup, hummus, and bean salad aren't out of the question if you're eating healthfully to reduce inflammation and keep blood sugar levels stable. As long as they don't lead to cravings and dips and peaks in mood and energy caused by uneven blood sugar, go ahead and eat them. You can consider them like root vegetables such as carrots and beets (which have a lot of sugar): they may not be your top choice, but in moderation they're probably fine for you. Tofu and edamame are made from soy, and they can be very healthy for most women. Refined soy is a problem for some—not all.

AGELESS EATING

The truth is that we're really designed to eat vegetables, some meats and fruits, and some nuts and seeds. Try to make sure vegetables take up most of your plate. Fortunately, there are an infinite number of ways to prepare them so you don't get bored and order up pizza to be delivered (although organic, whole-grain-crust, all-vegetable pizza can be a delicious, occasional treat). You can even make pizza dough and pasta from ingredients such as zucchini, cauliflower, and coconut flour. I'm a big fan of quinoa, which is a seed, not a grain. And it's gluten-free.

If you're not used to eating a mostly plant-based diet with healthy proteins and fats, here are some ideas for what to eat:

Instead of Eating This	You Might Eat This
cold cereal with milk	an omelet made with high-omega-3 eggs from free-range chickens, some vegetables, and a little cheese, cooked in a little coconut oil or extra virgin olive oil
toast with jam	a muffin made from ingredients such as nuts, ground flaxseed, carrots, almond or coconut flour, and coconut oil (for this recipe and other Paleo diet recipes, see www.fastpaleo.com)
spaghetti with meat sauce	small organic veggie burger or meat burger along with a fruit salad containing berries, melon, and other whole fruit
chicken salad sandwich	organic, free-range chicken and grilled eggplant or zucchini cooked with olive oil and fresh herbs
chocolate cake	1 oz. of fine dark chocolate paired with fresh fruit and 1 oz. of organic cheese
potato or corn chips	kale or seaweed chips or a handful of nuts or seeds

| chips and dip | vegetable sticks or gluten-free organic crackers dipped in hummus, bean dip, or baba ghanoush (made from eggplant) |
| pizza | a tomato-basil-cucumber-garlic-olive oil salad plus 2 oz. of meat or cheese |

Notice the pattern here: fill up on cruciferous (crunchy and fibrous) vegetables with plenty of texture, color, and flavor, and use moderate quantities of healthy fish, meat, dairy, eggs and fruit. Use the highest-quality, freshest ingredients you can for the most flavor.

Don't forget to drink plenty of water—cold or room temperature, whatever makes you more likely to drink it. Enjoy tea, and if you like a little caffeine and your body can handle it, upgrade your coffee to be the least processed type or switch to green tea, which is loaded with antioxidants that prevent inflammation and oxidative stress.

WHERE THE FOOD IS

More and more, you can find healthy foods in the most unexpected places. I'm thrilled with the new fast food options that are springing up around the country: Chipotle Mexican Grill, Tender Greens, and Elevation Burger are examples. Even that fast food chain with the clown mascot is having to change what it offers on the menu because people have come to realize that "cheap" food isn't cheap in the long run. When it leads to poor health, it's just not a happy meal. You can also find healthy food at farmers' markets, or sign up for what's called a CSA (community supported agriculture) share. With CSAs, you pay at the beginning of the growing season to get a weekly delivery of fresh produce right off the farm. This is a fantastic way to get the best of local, organically grown produce and support the farmers in your area. I adore my local farmer Justin, who also happens to be a very accomplished salsa dancer. Get to know your farming neighbors! CSAs are also a great way to get creative about your cooking because you'll get a box full of vegetables you've never eaten or prepared before. Search online for "recipes kohlrabi" or "recipes beet greens." You can also grow your own fruits, vegetables, and herbs in your yard, in containers on your porch, in a rented garden plot—you can even grow them in hay bales or in your basement. Eat up and enjoy!

Regardless of where you buy packaged foods, it's important to read the labels. Sauces, salad dressings, and frozen foods often have hidden ingredients. Gluten's a common one, but sugars, MSG in all its many guises, and extra salt are added too. Watch how much you use.

The "slow food movement" is all about slowing down to savor your food and be mindful of how it comes from the earth, through animals and farmers and people who sell and distribute food, so that you support sustainable ways of growing food and consuming it. When you slow down to eat, instead of grabbing something on the go or distractedly plowing through whatever's on your plate while thinking about what's next on your To Do list, you're less likely to overeat. You start to realize how ridiculous food portions in restaurants can be and how little food it takes to fill up if you're eating good food slowly, enjoying every bite.

Remember, ageless goddesses take pleasure in food. When you talk to people about food and healthy eating, watch your language and your tone. Are you turning into the food police and judging yourself and everyone else? That will just give everyone indigestion. And don't get into an organ recital about how you can't eat this anymore because of your heart troubles and you're supposed to eat that now because of your stomach issues. Make it easy for someone to invite you over for a meal by bringing the foods and condiments and digestive supplements you need without having to rattle off a list of foods you can't eat. A funny cartoon I saw recently made the point—and cracked me up. A woman is talking with a friend, saying, "I've been gluten-free for a week. And already I'm annoying." Don't be that person. When you're with friends and family, talk about a new food or recipe you tried. Go apple or berry picking with your friends and their grandchildren. Walk over to the neighbor's with some extra basil or peppers, and when she hands you some tomatoes, swap growing tips. Food growing, buying, preparing, and enjoying can all be communal experiences.

So try to "break bread" with others even if you're not actually eating bread! There's a folk tale about stone soup, in which a village of people come together to add something to a pot on the fire that contains only a stone. It's not the stone that makes the soup delicious but what everyone adds: the love that forms a community. That's the best kind of nourishment.

SUPPLEMENTS TO AGELESS, HEALTHY EATING

Eating whole, healthy foods will nourish your goddess self, but for truly optimal nutrition, food supplements are important. They'll bring balance back to your body and replenish it more quickly. They'll also improve your brain chemistry, which affects your moods and outlook, so it will be easier to plan for healthier eating and stick with your program for self-nourishment. In Chapter 12, you'll find specifics on what supplements to take to quickly replenish yourself—and you'll be familiar with some of them, such as vitamin D3, from reading this book. But let me give you information on a few more that are important and that you should be taking along with the supplements I mentioned already. (You'll find a full list in Chapter 12.)

The first is turmeric, containing the active compound curcumin. This spice is found in many Asian foods, including curries, and is an incredible anti-inflammatory. In fact, it turns on the body's ability to produce the super anti-inflammatory biochemicals BDNF (brain-derived neurotrophic factor, a type of enzyme) and glutathione (a combination of three amino acids). You can cook and prepare foods with turmeric, but think seriously about supplementing with it too. (By the way, if you want to help your brain produce BDNF, cut the sugar in your diet).[9]

Another important nutrient is magnesium, which most women are low in. You can't accidentally overdose on magnesium because too much results in loose stools, which you're bound to notice. (You've heard of the laxative milk of magnesia, right? Enough said.) Still another nutrient that women need is iodine, which helps alleviate breast pain and contributes to healthy hair, nails, and hormone balance. Most women in the U.S. aren't eating sea vegetables or kelp, which are good sources of iodine. In the U.S., the average woman consumes 240 micrograms a day compared to Japan, where the average woman takes in 45 *milligrams* a day (a milligram is 1,000 micrograms). It takes about 3 milligrams a day to support healthy breasts, so clearly most American women don't even come close to getting enough. But according to some sources, the typical Japanese woman gets about *six times* what a woman in the U.S. gets through her diet because of seaweed consumption.[10] (Note that organic eggs are another good source of iodine.)

To ensure you're getting enough iodine, I recommend supplementing. Be sure to add iodine to your diet slowly, *especially* if you have a thyroid condition such as Hashimoto's disease or you are taking a prescription drug with bromides. Otherwise, you might experience rashes, increased heart rate, and hyperthyroidism (overactive thyroid). The best website for thyroid information I've found, by the way, is Mary Shomon's http://thyroid.about.com.

A good multivitamin is important too. The label should say "guaranteed potency" and "manufactured in a GMP facility." GMP stands for "good manufacturing practices," and for a facility to make this claim, it has to check out with NSF International, a public health and safety organization. There is also a very good resource called *NutriSearch Comparative Guide to Nutritional Supplements* by Lyle MacWilliam, M.Sc., F.P., that rates supplements for quality.[11]

I also recommend that you start taking some probiotics. As I said earlier, probiotics are in yogurt and other fermented foods such as tempeh, tofu, miso, sauerkraut, and pickles, but most women need to supplement with them. Let me explain a little more about what they are and what they do for your gut.

PROBIOTICS, PREBIOTICS, AND A HEALTHY COMMUNITY IN YOUR GUT

Your gastrointestinal (GI) system, or gut, plays a crucial role in your health at every level. It's actually part of your brain, making neurotransmitters such as serotonin—in fact, most of that's

A Word about Iodine

The amount of iodine (in the form of both iodine and iodide) that the body needs for optimal health is about 12.5 mg per day. Some individuals require more. A combination of molecular iodine and iodide is best. The current RDA for iodine is only 150 *micrograms* per day—just enough to prevent goiter but not nearly enough to provide optimal health for the rest of the body, including the thyroid. Iodine is known as a halogen; the other halogens—chlorine, fluoride, and bromide—compete with iodine, and when you first add iodine to your diet, your body may detox those other toxic halogens in the form of a rash. Many mistakenly take this for an allergic reaction to iodine instead of what it is—the body healing itself. The problem is easily fixed by simply replenishing iodine more slowly. Thyroid hormone is made up of iodine—the symbols T3 and T4 refer to the number of iodine molecules in the hormone itself. Many people who take adequate amounts of iodine find that their thyroid function normalizes by itself. But the thyroid isn't the only gland that requires iodine. Breast tissue requires 3 mg of iodine per day for optimal health and prevention of cysts and pain, and the ovaries also require it. Iodine deficiency is a worldwide problem at this point, and iodized salt doesn't contain enough of the right kinds to provide what is needed. Given that adequate iodine is absolutely essential for nearly every function in the body, I highly recommend adding it to your diet in some form.

made in your gut. Your gut is also part of your immune system, protecting your body against foreign microorganisms, whether they're bacteria or viruses. We don't live in a sterile world, so your GI tract is actually filled with microorganisms. You have more of them there than you have cells in your entire body! In other words, your belly is a community. Are the neighbors getting along? Or do you have an imbalance where the bad flora, like yeast and unhealthy bacteria, are crowding out the good flora?

The best way to make sure you've got enough good flora is to eat plenty of cruciferous vegetables, such as broccoli, cauliflower, kale, and collard greens, because the fiber in them serves as a breeding ground for the good bacteria in your gut. You also want probiotics—the good bacteria—to enter your GI system and flourish there. A good probiotic supplement should be packed with beneficial microorganisms that support digestion. If you have frequent yeast infections in your vagina or your mouth or both, there are probiotic supplements with bacteria that are especially good for clearing them up. Getting the sugar out of your diet will help too. A recent study showed that a cup a day of Activia yogurt, which has a relatively small number of beneficial bacteria in it and far too much sugar in my opinion, can boost a woman's mood because of the relationship between gut health and the brain. If a little bit of sugary yogurt can do so much, imagine what high-quality probiotic sources can do. And you can support all those beneficial microorganisms (also known collectively as the microbiome) by eating your cabbage, greens, broccoli, and so on. It's easy to become overwhelmed by the idea of changing your entire diet, but you can significantly change your gut flora balance through changing what you eat in as little as 24 hours.[12]

Eating too many grains and sugars throws off the balance in your gut flora as yeast grows and good bacteria die off. You develop leaky gut syndrome and inflammation and oxidative stress, as I explained, and serotonin levels drop. You start craving sugars, and once you give in to those cravings, you make the situation worse. So while taking the probiotics is good, it's not a panacea. You have to cut out the sugars too.

If you've cut the sugars and the grain but your GI system is still off, it could simply be that you're not drinking enough water or you're eating too little fiber, or you ate something that doesn't agree with you. The problem could also be emotional. Remember, the gut makes more neurotransmitters than the brain does, so it's constantly talking to us! Pay attention to the subtle signs from your gut, because it responds to both food and feelings.

If you're anxious, angry, or depressed, you might have bowel movements that are too loose or too firm, or your intestines will cramp. Energetically, your digestive system is associated with your third chakra and issues related to personal power, self-worth, self-esteem, self-confidence, and feelings of responsibility. When you're nervous or insecure, afraid of being shamed for being yourself, feeling overly responsible for everything and everybody, your gut may respond by becoming agitated.

We say "listen to your gut instincts" and "I just can't stomach that situation" because on some level we sense the brain-gut connection—and scientists are now realizing it is stronger than we ever knew. Don't neglect your gut! Take your probiotics, and if you're having some digestive troubles, take an enzyme with your meal. For example, if you're going to enjoy an organic rice-and-beans dish, an enzyme supplement will help prevent excess gas.

HAPPY BELLY AND HAPPY BODY

If you're unhappy with the shape of your belly, know that cutting out the wheat will reduce it, but whatever your belly looks like, you can make it happy. Balance your gut flora. Nourish yourself with good foods and clear out the junk, including the shame, perfectionism, and emotional stress that are affecting you.

Let's make it a happy belly, one you're comfortable with, one that isn't holding on to toxins buried in fat and creating a body shape that makes you prone to diseases like diabetes. Show love to your belly as you heal your gut. You might even take a belly-dancing class and get back in touch with this part of your body. Belly dancing, like any sensual dancing, makes it easier to reconnect with your beautiful, divine, ageless inner goddess.

Give up the goal of achieving what our culture calls a "perfect" or "ideal" body shape. Only about 1 percent of women have that shape at any age. Besides, what is culturally idealized varies from decade to decade. It's time to simply accept that and get on with it. Embrace the changes that arise in your body, and think about what they're alerting you to. Do you need to make changes in your life? Have you learned to love yourself fully and embrace the physical manifestations that are your belly, your breasts, your face, your arms, your bottom, head, and feet? Pay loving attention to your body and nourish it. Trust your appetite and your body's desire to settle into a particular weight and shape when you're eating healthfully.

Delight is a crucial ingredient in agelessness. Ignore the food police. Be a laughing Buddha with happiness in your belly. And indulge your appetite for the pleasures of food shared with good company or eaten alone, in peaceful contemplation of the fruits of the earth.

CHAPTER NINE

GODDESSES
MOVE JOYOUSLY

You move and you live, you stop moving and you die. Simple.
— BOB COOLEY, AUTHOR OF *THE GENIUS OF FLEXIBILITY*

I have a habit of mindfully noticing moments in my life that represent the fulfillment of long-cherished dreams that took some real effort to manifest. One of those golden moments was dancing tango in Buenos Aires with an Argentine native while listening to Color Tango, a live tango orchestra playing at Salón Canning, a well-known venue. Dancing there marked a completion of epic proportions because it represented that I had, for the first time ever, found a form of movement that truly spoke to my soul. Movement that is in tune with our core being is movement that is sustainable—and it's the type of "exercise" we all need to do.

I'd wanted to dance for my entire life, but I grew up in a family of sports enthusiasts who skied, hiked, and played golf and tennis. Dance wasn't on the agenda. At seven, I gleefully watched my father walk up the driveway with a special package that contained tap shoes I had ordered by mail, but the one dance teacher in town moved away shortly after my cherished dance shoes arrived. I made a few attempts to try ballroom dancing over the next several decades, always with an unwilling and sports-oriented partner. Finally, I realized that if I were ever going to fulfill my desire to dance, I would have to make it happen myself. I would simply sign up for ballroom dance lessons again. But then, while standing in front of the huge storefront window of Maine Ballroom Dance Studio one snowy and cold January night, I watched a couple dancing Argentine tango in close embrace. The dance was so sensual, so moving, that it called to me. My heart said, "That's what I want to do."

It's one thing to be inspired by watching a couple dance skillfully. It's quite another to show up as a clumsy beginner at a dance class or practice session, especially when you've already mastered your own career and inhabit the comfortable realm of being an authority in your own sphere. How many of us have held back from trying something our hearts called us to do, fearing that we would be laughed at or shamed? There is always a reason to stay home and not take the risk of embarrassing yourself, but this is an obsolete voice you need to resist. That's what I decided to do, and that choice changed my life.

Despite my nervousness, I showed up at a tango class as a total beginner and slowly and self-consciously began to learn the art form. There were far more women than men at the dances and practice sessions, and my fellow female dancers were all waiting to be asked to dance. I thought, *Oh, good. Just what the world needs—another single, middle-aged woman who wants to learn how to dance. There aren't enough men to go around. And now I show up and make the ratio even worse!*

But I had a burning desire to feel this romantic dance in my body, mind, and spirit. I wanted to feel the thrill of surrendering to the lead of a skillful man. I wanted my body to know how to express the way the music felt inside me. To do all that, I had to create new pathways in my brain and body and completely redo my wiring diagram. I had to work at making my body bring sacred pleasure into every nerve and muscle while I was connecting with the heart of my partner. Doing this was, quite frankly, much harder than medical school and residency had ever been. Why? Because learning to dance tango as a single woman over 40 with no dance background whatsoever uncovered all of my insecurities about my desirability as a woman. Argentine tango—that dance of connection and passion that was born out of the pain of so many displaced Africans and Europeans coming together in Argentina more than a century ago—became the crucible in which all my own pain and insecurity were forged into a new, more vibrant, ageless body and, indeed, a whole new life.

Do you have a secret desire when it comes to how you want to feel in your body? If you're not feeling exquisite in your body now, when will you allow yourself that experience? Each of us is designed with a unique approach to movement that feels satisfying. To remain ageless, you need to remember how you moved as a child, before you internalized other people's ideas about when you should move and sit still, and how you should express yourself and feel joy in your own skin. Back then, you were moved by enthusiasm, not a relentless drive to push your body through something called "exercise" that was "good for you."

In your ageless years, you don't need to go back to those junior high school days when you had to compete against your friends, do specific movements the way your teacher told you to, wear an ugly and uncomfortable uniform, or allow people more skilled than you were to have all the fun. Instead, you can bring pleasure into your movements as you embrace a sense of adventure, stretching yourself in new ways. Ask yourself: What is possible with my body today? How can I move differently than I did yesterday and have more fun doing it? How can I keep moving more joyfully, more freely, and more fully?

Rx FOR AGELESSNESS: MOVEMENT AND FUN

I dislike the word *exercise*. It has become synonymous with *all* movement. We get injured because we've been taught "no pain, no gain," "push yourself," and "pain is weakness leaving the body." Injuries can plague us for the rest of our lives if we don't know how to change the connective tissue in our bodies—the fascia that connects everything to everything else, which I described earlier in the book. The energetic impact of physical injuries is usually stored in this connective tissue, but what's stored can be released, as you'll learn. Bringing a sense of dread and obligation to moving your body is simply unsustainable. Over time, you will find that you can't force yourself to do something you really don't want to do.

Can you remember the first time you did a somersault? Rode a bike? Swam in a pool? Ran along a beach? Jumped rope? We're designed to move. When you were a young child, no one had to push you to exercise. In fact, it was just the opposite. You moved joyously in your body and had energy to burn. If you've forgotten what that was like, make a point of watching some kids under age five. There are plenty of videos online of adorable children who can't stop moving. Watch what they do when they're supposed to be sitting or standing still or following the careful choreography of their tap dancing teacher. When they're excited, they're like whirling dervishes, those Sufi mystics who spin with the sheer delight of being connected to Spirit while in their bodies. Like every child, you were taught to stop squirming and sit still to fit in at school or church, or in a car seat. And now, of course, the authority figures are telling you to stop sitting still and start moving!

How important is movement? Here's an example. I was on a family trip with my siblings and my mother a couple of years ago, and we ended up having to use a moving walkway in the Istanbul airport to get to our flight on time. My mother, who was 87 then, was looking back when the moving walkway suddenly ended. She stumbled onto the floor in front of it and instinctively reached out to try to catch herself, but there was no railing. She started to fall off the side, and there was a two-foot drop down to the sidewalk. Realizing she was falling, she sprang off the end of the walkway and landed two feet below, then ran forward to work off the momentum resulting from losing her balance. Very impressive. Very athletic. I swear, if she had been less fit and agile, we'd have spent the next month in a Turkish hospital standing by while she recovered from a hip fracture. Her instinctive self-preserving physical motions were the result of a lifetime of physical prowess and movement—which in my mother's case had involved hiking and skiing. Being present in your body, having good balance, and being aware of your movements can save your life—and joyful movement can certainly make your life worth living. Remember—muscle strength and balance do not deteriorate with age. They deteriorate with lack of use resulting from a sedentary lifestyle.

Improve Your Balance

Dr. Joan Vernikos, formerly of NASA, has noted that after being in space, healthy young astronauts often have trouble walking when they return to earth. They walk with a wide-based gait like old people because the vestibular systems in their brains have atrophied from lack of gravity. Likewise, when we sit all day and do not move regularly against the forces of gravity, we too lose our balance. The astronauts regain theirs in a couple of weeks. All of us, regardless of age, can do the same. Here's what to do. At least three times a day, stand on one foot and close your eyes. See how long you can balance without needing to steady yourself with a hand or your other foot. I do this in the shower each morning, at least once during the day, and before going to sleep at night. When I started, I could scarcely stand for even ten seconds before needing to catch myself. Within about a week, I was up to 30 seconds. And here's the fun part. My balance just keeps getting better and better! Know that your balance and vestibular system can always be improved with practice.

If you do exercise, be aware that it's not enough to simply sit all day and exercise before or after that long stretch spent in a chair. New research shows that if you have a sedentary job, even if you work out for an hour, all that nonstop sitting increases your risk of cancer, diabetes, stroke, and heart disease—and increases your risk of dying in the next three years by 40 percent.[1]

You have some options, however. You can sit on an exercise ball with or without a holder supporting it (I'm doing that right now!), or set a timer and stand up every 15 minutes to stretch and move (even standing up and sitting right back down can be very effective). You can also use an adjustable desk that lets you go back and forth between standing and sitting. In the future, we'll probably have holographic computer "screens" that we can interact with using our bodies, hands, and voices. There are already devices that allow you to do this to some degree. Until then, if you're sitting for long hours every day, you need to find ways to get up and move regularly while you're working—as if you were a squirmy child!

Everyone has different physical abilities, but too many of us learned in childhood that movement meant competitive sports. Often, we have been judged according to sports skills that aren't synonymous with fitness at all. There's nothing wrong with a baseline of strength and flexibility, but even today schools' standards of fitness are based on acquiring boot camp skills, not moving the body in rhythm or exhibiting flexibility, balance, grace, or sensuality. The same standards are found in the larger culture too, which is why so many women end up hating "exercise" and give up on finding ways to move their bodies.

For a long time, moving my body to get exercise wasn't very joyful for me. I associated exercise with trying to fit into a family where everyone, including my mother, played competitive sports. Whether we were hiking, skiing, or playing tennis, movement always seemed to be about winning a game, keeping score, or conquering a steep hill. I went along with everyone else, and I enjoyed zipping down a mountain or hitting a tennis ball occasionally. But overall, none of these activities was satisfying to me. I'm very glad that I grew up in a family in which fitness was an important part of daily life. However, like many women, I found it took me many years to discover the physical activities that are truly satisfying for my particular body, mind, and spirit. Too many women spend decades feeling guilty that they aren't "exercising" and unaware that there are forms of movement that feel natural to them—forms they've forgotten about, in many cases.

By returning to the movement that simply makes them feel good, they can get the "exercise" they need to be healthy.

To maintain a healthy, flexible body for life, you need a joyous expression of your life force that gets your heart pumping and your bodily fluids and chi circulating. You don't have to join a gym and work out on a stair machine while staring at a 24-hour news channel, or join a competitive sports team—you only need to do that if that's what your heart is telling you to do. There are many options for movement. What you need is a sustainable form of it. It has to be fun and it has to work for your body given your physical state. If you're not moving your body regularly, you need to start identifying ways to do so that get your juices flowing. If you're moving your body regularly but experiencing pain or finding it hard to motivate yourself, then your form of movement has to change.

No matter how many calories or how much fat it burns, how good it is for your heart, or how much muscle it builds, if the way you're moving is not something you enjoy, you're eventually going to run out of willpower to force yourself to do it. The more stress you're under, the more quickly you deplete your willpower reserves. Kelly McGonigal, Ph.D., author of *The Willpower Instinct: How Self-Control Works, Why It Matters, and What You Can Do to Get More of It* (Avery, 2011), has written extensively on willpower being a limited resource that has to be replenished regularly.[2] It's when you're the most stressed out and pressed for time that you most need to have fun moving your body. So let's throw out the word *exercise* altogether and talk instead about how you are going to move your body joyously, like the divine goddess you are.

THE PLAYFUL, DANCING GODDESS

As I've already mentioned, one of the ways that I and millions of other women love to move joyously is through dance. In the U.S. when I was growing up, a girl just didn't ask a boy to dance, which meant most girls did everything they could to signal to a boy, "Pick me!" A friend of mine remembers the joy of growing up in a place where the girls gave up on the boys who weren't into dancing and simply danced with each other, with no social stigma. She has a middle school–age son whose experience is very different. He says at his school dances, the girls ask the boys; it's the boys who wait to be asked. The fact is that many of us need to leave behind the strict ideas we grew up with about how men and women dance, along with the fear of being judged.

Dance is a part of every culture around the world. It's the way we connect with our pelvic bowl, which is why the power structure in a dominator society tries to control who dances and how they dance. When we allow our bodies to dance with wild abandon and joy, we nourish our spirits and help our brains and hearts experience optimum health. In my tango group, we've given up on all those rules about who gets to dance. Everyone dances with everyone—men with men, women with women, men with women. We don't assign roles by gender or height. Some women have awful memories of getting stuck always having to lead in partner dancing in classes simply because they were on the tall side, and they don't want to repeat that experience—so we don't make them. We just dance.

Dancing is good for your brain and cognition. A major longitudinal study of people over age 75, conducted over a period of 21 years by the Albert Einstein College of Medicine in New York City, looked at whether activities from playing cards to swimming to doing housework affected cognitive ability. Almost none of the physical activities had any effect on dementia rates except for one: partner dancing, which lowered the risk by 76 percent. No other activity came anywhere near being as effective at protecting people from cognitive decline![3]

Let's look at why that is. For one thing, it's fun to dance if you're not afraid of people judging you or of being imperfect. And we've established that joyous living is good for brain chemistry. Also, dance, especially with partners, is a way of moving that's both creative and responsive. If your partner suddenly cues you to dip or twirl, you have to quickly adjust your own movements. Studies on dance and cognitive abilities suggest it's the need to make rapid decisions while dancing with a partner that makes it so effective in keeping our brains sharp. Learning new moves supports the health of the hippocampus, a structure in the brain associated with learning and memory that becomes damaged when you have Alzheimer's. So when it comes to dance, going through the motions of sequences you've already mastered won't cut it; you have to move in novel ways. In other words, go ahead and do "the Robot," but don't do it robotically—be spontaneous with your moves, and do it with a partner![4]

Dance is also social, and we know sociability is health protective. Researcher Patricia McKinley of McGill University in Montreal has found that Argentine tango in particular helps with sociability and mobility.[5] Dance also helps with balance and co-ordination, which often falter with advancing age. This happens in part because we stop moving in new ways and in part because of the accumulation of dense fascia, which builds up over time when muscles are used in limited ways. When balance deteriorates, people often walk staring at their feet to prevent tripping. You don't want to end up doing this. There are many ways, including dance, to regain good balance as well as coordination. Argentine tango is particularly good for all these skills.[6]

More and more, video games are starting to simulate dancing, including dancing with partners, although the spontaneity and physical touch aren't there as they are in real dancing. They can be a part of your joyous movement mix, especially if you use them with other people. Make them part of family life. Bring them out when you've got friends over. Play some music to get yourself moving. Music inspires us to move our bodies pleasurably. With some pieces, you might feel the need to sway your hips, while others might get you doing specific dance moves that work out your arms, neck, lower back, and so on. Check out some online videos of people dancing in different eras and remind yourself of all the ways you've moved your body and could move it again.

MOVEMENT FROM AND FOR THE HEART

Although your brain uses more energy than any other organ in your body, it's your heart that's the biggest generator of electromagnetic activity. Move your body and your blood and fluids circulate, your heart muscle is worked out, and you get into shape and foster heart health—that's the idea behind aerobic exercise. But the heart is more than just a self-propelled muscle the size of your fist. Your heart is the center of your emotional expression, and what it sends out can be felt by those around you. And this is most likely why partner dancing is so effective at maintaining physical prowess. It is quite literally two hearts in two different bodies, moving as one. Twice the joy. Twice the pleasure. And, I admit it, twice the vulnerability when you're first learning.

You've heard the phrases "Her heart just wasn't in it" and "She's all heart." Our hearts thrive when they're not being controlled by others. And they're powered by Divine Love, the most powerful healing force in the world. Say this regularly: "Divine Love manifests in my heart now."

One of the more sustainable ways to get movement is to make it heart centered. Move to music you love, as in the dance we've just discussed. Exercise in nature can open your heart chakra, making it easier to get out and move. In the summer, I love to take my yoga mat out onto the back lawn and do Pilates under the oak trees overlooking the tidal river there. Find a movement partner or a group of people willing to bicycle with you, hike with you, or play golf with you so that the activity is social and enjoyable. Take a class with a friend. And honor what makes you happy and what doesn't. I'll hike a steep mountain trail as long as I don't have to spend the night in a tent, sleeping on a surface that doesn't support my bones and joints the way I like them supported. A woman I know says she "doesn't do mosquitos," so she does outdoor exercise at times other than dawn and dusk in the summer when the mosquitos are most active. Whatever it takes to get your heart pumping with excitement and full of the joy of movement, go for it and don't apologize to anyone. And while you're at it, give yourself permission to spend money on exercise gear that makes you feel strong and like a "real" cyclist or dancer if that helps you emotionally connect to the activity.

Movement doesn't have to be confined to long, scheduled sessions. Move your body throughout the day, whether it's taking a little dance break or lifting some free weights or doing some stretches or yoga moves while you're watching television. A mini-trampoline, also known as a rebounder, is great for getting weight-bearing exercise and getting your lymph fluids flowing. It also applies g-forces to your whole body with minimal impact on your joints, making it very effective for combating the effects of "weightlessness"—sitting. You can get one with a handle for stability if you like. When I was pregnant with my second daughter, I regularly danced on the rebounder to Donna Summer singing disco songs. I got a good, safe aerobic workout, and a daughter who came out of the womb loving dance and movement!

You can also swim, which is a marvelous way to reconnect with your breath and with water. Swimming in a natural body of water is ideal. Failing that, you can try to find a pool that's cleansed not by harsh chlorine but by ionization or salt. Make swimming a delightful sensory experience if you can. Swim in the sunlight, with music playing over the pool's loudspeakers, or just enjoy the sound of your body moving in the water, the seagulls overhead, and the far-off chatter of people on the beach. In some spiritual traditions, water represents deep emotion and the mother force. In fact, goddesses were often associated with rivers and lakes. Swim laps if you like, but also dive in and out of waves, do somersaults and handstands, and frolic like a fish or dolphin in the mother energy of the water. In this way, your whole body gets movement. And if you touch the earth by doing handstands or stepping on the floor of the ocean, lake, or river, you are grounding yourself on Mother Earth. Even walking on the beach, especially if you do it barefoot, and looking out across the water at the horizon can be very calming and an enjoyable form of movement.

In fact, walking is a great way to move if it feels good to your body. There's nothing like a good walk with friends, talking and laughing and looking at the scenery—and walking alone can clear your head and put you back in touch with your body and spirit. Paul Dudley White, the famous Boston cardiologist who brought the first electrocardiogram (EKG) to the United States, used to walk and bike along the banks of the Charles River in Boston regularly. He was fond of saying that he had two physicians: his right leg and his left. I couldn't agree more. On average, regular exercise adds seven healthy years to your life. So when someone tells me she doesn't have time to exercise, I always reply that being dead seven years prematurely really eats up a lot of time too!

FASCIA FACTS

One of the most amazing innovators when it comes to the integration of movement, muscles, mind, body, and spirit is Bob Cooley, author of *The Genius of Flexibility: The Smart Way to Stretch and Strengthen Your Body* (Touchstone, 2005). After being hit by a car going 70 miles an hour while he was crossing the street, Bob suffered a broken pelvis and many other injuries as well. The usual physical therapy, massage, and orthopedic surgery didn't help, even though Bob already had a background in anatomy, physiology, and biomechanics. It was through his own experience of trying to get comfortable in his hurting body that he discovered how to change fascial patterns in the body through resistance stretching.

Fascia is a dense material that surrounds our tissues and muscles in a secondary nervous system that links all our organs and muscles in a seamless web. The fascia is where we store all of our traumas, whether physical, mental, or spiritual. These traumas all create thickened, dense fascia, which impedes full functioning and causes aches and pains we mistakenly believe are a normal part of aging. John Barnes, a physical therapist and pioneer in myofascial release therapy, points out that restrictions in the fascial structures of our bodies—which do not show up on X-rays, MRIs, or any standard medical tests—can exert up to 2,000 pounds of pressure per square inch on pain-sensitive structures in the body. In fact, I've come to believe that most of the muscle and joint restrictions we associate with aging are nothing more than dense fascia that needs stretching!

Bob discovered that he could actually lengthen and contract a muscle at the same time. In this way, he could remove the dense fascia from an injured muscle so that the muscle could shorten as it should. The result is a muscle that functions optimally through its full range. Each of us can do the same thing!

Here's how you can experience what it feels like to stretch your fascia: Start with a cat stretch. Kneel down on all fours. Now arch your back and tense your arms just like a cat that has just gotten up from a nap. Repeat six to ten times. Here's another: Lie down on the floor. Bring your knees to your chest and lift your head and chest. Pull your thighs into your chest with hands behind your thighs. Kick your legs away from your chest while resisting the kick with the hands on the back of your thighs. Notice how this feels in the small of your back. You can also use resistance while doing yoga poses, tensing your muscles to get a better stretch. You'll be able to feel the areas where you have dense fascia. It will feel tight and restricted and maybe a little painful. If you mindfully tense your muscles and stretch, you will soon find that you can move in new, freer patterns. And as you tense your muscles and stretch them in these planes over time, you'll see that the dense fascia remodels. The only way to make muscles more flexible is to learn how to stretch them at the same time you're contracting them, thus breaking up dense fascial patterns. Notice that animals do this all the time!

Bob Cooley trained Olympic swimmer Dara Torres, who won three silver medals in the 2008 Beijing games—at age 41, making her the oldest swimmer ever to compete in the Olympics. Now that is an ageless woman! Cooley has also worked with many other athletes, including speed skater Eric Flaim. But the real genius of his Resistance Flexibility work is that using it to change fascial structures is the key to ageless flexibility in body, mind, and spirit. Though there are many systems that address the fascia, including Yamuna Body Rolling and myofascial release techniques, Cooley's is the fastest and most effective method I've ever worked with.

Resistance Flexibility, or Cooley Yoga, has to be experienced to be understood (which, as you've learned, is true of the pelvic floor muscles too—those make up another important internal structure that most of us can't feel without some direction). Resistance stretching, unlike passive manipulation of the fascia by another person, is active and you can do it yourself. It works your fascia by shredding it as you would shred cotton candy or steel wool to stretch it—and you have to do this with your full attention and strength. Now, "shredding" your fascia may sound painful and damaging, but it's not, because you don't have nerve endings in these structures. In fact, if your fascia is dense and tight and in need of shredding, it can *cause* chronic pain. The pain is experienced not in the area of the dense fascia but in the muscle group that opposes it. Yes, your muscles can become fatigued in stretching and contracting them simultaneously, but the fatigue and pain won't be intolerable if you go slowly and pay attention to your body's signals. You can do this yourself following Bob Cooley's program as outlined in his book or go to his website to learn more: www.thegeniusofflexiblity.com. And if you're really serious, I highly recommend undergoing some assisted stretching from one of Cooley's elite trainers, whom you can reach via the website.

Earlier I explained how working certain pelvic floor muscles and not others can be a problem because it results in the opposing muscles being underdeveloped. It's the same idea with resistance training. You want to work the complementary muscle groups. Think about your calf muscles: If you're used to walking in high heels, your calf muscles have become shortened because they're used to being in a contracted position. As a result, walking in flats can be uncomfortable. Of course, the opposite is true too: if you're used to flats, it's hard to balance when you're wearing high heels, and you'll feel uncomfortable contracting your calf muscles to walk in them. The ideal is to have *all* your muscles strong, flexible, long, and supporting each other. That's what you can achieve with Resistance Flexibility.

Yoga, tai chi, qi gong, and other martial arts, along with Pilates, are other whole-body movement disciplines I recommend. But if you add resistance stretching to your movements, as explained by Cooley, you're less likely to become injured by too much stretching without resistance to balance it. I have met one too many yoga instructors who needed a hip replacement. If you have naturally flexible joints, you're likely to overstretch your joints doing yoga, and injury occurs when the body creates dense fascia in the joint capsule to protect it after it has been overstretched. Over time, this can result in all kinds of joint problems. You want to stretch your muscles and fascia, not your joints.

After doing a series of assisted stretching sessions with Bob and his trainers, I now have a series of stretches I do daily to maintain the changes in my body I've experienced from his program: improved sleep, much better digestion, a flatter abdomen, improved breathing and stamina during exercise, and an en-hanced sense of well-being and body confidence. This kind of training simply removes the blocks to the optimal functioning of the body. Hence, Bob calls it "training that leaves no residue." You naturally stand up straight and breathe fully as the body was designed to do. You don't need to think about it and "will" your-self to do it. And there's something else that happens with this work. I feel as though I'm a new person—emotionally, mentally, spiritually—as though I'm now living the life I'm meant to live, in the body I was always meant to have.

MOVEMENT FOR HEALTHY BONES

Any movement that puts healthy stress on your muscles and tendons supports your bones in several ways. Pilates can keep your bones aligned properly, and two 40-minute sessions of weight-bearing exercise a week can prevent osteoporosis because of the pressure your bones experience. Bob Cooley's Resistance Flexibility will do the same thing, as will yoga because it in-corporates stretching with muscle contraction. Miriam Nelson, Ph.D., director of the John Hancock Research Center on Physical Activity, Nutrition, and Obesity Prevention at Tufts University and author of *Strong Women, Strong Bones* (Perigee, 2006), has said that high-impact aerobic exercise (think hiking, climbing, and jumping) builds healthy bones. However, do these move-ments in moderation. Listen to your bones, joints, and ligaments. Don't try to conquer your body and force it to do a certain num-ber of jumping jacks, or push yourself to hike if it doesn't feel right in your bones. Work in harmony with your body. It's not that you're too old to move "that way"; you just have to be in tune with your body and listen to it when it says, "Enough of that movement for now—I need rest." What it might be saying, too, is "Shred my fascia!" Getting older doesn't mean deterioration, but it does mean that you have to pay attention to the wisdom of your bones and tissues, not your preconceived notions about how you're supposed to move at a certain age. Bones are designed to be flexible and regenerate for a lifetime. And remember that every structure in your body has to be subjected to the forces of gravity to continue to function well. Enough sitting! Just standing up regularly and doing tasks around the house can help you reap extraordinary benefits.

Speaking of bones, keep in mind that we've been oversold on the risks of calcium deficiency. It's usually not that we're calcium deficient so much as deficient in the nutrients that help us use the calcium in our diets. Take regular Epsom salt baths, which contain magnesium sulfate, or magnesium supplements. One of my favorites is CALM magnesium supplement, which comes as a drink containing magnesium citrate. Calcium and magnesium need to be present in amounts that are balanced. I strongly recommend that you avoid drugs that protect against osteoporosis, such as Fosamax. They can result in bones that are so dense and brittle that blood can no longer get into them and remodel them.[7] Hence, women on these drugs have an increased risk for needing root canal work or suffering hip fractures in the mid-femur that don't heal.[8]

Bones and connective tissue form our skeletons, but we also each have an energetic cytoskeleton that runs through our fascia, where the wiring of our secondary nervous system is. This energy field connects back to the heart and its strong electromagnetic field. And every energy meridian you have running along your fascia is connected to a major organ system. When you work with your muscles, fascia, and connective tissue to affect the energy flow along that meridian, you bring energy and health into the corresponding organ system. According to traditional Chinese medicine (TCM), bone health is governed by the kidneys, where chi is stored. The kidneys keep your blood clean and your bone marrow healthy and flowing. When your fascial tissue is well hydrated and you do stretches related to the kidney meridian, it helps your bones stay healthy.

Keep in mind that when you try to get flexible by focusing on a particular muscle without simultaneously engaging its corresponding muscle, you put too much pressure on the joints. If you're feeling muscular pain in your body, pay attention to the set of muscles opposite those where you're experiencing discomfort. Restricted pectoral muscles, which are common in people who have desk jobs, cause hunched shoulders and upper back and neck pain. You have to work on both sets of muscles, the pectoral and the neck and upper back muscles, to get relief. Fortunately, relief can happen quickly if you use a holistic approach that addresses all the muscles involved as well as the fascia. For 30 years I had discomfort and inflexibility in my right hip whenever I had been sitting for a long time. The problem lessened considerably when I started to do Pilates. In fact, without Pilates, I fear that I would have had a right hip replacement by now. That right hip got completely fine-tuned and back to normal after three or four sessions with one of Bob Cooley's trainers because the resistance stretching broke up the remaining dense fascia and lengthened and stretched all the muscles involved. Cooley also points out that almost all back pain and disc problems are due to the inability of the hamstring muscles to optimally shorten because of dense fascia. Stretching the hamstrings takes care of the real problem and removes the strain from the vertebrae in the back.

MAKE PEACE WITH YOUR WEIGHT

If you're worrying about not doing enough exercise to lose weight, or you're doing it mostly because you haven't made peace with your body, it's time to let that go. Love your body enough to move it the way it calls to you to be moved—don't try to browbeat it into submission so that you can regain the figure you had at 17. We've all been to the gym and seen women built like fireplugs sweating on the treadmill or doing decathlons yet not losing weight. If you don't change your diet and get your cortisol levels under control, no amount of exercise will help you lose weight. And if you've been dieting for much of your life, your body may simply say to you, "That's it. I'm done."

Several times in the past, I went on a 500-calorie-a-day diet for almost a month and lost a mere two pounds. When this happened for a fourth time, it marked my final attempt to force my body into submission. I couldn't believe that it was possible to restrict my food that much and not see the scale budge. "Calories in, calories out" as a theory for how to lose weight is dead wrong. Your metabolism shifts as your level of stress hormones becomes chronically high, and your extra weight wins. That's not to say you can't jump-start your metabolism, but focusing on diet and exercise as you've been told to do all your life is a very limited and inefficient way to do it. A friend of mine has a Ph.D. in exercise physiology and, like me, she did that strict 500-calorie-a-day program with no results. Then she left her house and kids for a couple of months to go on a trip she'd been anticipating eagerly for a long time—and lost 25 pounds. You can lose five pounds overnight if you release grief you've been holding on to. The key is to love your body into permanent changes. That involves changing your old trauma patterns about your body.

When it came to making peace with my weight, the final piece of the puzzle was using the Emotional Freedom Techniques (EFT, commonly known as "tapping"). Tapping helped me uncover and release some old beliefs about my body, exercise, and diet that needed to go. Give it a try and see if it works for you.

Exercise: Tapping to Release Painful Emotions and Beliefs about Food and Your Weight

Tapping, also known as the Emotional Freedom Techniques (EFT), releases the emotions bound up in your beliefs about yourself. You can use it to help you loosen up and discard old beliefs and feelings about anything. Research has shown that tapping reduces stress hormone levels by an average of 24 percent, with some subjects showing a drop of as much as 50 percent. Just ten minutes a day of tapping can increase your body confidence and end your battle with food. I learned tapping from Jessica Ortner, author of *The Tapping Solution for Weight Loss & Body Confidence*, in the weeks leading up to the photo shoot for the cover of this book—a time when I usually would have started starving myself to fit into the clothes I wanted to wear. The tapping allowed me to uncover a long-buried belief that getting my body into the shape I wanted was going to be grueling and hard, like climbing a mountain with a heavy backpack (which

I did in my childhood far more than was enjoyable). Tapping while recounting that memory of physical struggle and speaking about it really helped me overcome a program that had been going on in my body for years—namely, that I had to fight and starve and push myself as the only way to lose weight! I did not go on a diet before that photo shoot. And when the day came, I enjoyed myself thoroughly and felt very confident. I highly recommend checking out the videos Jess has created to see a demonstration of the technique, in which you tap your middle two fingertips rapidly on acupressure points on your body while acknowledging your true emotions, and then instill new beliefs by tapping while reciting positive affirmations about loving yourself.

You can watch Jessica explain the technique at www.TheTappingSolution.com. Then go to www.TheTappingSolution.com/Goddesses to find a tapping meditation she created exclusively for readers of this book, designed to address issues related to food and your weight.

THE TIME IS NOW

It's never too late to transform the old, outmoded beliefs about your body that have been keeping you stuck for years and replace them with updated ones while becoming stronger, more agile, and more movement oriented. The mother-in-law of a friend of mine never exercised after playing college tennis in her teens and 20s. When she had a hip replacement in her 90s, she took a look at the physical therapy exercises she was supposed to do to rehabilitate her muscles and said to her daughter-in-law, "I'm not doing these." Her daughter-in-law told her frankly, "If you fall, I can't pick you up. So you might be on the floor for some time and you might even die there. Can you live with that?" And the woman said, "Yes." So be it! Know the consequences of your choices about movement.

If you find your balance isn't what it used to be, you can't keep up with your grandchildren, or you bow out of social activities because of the amount or type of movement involved, decide whether you're okay with that. There's no age limit for flexibility or fitness. Research has clearly shown that people in their 90s can build muscle and improve balance and flexibility. Don't buy into the cultural myths about what you can do at a certain age. *Do* go slowly and respect your body's messages about what type of movement is right for it. You get to decide how, when, and how much you move. Healthy centenarians can be found doing tai chi in the parks every morning. That can be you!

I go to Pilates class twice a week, walk a couple of miles three or four times a week, dance the tango, and do Resistance Flexibility regularly. I'm also doing something called Sprint 8 for cardiovascular fitness. It's a form of high-intensity interval exercise that is proving to be not just a timesaver but a way to boost metabolism. Using an exercise bike, a treadmill, or an elliptical trainer, or doing intervals of sprints and walking, you work out to your maximum intensity for 20 to 30 seconds, then move gently for 90 seconds, then repeat the sequence for a total of eight cycles. It only takes 20 minutes once or twice a week but leads to dramatic increases in growth hormone, and it's far more effective than an hour of regular aerobic activity. It also takes away the excuse "I don't have time to exercise." At first, I found myself gasping for breath when running on the elliptical as fast as I possibly could. But after a couple of weeks, my cardiovascular fitness increased dramatically, and Bob Cooley's resistance stretching made the movements easier than ever. (You can learn more about Sprint 8 and its benefits at http://fitness.mercola.com.)

Although I do enjoyable movement every day, I now find I'm unable to sit for long periods like I used to. Conventional wisdom would say that this is because of arthritis in the spine due to age, but that's not it. I'm more embodied than I have been since I was a child, and I can no longer disconnect from my body as I trained myself to do during college, medical school, and residency training. If I sit down to work at the computer, I find it very hard to sit there for more than 30 minutes before I have to take a movement break. I also sit on a yoga ball to keep my hips and spine mobile during the sitting time. Don't wait until your body screams at you to do this. Instead, take regular dance breaks and stretches—there are plenty of apps you can use to remind you. And if you have a cat that jumps onto your keyboard, interpret it as a sign from the universe that it's time for a movement break!

MANY BENEFITS OF MOVEMENT

An increasing amount of research is showing that regular exercise is brain protective (and as I mentioned earlier, partner dance is particularly good for this purpose). Exercise improves cognitive function in older people with or without Alzheimer's.[9] Two 20-minute periods of aerobic exercise weekly have also been shown to increase the size of the hippocampal memory area in people in their 60s.[10] Weight training has been shown to improve cognitive abilities in women in their 70s who had mild cognitive impairment, according to research done at the University of British Columbia.[11]

Be smart: Move your body, and when you find you're falling back into sedentary habits, self-correct. Love your body so that the changes you make in your movement routine are permanent, and so that your attitudes change and aren't overridden by old beliefs about conquering your weak body, or about certain types of movement being womanly or not womanly. Here's a prayer you can say: "Divine Beloved, please change me into someone who loves to move my body!" And consider those quintessentially feminine ways of moving that are part of belly dancing.

You may well find that emotions, memories, and thoughts stored in your fascia and muscles come up as you begin moving your body. Any massage or yoga teacher will tell you that it's common for people to burst into tears when certain fascial tissues are stretched or touched. Past trauma—and all the memories associated with it—are stored in fascia. If this happens, don't try to stop it. You'll be surprised at how often you end up laughing at the end of a good cry. Congratulate yourself for letting your old feelings and thoughts come up and out of you so that your body's self-healing processes could be turned on.

You might find that, as for many women, your beliefs about your body and how to move it are based on old ideas that you thought you had rid yourself of long ago. The shaming of women so prevalent in a dominator society can lodge itself deep in your tissues. So if any of these old shame patterns arise, know that you are right on track. When I was working with Tami Lynn Kent, a physical therapist who works with pelvic bowl energy, she "heard" my mother say, "I hate this part of my body" when she was working on the fascia of my left pelvic side wall. Together, we consciously released this old shame from my body. The shame wasn't even mine—it was my mother's—but I had been carrying it in my fascia for years.

Shame keeps a constant supply of inflammatory chemicals in the body. When you remove shame energetically, it feels as bad going out as it did when it went in. The discomfort is only temporary, however. And it bears repeating here that shame can't exist in an atmosphere of light, consciousness, and humor. It lurks only when it's kept secret. So if you find shameful memories coming up and out, talk about them. Air them. Take them into the sunshine of awareness. You'll feel ten pounds lighter. Release any old self-hatred and any fears that you aren't enough—beautiful enough, sexy enough, young enough, and so on. Instead, bring the vast, ageless energy of the Divine into your heart and your pelvic bowl. Move your hips and your whole body with sensual abandon. Dance like the goddess you are.

CHAPTER TEN

GODDESSES
ARE GORGEOUS

The sense of being perfectly well dressed gives a feeling of
inward tranquility which religion is powerless to bestow.

— RALPH WALDO EMERSON

A s I was leaving the bus station the other day, a stylish
woman with flowing long gray hair was hurrying up the
steps. I smiled at her with approval. *Ah—another ageless
beauty.* Over the past decade or so, I've made a habit of noticing—and really taking in—the beauty of women who are over
50. Here's what I've found. The more I look for ageless beauty,
the more I find it. Of course, there are the famous gorgeous goddesses: Helen Mirren, Meryl Streep, Jane Fonda, and Barbara
Walters, to name a few. But when you decide to pay attention,
you too will begin to notice more and more incredibly attractive
ageless beauties in your day-to-day life. Believe me, they are out
there, and you can be one of them.

You have to let go of the myth that to be beautiful, a woman has to be young. To be beautiful, a woman needs to be youthful and supple in mind and spirit. Then she has inner beauty that radiates outward. As Tosha Silver says, "The true depth of your own value, beauty, and worthiness has already been conferred by the Divine. It is set. No one else's behavior or opinion can honestly *ever* minimize it. It's like clouds trying to eradicate the sun. It always reemerges."

UNCONSCIOUS PROGRAMMING ABOUT BEAUTY AND AGE

As I said at the start of the book, the first step to becoming an ageless goddess is to become aware of your cultural programming so that you can step out of it. For example, have you ever noticed how women's magazines tend to run stories on what to wear or how to style your hair based on your age? "Your Best Hair in Your 30s, 40s, and 50s" is a typical one. I have yet to see one that reads, "Your Best Hair in Your 60s, 70s, and 80s," nor have I ever seen men's style advice broken down according to age. Instead, a recent issue of *GQ* called the Style Bible had a headline on the cover that said, "Look Your Best in 2014"—period. The message is clear that we women are not supposed to care how we look after 60 or so and that our age determines what our style should be.

Mindfulness expert Dr. Ellen Langer suggests changing your "priming," that is, your expectation of what you are supposed to experience as time goes by. I want you to forget about which hairstyles are appropriate "for women over 40." Rejecting this sort of priming helps you feel beautiful as you enter your ageless years.

Yes, I'm fully aware of the ageism all around us. In the editorial from *AARP: The Magazine* I mentioned earlier entitled "The Smart Money Is on the 50+ Crowd," editor Robert Love writes, "Older Americans are virtually ignored by marketers mired in last century's obsession with youth. In fact, only 5 percent of advertising is directed at older consumers, according to Nielsen, which has been tracking Americans' habits for decades.

It's insulting. As veteran ad man Bob Hoffman put it recently, 'Almost everyone you see in a car commercial is between the ages of 18 and 24. And yet, people age 75 to dead buy five times as many new cars as people 18 to 24.' Nielsen calls people 50 and up 'the most valuable generation in the history of marketing.'" I personally see this as a huge opportunity to turn ageism right on its head. So I, for one, am no longer buying into the ageism agenda. And I hope you'll join me. After all, I was part of the strike generation. Why not keep that new energy going? The baby boom generation has changed every stage of life it has gone through. Watch us change this one!

It's also true that as women get into their ageless years, it's often hard for them to accept their changing looks, especially if they've been used to heads turning when they enter a room. It's a real loss if you've never developed a true inner sense of self and all the gifts of wit and wisdom that come with the years. For those of us who never had that "turning heads" experience in our youth, the transition to a new kind of beauty is often not as difficult. That's especially true when you've developed "centenarian consciousness" and believe that your best years are all ahead! To do this, we must change our thoughts and beliefs. The nuns' study and studies by researchers such as Becca Levy that I've mentioned have proved beyond a shadow of a doubt that acting as though we are in our prime has a huge impact on our health and physical appearance—so pay attention to your self-talk! In our ageist culture, even 25-year-olds worry about one gray hair or a laugh line that you can see if you position yourself just so in front of a magnifying mirror. Women reaching 30, which is probably our first shared cultural portal about beauty in the West, can start panicking about looking old. But what if you had no notion of what you're "supposed" to look like on any milestone birthday? Forget the number of candles you're "supposed" to put on your cake and your notions of beauty can change.

Instead of fretting about your age, make an empowering change such as quitting a job that's draining you and making you feel disrespected. This alone can make you look healthier and younger almost instantly. You might find people asking you if you "had something done" (as in plastic surgery) after you've walked away from a stressful, overly demanding job. And there's nothing more beautiful than deep contentment and happiness, the kind of happiness that comes only when you have connected with the ageless goddess within. When you're a happy, joyful, ageless goddess, people see you in a different light. They aren't noticing the lines in your face or the skin on your neck. They're seeing your sparkling eyes as you laugh.

OWNING YOUR BEAUTY

An ageless goddess rejects ageism and owns her beauty. One way you can do that is to acknowledge it through affirmations or a Divine Beloved Change Me prayer, such as "Divine Beloved, change me into someone who sees, appreciates, and cultivates my own beauty."

Another way to own your beauty is to adorn it in your own personal style. Don't think of clothes as "fixing" a "figure flaw" but as flattering you and bringing out your natural beauty. Spend money on clothes that make you feel beautiful. How a jacket or dress is cut can make a huge difference in how you feel in an outfit. A friend of mine jokes that at 50 she dresses pretty much the same as she did in the second grade: turtleneck or simple long- or short-sleeve shirt or sweater, jeans or trousers, and flat black shoes. The look works for her and she is happy sticking to it. But now she's meticulous about choosing the cut, color, and style of every item in that simple list. She can spot in an instant whether an item is even worthy of trying on her Aphrodite body. And she feels great and is often complimented on her looks and style. Where she sometimes gets daring is with jewelry and lipstick. She says, "I take chances with accessories or makeup when I feel like it, not because I'm trying to please other people and be trendy and fashionable. When I was younger, my look said, 'I can fit in and be anything you need me to be.' Now my look is classic *me*." She doesn't worry about whether her look is trendy, or "too young," "too old," "too conservative," or "too" anything else.

As Shirley MacLaine has said, "I don't think you go out of style when you're living in the present most of the time." Don't be embarrassed about developing a style that's right for you right now—and asking someone to help you if that's what you need. Agelessness means being daring and courageous, so take some chances. I know this can be hard to do because we live in a shaming culture, but don't give in to other people's limited ideas about how you should dress or style your hair. If you want to keep your hair long, go for it. If you want to dye it purple, don't let anyone stop you. If you're a bold lipstick kind of woman, choose a shade that can be seen across a room. Do you love stilettos? Find yourself a pair that's five inches high, and develop the muscles in your feet and ankles so that you can wear them proudly and skillfully—at least for an hour or so. And if you want to get your eyes done or have a facelift, go for that too. That is how an ageless goddess owns her beauty—no shaming, no apologies.

And if you don't know who you are in terms of your personal style, use adornment to help you figure it out. Push yourself out of your comfort zone and see how it feels to own a new way of doing your makeup (or going without), a new way of dressing (or merely tweaking the way you have always dressed), or a new way of styling your hair.

Is your appearance highly valued in your line of business? If so, I encourage you to invest in hiring a personal stylist. A good one will help you own your beauty rather than try to pressure you to dress a certain way because "everyone's wearing this now." It's completely worth the money to find clothing that works for you and makes you feel beautiful and confident. Some women just have the gift of personal style, but for those of us who don't, a hired advisor—or a good friend who has the gift—is a marvelous thing. When you work in the public eye, it's especially important to let go of any fear of asking for help in this area. That said, if someone tells you that you shouldn't wear something, but it feels right when you put it on and you like how it looks, don't take her advice.

Do you have self-nurturing beauty rituals? I don't wear a lot of makeup on a typical day, but I do get a blowout at a salon every Friday. It's a beauty ritual that says, "Bring on the weekend!" and makes me feel like a goddess. I mentioned the benefits of massage earlier, and it can be a marvelous beauty ritual too. So can facials, manicures, and pedicures. If you don't have a lot of money, do it yourself at home or with your daughters, grand-daughters, or girlfriends. Go to a spa or a beauty school. I like the new Shellac manicures done with UV light that last for a couple of weeks. Something as small as having lovely nails, or glowing skin after a facial, can boost your confidence too. It can be fun to choose outrageous colors or match them to an outfit that flatters you. If you don't want color, you can get a manicure and get clear polish or no nail polish at all, and enjoy the sensation of warm paraffin on your hands and a hand massage.

If the very idea of self-nurturing beauty rituals feels uncomfortable for you, think about why that is. There's nothing wrong with wanting to be pampered and owning the fact that you are a beautiful, ageless goddess.

One very specific way to "own" your beauty is to invest in glamour or boudoir photography. The photographers who specialize in these services are often women who genuinely want to help other women reclaim their confidence in their attractiveness. A good photographer will do her best to put you at ease so you don't look stiff and uncomfortable and will adjust lighting, props, and your positioning to make you look great. She can help you come up with flattering poses, but if you do an Internet search, you can find plenty of ideas too. Having a good music soundtrack during a photo session and friends to make you laugh also really helps. When you're relaxed, it's easier to own your beauty and prevent any negative self-talk about not being attractive. Let go and feel like a gorgeous goddess posing for the camera. Also, a photographer told me to have someone make you laugh, or to think of something funny, just before the shutter is snapped. The best photographs capture your genuine emotion. There's a huge difference between a forced smile and a genuine one.

Even if you're sticking to snapshots rather than professional photos, keep in mind that a few tricks can enhance what you look like. Remember the Hollywood actress tip of paying attention to lighting: natural lighting or soft, full-spectrum lighting indoors is very flattering. The light at dusk is so forgiving that photographers sometimes call this part of the day "the magic hour." In the days before cosmetic surgery, Botox, fillers, and collagen boosters, Hollywood actresses like Bette Davis insisted on having control over who set up the lighting for a movie—or even for a personal appearance. Davis could even tell when one of the many lightbulbs on a movie set had popped because she was meticulous about how she looked on camera. You don't have to go as far as hiring a lighting designer to follow you around, but you can be more conscious about lighting and how you appear in photographs and video.

Once I was having some old slides scanned and made into digital files, and I found a picture of me on my honeymoon. I was stunned by the beautiful young woman smiling into the camera—I mean, really stunned. Back then I thought I was too fat and not all that attractive. I had been ignorant enough about my worth to have asked the man I married what he thought about my weight. His reply? "You could stand to lose five pounds." I weighed 125 pounds, a weight I most likely will never come close to again. It's amazing to me that I feel more attractive and happy now than I ever did back them. What a relief! Have you had a similar experience of having your insecurities solidified by the people around you? It's so common! That's why I want you to take the following pledge. Raise your right hand and say the following aloud: "I promise to never, ever, ever doubt my own attractiveness and worth again. And I will never again ask anyone what he or she thinks about my weight, or whether he or she thinks I look fat in an outfit." If you've gained weight, what's important is whether it's healthy weight for you, not whether it makes you look different than you did in your 20s. *Of course* you look different! You're an ageless beauty now. Own it without apology.

MY EDUCATION IN THE ART OF ADORNMENT

Years ago, I did a lecture at the famous Chautauqua Institution that was carried on NPR. A couple of television producers in Chicago heard the lecture and wanted to put me on a show, but said they needed to see photos of me first. As they put it, "We had to find out what you look like. Television is, after all, a visual medium."

Thus began my education in the art of makeup, clothing, and appearance—and all the tricks of looking better. Until then, I had never even had a professional manicure or pedicure, let alone professionally done hair, makeup, or styling. It never occurred to me that my nails could be seen on television. I do a lot of public speaking and appearances now, and over the years I've become well aware that "the medium is the message," so I take a lot of care with my clothing and appearance. Once that's taken care of, then I can forget about how I look and just deliver my message. But I know that the two are inextricably linked. And instead of resenting that I have to dress up and make up for the camera, I accept this as part of my work and I take pleasure in it.

For much of my life, I paid no attention to my looks. My natural love of clothing and beauty was deep-sixed by my medical training. I couldn't even see myself as an attractive woman on any level. Luckily, when I needed to do something about my appearance and style, I attracted a lot of help, especially from gay men! A while back, while speaking in the Cape Cod area, I stopped into a local hair salon in Provincetown. A hairdresser told me, straight out, "Honey, your hair is doing nothing for you." He suggested that with my fine hair and facial features, I needed something called an "A-line bob." Who knew? Clearly, he did. He gave me the best haircut I had ever had. Another time, when I had to buy an outfit for a big TV appearance, Joseph, a sales clerk at a Boston boutique, put me in a dressing room and began to bring in outfits, many of which were way out of my comfort zone. The stilettos in particular were a stretch. When he saw my uncertainty about wearing an item that was blatantly sexy, he told me to "get used to it." Another time, when I was visiting a friend in Boca Raton, Florida, I went into a high-end department store with her and tried on a designer black dress and heels. She told me I looked fabulous, but I couldn't see it. I was afraid that my friends and family would make fun of me for daring to wear anything that stylish or sexy. We often don't see ourselves in our finest light, so we need others who can reflect our beauty back to us and remind us we're gorgeous goddesses.

That said, some of our closest associates will actually work to keep us down when we begin to upgrade our looks, because they feel threatened by our beauty in a dominator culture where women are supposed to compete with each other in the realm of physical appearance. This is known as the "crabs in a bucket" syndrome. When one crab starts climbing over the top of the bucket, the others will drag it back down. If you're in a bucket with a bunch of crabs dragging you back down, get a new bucket. If you, like the old me, are worried about what your friends will say when you suddenly start to look better, that's a sure sign that you need a friend upgrade. We all need what I refer to as a "placenta of support"—women and men who uplift and nourish our expression of our best selves. Without that, it's hard to reject the cultural idea that we'll never be adequately pretty, and that we're always lacking somehow.

When I saw myself in my designer suit and stilettos on camera after that first PBS television show was taped, I realized that the outfit Joseph had chosen for me made me look not just serious and professional but stylish and even sexy too. I had to admit that the look worked for delivering my message. For years, I'd seen myself as a frumpy doctor, so the idea that I could be attractive in a daring way yet still be taken seriously was liberating. I had taken an important step toward becoming an ageless goddess.

I have had to learn to own my beauty and not feel awkward and insecure when I have to present myself in public or have a photo taken. The professional photo shoot for the cover of this book took an entire day, a clothing stylist, an amazing photographer and studio, and a skilled makeup artist. And I had a ball doing it. Why? Because I know how all that magic in magazines happens, and I enjoy being part of it. I arrived at the studio with wet hair and no makeup, had fun all day changing outfits and smiling for the camera, feeling confident and happy, and ended by hugging all the wonderful people involved.

Have you been afraid to step into new shoes—literally—or style your hair differently? When was the last time you let yourself take chances with fashion, hair, or makeup? Give up the absurd expectation of perfection when it comes to your looks and have fun with adorning yourself. Claim your beauty, enhance it, and enjoy it. When you do, everyone benefits. And there are many healthy, natural, easy ways to do it that may not cost you a cent!

SECRETS FOR LOOKING FABULOUS AT ANY AGE

You don't have to invest a lot of money in clothes, hair, and makeup to feel good in your body if you expand your ideas about what constitutes beauty. What's most important is to feel beautiful, even if you don't match up with someone else's limited ideas about what's attractive. Remember, your ageless years are the time to give up for good your addiction to pleasing other people and focus instead on pleasing yourself. There are many simple things you can do to look better and boost your confidence in your beauty.

Ageless Hair

With hormonal changes, hair can change texture and color. You can use dye, wigs, extensions, and chemical or natural curlers or straighteners to change your hair if you don't like it, or you can come to love the way your hair looks and feels now. If your hair is breaking off easily, or not growing past a certain length, it could be that you're under a lot of stress or not eating and sleeping well. It could also be that your hair can't handle the amount of punishment it's taking. Consider taking a break from the chemicals and hairstyles that put stress on your hair follicles. You can also enhance your personal style with hats, scarves, or a radical short haircut. I always find that look really stunning!

If you're losing your hair, it may be because you have a hormonal imbalance, particularly one brought about by thyroid imbalance, too much sugar and insulin, and a lack of iodine. When you have too much dihydrotestosterone, or DHT, in your system (which results from a combination of too much insulin and too much estrogen), you may experience male pattern baldness and even some darker, heavier hair on your upper lip and chin. Very often, the problem is sugar in the diet, along with iodine deficiency. The hair follicles on the head have a receptor for testosterone, and when there is too much sugar in your system and not enough iodine, you end up with metabolites that fit in those receptors and shut down the testosterone-sensitive hair follicles. On your head, too much testosterone shuts down hair growth.

But on your face, the opposite is true. I have seen iodine supplementation restore hair—not to mention energy, breast health, and thyroid health—in many.

Shoe Beauty

For me, beautiful shoes are key to feeling good about how I look. High heels make a woman's legs appear longer, and the right pair can be incredibly sexy. In the Broadway show *Kinky Boots*, there's a whole song about how "sex is in the heel." Llorraine Neithardt of the radio show *Venus Unplugged* designs shoes as an offering to Aphrodite (you can see some of her designs at www.shoefineart.com). Her glamorous shoe designs were used in the movie *P.S. I Love You*. They capture the aesthetic of sexy shoes.

I am quite new to the allure of shoes, having been born with very wide feet and a condition called metatarsus adductus, in which the fronts of my feet turned in. When I was a child, they thought I had clubbed feet. However, cool shoes are now available in wider sizes than ever before, and the Internet has made it easier than ever to find shoes in a variety of sizes. For the first time in my life, I can actually find shoes that fit.

That said, I consider wearing high heels an "athletic" event. I can keep them on for about two hours, tops, which is long enough to dance the tango until I feel full of pleasure. No woman should wear heels all day long because they're awful for posture and pelvic health. Women's heels, worn constantly, keep podiatrists in business. If you enjoy heels, there are exercises you can use to keep your feet in good condition so they support you and make those problems less likely. One, which I learned from Pilates, is to roll the bottoms of your bare feet over tennis balls while you're sitting. After dancing, I always do a self-massage of my feet in the bathtub and a series of foot stretches and exercises while soaking in Epsom salts in the water. In fact, foot reflexology is, hands down, my favorite spa treatment. Do an Internet search for Pilates foot exercises. You'll discover some good techniques for keeping your feet flexible and pain free. Bunions can be stopped in their tracks or even reversed through these techniques. Try them before you consider surgery.

Ageless Skin

Whether it's the skin on your face or anywhere else, you can make it look younger by making it healthier. In fact, your skin is simply a reflection of your overall health. And that means that the things you do to maintain optimal heart health, for example, will also show up as radiant skin. I think by now you know that joy is a real beauty secret too.

Most skin damage is due to cellular inflammation caused by too much sugar and trans fats in the diet along with too much of the stress hormones cortisol and epinephrine. The levels of these hormones increase when you eat poorly, which interferes with the self-healing mechanisms of the body, including the mechanisms that keep skin looking healthy and vibrant. Quality sleep will improve your skin's health and appearance too. "Beauty" sleep is no joke. Everything is connected, so as you change your diet, combat stress by learning methods to relax deeply, breathe fully, release old resentments and anger, move your body joyously, laugh more, and replenish yourself with a good night's sleep most nights, you'll look and feel better in every way.

If you want your skin to be repaired and look better quickly, try this three-day nutritional facelift from Dr. Nick Perricone, author of *The Wrinkle Cure:* eat nothing but wild-caught salmon, watercress, blueberries, and cantaloupe for three days. All of these foods are rich in antioxidants and other micronutrients that will help heal your gut, reduce inflammation and oxidative stress, and contribute to glowing skin. In the long run, a low-sugar, nutrient-dense diet with healthy fats will also promote healthier skin. And if you have rosacea, you'll see it reduced when you clean up your diet because sugar and alcohol exacerbate the condition. My company A-ma-ta also makes a wonderful skin care line called Performance[3] that contains the herb *Pueraria mirifica,* which is known for its skin-enhancing effects.

The production of the collagen that provides the underlying structure of skin is reduced as we age, thanks to years of stress, poor diet, environmental toxins, and gravity. African Americans have the most hearty collagen-making ability. (I've heard Whoopi Goldberg say, "Black don't crack" with a smile, and yes, there's truth to that!) Asians have the next largest amount of collagen-making capacity, and then Caucasians, with blonde and red-headed women making the least.

Whatever your complexion, you can increase your body's ability to manufacture collagen that will make your skin healthier and younger looking. Eat a low-glycemic diet and take supplements such as vitamins C and D3. Skin care products with ingredients such as *Pueraria mirifica* can help prevent collagen breakdown. If you live in the northern hemisphere and are entering your ageless years, you probably need 5,000 IU of vitamin D3 in winter to keep your levels where they should be.

If your skin is discolored from sun damage, there are ways to reverse the damage. The most effective method is IPL, or intermittent pulse laser, a treatment you can get from a dermatologist or plastic surgeon. This procedure also works beautifully for spider veins. If you don't use it already, start using sunblock daily. It's often added to makeup, but don't forget to use it on your neck and chest, arms, ears, and other exposed areas as well.

Acne is often the result of a diet high in sugar, especially after the teen years. What's going on in your body can often be read on your face. You might find, for example, that consuming certain foods results in pimples in specific places. A friend of mine found that she broke out in the same place on her chin every time she drank diet cola. Pay attention and make the connection between what you're eating and what is going on with your facial skin. If you have hormonally related acne, detoxify your body nutritionally to balance your hormones.

If you're very uncomfortable with your skin's appearance, new types of cosmetic surgery and procedures you might want to consider are always becoming available. For example, I had a lot of spider veins on my cheeks that completely disappeared with IPL treatments. I get a treatment every six months. Work with an esthetician, dermatologist, or cosmetic surgeon who specializes in working on skin, but beware of the ones who start ticking off all the things you can change about your face. If you go in because you want to do something about the lines near your upper lip and you start hearing about every other part of your face or body that "could use a little work," walk out of the office. You don't need to feel pressured by an "expert" to suddenly see "flaws" in your appearance that never bothered you before.

The lines on your face represent the wisdom you've acquired. Don't get cosmetic procedures to try to look like you're 22— you'll just end up looking artificial. A woman once came up to me at a tango event and said, "Look at your daughter's skin! It's so beautiful! I wish I could still have skin like that—don't you?" And I thought, no. I spend no time wishing I could regain the skin or looks I had years ago. That's because I feel better and more confident now than I ever did at 18, or even at 45! Let divine energy flow through your body and you'll look vibrant at any age, whether or not you decide to have plastic surgery, get laser treatments, or let your hair go gray. You get to decide.

An Ageless Smile

As a dentist's daughter, I know that you can tell the state of someone's health by looking in her mouth. Our teeth naturally fade from a bright white to a more ivory tone as we age, but it's possible to whiten teeth somewhat through peroxide treatments at home or at a dentist's office. As you enter your ageless years, you might want to think about doing the dental procedures that will give you a better smile that you've put off because it felt frivolous to invest in your own beauty. Veneers, caps, and whitening can all make you feel more confident as you smile.

Whatever your age, good dental care prevents you from experiencing gingivitis that can lead to periodontal disease and tooth loss. It's important to stay on top of dental hygiene because periodontal disease puts you at higher risk for heart disease and diabetes. The bacteria that build up in your mouth enter your bloodstream through your gums, causing inflammation. Take the time to floss and stimulate your gums, and get cleanings regularly. Don't bathe your teeth in sugar by snacking throughout the day—and drinking coffee or tea with milk counts as snacking.

Milk and cream, of course, have sugar (though cream has less), and constantly drinking any beverage with sugar in it contributes to tooth decay as well as the buildup of bacteria. To reduce bacteria in the mouth, you can use a technique called oil pulling: put a spoonful of coconut oil in your mouth and pull and push it through your teeth, using your tongue, for about 20 minutes a day. You can also reduce bacteria by brushing with red clay. If you like to chew gum, choose a gum with xylitol, which has been shown to reduce tooth decay.

Teeth, like bones, require calcium, magnesium, boron, and other trace minerals to be strong and healthy. But again, it's usually not a calcium deficiency that causes problems so much as a lack of magnesium to help you use the calcium in your diet. Osteoporosis usually begins in the jawbone and can be spotted by a dentist long before you're at risk for a broken hip. As I said earlier, I don't recommend drugs such as Fosamax for treating osteoporosis because they make bones denser and impede circulation to the roots of the teeth, leading to the need for root canals.

Ultimately, the most beautiful smile is one that's genuine. It is an expression of sheer pleasure that comes from the heart. As you let go of constricting ideas about beauty and the cultural shaming that affects almost all women, your smile will come more easily. You'll laugh heartily, without fearing that someone might think you're too brassy or that you shouldn't draw attention to yourself. You won't care about what anyone has to say regarding your personal style because you will have owned that you are a gorgeous, powerful, and ageless goddess—an expression of the life force that can't contain its joy. That is your birthright. Claim it and celebrate it and you'll be ageless!

CHAPTER ELEVEN

GODDESSES EMBODY THE DIVINE

The strongest, surest way to the soul is through the flesh.

— Mabel Dodge Luhan

In *Riding Giants,* a documentary about big-wave surfers, surfer Laird John Hamilton explains that his soul comes to him when he's at one with these waves, actively engaged with every muscle in his body. When they're not running, when he is not out there in the water, he's depressed. Another surf legend, Greg Noll, describes surfing as a lifelong love affair with an extraordinary woman called the ocean. He notes wryly that if someone spends a lifetime in a monastery praying all day, we don't call him or her a "prayer bum," but if a person has a deep, sacred relationship with the ocean, which is embodied in the practice of surfing, we apply the label "surf bum." What both surfers describe are just two of thousands of examples of how thoroughly we've separated spirituality from the pleasure of living in a physical body—as though experiencing the ecstasy of being in our bodies is not sacred or useful, but removing ourselves from them in hours of meditation is. Many of us have internalized the message that our bodies are some kind of burden that must be subdued and transcended.

Unfortunately, many people have mixed-up ideas about divinity and God. God isn't confined to a book or a church or mosque or synagogue. Divinity is the creative, loving, vital flow of life force that we're all part of and connected to. Our Spirits serve as a direct phone line to this loving force that actually *is* us. Our bodies are exquisite containers meant to embody, not deny, our spirits.

If you were brought up in a religion that taught you that God is vengeful and punishing—and that if you don't please God, you'll be damned with eternal punishment—you might find it challenging to not feel ashamed of your body and its functioning. After all, the roots of Judeo-Christian religions link the downfall of humanity with a woman, Eve, who was seduced by the serpent and tempted Adam with food and sexuality, causing him to eat the fruit too and ensuring that we were banished from paradise. Thenceforth, all women brought forth their children in pain and suffering as penance for Eve's sin. Talk about adverse programming! But it is from this myth at the heart of our belief system—a system that for many of us goes unexamined—that we've come to think that to be spiritual and "good," we have to deny our bodies and sacrifice ourselves. Dr. Mario Martinez calls this the "atonement archetype," and believe me, our society is awash in it. We've all heard the saying "The spirit is willing but the flesh is weak." This statement alone is a setup for suffering and the denial of the very exalted emotions and experiences that make life worth living. We don't have to separate out the desires and needs of the flesh from our spirituality. They're an expression of the creative life force.

Our bodies require regular touch and pleasure to truly flourish. When you hear the word *pleasure,* do you instantly think of sex? Many do—and this is so limiting! Our culture has focused the enormous range of delights available to humans into the narrow range of sex and slapped a big label on it: SIN!

Yes, sex is highly pleasurable. But there's an infinite range of pleasure available to us when we're in a human body that is consciously connected with divinity and our goddess nature. In the movie *City of Angels,* this pleasure of the senses is beautifully depicted in a scene featuring an angel (played by Nicolas Cage). When the angel becomes mortal and is finally able to experience the exquisite taste and juiciness of a pear, he recognizes a simple yet divine pleasure of the earth. Watch it and see what I mean! As long as we have a body, we're meant to enjoy it with every one of our senses.

As you uncover your pleasure and transform your spirit-denying beliefs, you'll find that sustainable pleasure is a conscious discipline, not an invitation to addiction and sloth. When you experience pleasure, God comes through you. As you become aware of your divine nature, you'll find that joy comes to you in ways that are unique to you. One person may express her spirituality through the pleasure of dancing, while another may express it through a love of riding and working with horses. When I was growing up, no one in my family played the harp, and I'd never seen one, but I was desperate to play this instrument and eventually I did. That gold harp is sitting right in front of me now. Although I haven't played it for years, it symbolizes a very strong connection with my own spirit.

When you have a calling that strong, it's coming from your soul. You're hearing the cry of your spirit yearning to express itself. When you answer that call, everyone benefits, because whatever you do personally to bring Spirit into matter and bring joy into your life changes the whole universe. The word *matter* comes from the root word *mater,* meaning "mother." When we refer to Mother Earth, it's more than a metaphor. Our physical bodies are made from the same elements as the earth herself. Our bones are made from minerals. Our blood and amniotic fluids are very much like seawater. Matter is the densest thing in creation. When we bring Spirit into dense matter through the discipline of connecting and reconnecting again and again with Spirit-drenched joy and pleasure, we bring heaven down to earth. We help lighten and lift the heavy vibrations of shame, anger, and resentment—not just for us, but for everyone!

You're a divine being who is designed to live agelessly. Honoring the "vessel" that is your body, and savoring every moment of life that you can—that's the whole point of being here. Your very conception and your presence here in this particular time and space was not a mistake. It is a miracle that was orchestrated before you were born by your spirit, the part of you that is eternal.

We are the leading edge of creation, and we are God dancing in flesh. We are not lowly, sin-ridden creatures who require redemption for the original sin of being born human. We and God are one. If you reclaim your goddess nature and express it as joy and passion for living, you experience what it is to be a divine creation—and you experience it now, without having to wait to make your transition into the nonphysical world. And when you experience divine creation here on earth, you flourish.

YOU ARE AN ANTENNA AND A CRYSTAL

We've forgotten that everything is connected to everything else. This is scientific fact. In our bodies, braided collagen strands make up our connective tissue, or fascia, which weaves through our organs and tissues and connects our muscles to our bones and skin, serving as a cytoskeleton. Electricity is conducted along the fascia by water molecules that sit atop the collagen molecules and act as liquid crystals, receiving and sending out energy (including energy that is bound up with information). This is why massaging your feet, for example, actually rejuvenates and relaxes your whole body! Acupuncture meridians lie along the fascia like a highway for subtle energies and the messages they contain.[1]

In tribal cultures, the wisdom of our connection with everything is taken for granted. That ancient wisdom is now being documented scientifically because we can finally measure it rather than simply intuit it. For example, research by Thomas Zwaka, M.D., Ph.D., of the Black Family Stem Cell Institute at the Icahn School of Medicine at Mount Sinai Hospital in New York, found that p53, a tumor-suppressing protein, prevents cancer cells from replacing healthy cells. When p53 mutates, cancer grows.[2] He says his study suggests that our evolution required co-operation, so we're actually wired not for cheating, manipulating each other, or fierce competition but for working in concert. And in her blog post "Cancer Is a Selfish Gene," researcher Lynne McTaggart notes that this protein or gene acts like a "keeper of the peace, much like the queen bee in a hive." Darwin seems to have overlooked the cooperation aspect of nature that underlies the competitiveness obvious on the surface.[3]

Another example of how connected we all are, and are meant to be, is the story of the "elephant whisperer," the late Lawrence Anthony. He was a conservationist who saved the lives of countless elephants—many of them rogues that had left their herds and were destined to be destroyed by humans. After Anthony's death, two separate herds of wild South African elephants that he had saved slowly made their way through Zululand, a 12-hour journey, without eating or drinking, arriving at the Anthonys' compound a day apart from each other. Each herd stayed for two days to mourn and pay their respects to the man who had saved them before slowly making their way back into the bush. How is it that two separate herds of wild elephants knew that the heart of a great man who had loved them had suddenly stopped?[4]

Whether we're discussing the behavior of the cells within our bodies or herds of elephants that somehow know a friend has died, both are examples of a profound truth: the hermetic philosophy of the harmony between man and nature contained in the phrase "As above, so below." We're now at a crossroads in our understanding of our place in the universe. We are finally coming to see that we are designed not to dominate nature and each other but to live in cooperation. We have to cultivate a relationship with something far greater than our egos. Until we do, we can't flourish.

A relationship with the Divine allows you to trust in and align with Divine Order. We all come to realize that change is constant and we can either go with the flow or spend our lives fighting it until we tire ourselves out. Aligning with Divine Order has nothing to do with passively waiting for something to happen *to* you. Instead, it's about surrendering your will to Divine

Will, knowing that the divine part of yourself knows your heart's desire better than your conscious mind, conditioned by cultural expectations, ever could. Your authentic, true self doesn't lie to you, mislead you, or take you away from your power source. It's a relief to turn your life over to Divine Will, or God. Remember, God is not some external force you're disconnected from, but the life force itself, which lives in you—not on some cloud somewhere.

Once you've aligned with Divine Order and Divine Will, you're free of the need to micromanage your life. You stop striving after perfection. The addiction to control and people pleasing ends. Instead, you make your life an offering to the Divine and ask God to use you. Then you follow the signs as they appear and act accordingly.

DIVINE ORDER: THE KEY TO LIVING AS A GODDESS

In her exquisite book *The Game of Life and How to Play It* (first published in 1925), writer Florence Scovel Shinn says that the perfect outcome for every problem or desire in our lives has already been chosen for us and will be revealed when we call in Divine Order. Years ago, before I was an author, I was reading an old edition of Scovel Shinn's book and a particular passage resonated for me. It was a Friday at 11:00 A.M., and I stood in my bedroom and read the text out loud: "Infinite spirit, show me a sign. Show me the next best use of my gifts and talents." At 2:00 P.M. that same day, I received a call from a literary agent who said, "I think you should write a book." *That* is Divine Order at work.

Divine Order works for the small stuff too. The more you align with it, the easier it is to get pointed in the direction of *exactly* what you need (and not always the way your ego wants it at the moment). The key is to loosen your grip. This past summer, I suggested to my daughter, who had just become engaged, that we shop for her wedding dress. I had no idea where or how to go about this, given that when I'd gotten married, I had borrowed a wedding dress and returned it to its owner the very next day. I was in medical school at the time and under the mistaken impression that taking the time to really get into something as frivolous as a wedding—including all the drama about the dress—was silly.

Anyway, unlike me back in the day, my daughter had given her dress a lot of thought, and had even created a Pinterest board I had never seen, which included a photo of her dream dress. She was aligned with what she wanted to manifest, and I was just plain open to whatever needed to happen. The first two shops we checked on the day we had chosen were closed. Late in the day, without any expectations at all, we went to a third one without an appointment—I didn't realize they often turn you away if you don't have an appointment. Who knew what a big deal buying a wedding dress at a wedding boutique is? Kate spoke briefly with the owner of the shop to convince her to let us in, and then tried on the first dress she pulled off the rack. It fit perfectly and was exactly what she had always envisioned. In fact, it was so perfect that when she emerged from the dressing room, stood up on the pedestal, and saw her reflection in the mirror, she wept with emotion. It was a beautiful example of what can come when you align with Spirit and don't get in the way. Nothing is too small for Spirit to care about—not the hair on your head, not the lilies of the field, and not the perfect wedding dress. Sometimes the manifestation is quick, and sometimes it takes years. The key to remember is that the Divine knows exactly what you need. And yes, the gown looked almost exactly like the one on Kate's Pinterest board!

The other thing about being aligned with Divine Order is that once you have some life experience, you can look back and see how those so-called obstacles turned out to be opportunities, and those lost opportunities turned out to be the greatest blessings. You say, "Oh, thank God I didn't stick with him!" and "If I hadn't been fired, wow, I would never have started my business!" The medical intuitive Caroline Myss says that when you pray for the angels to make your life better, you'd better watch out, because it's a day at the beach for an angel to wipe out a job and marriage within a week. It happens—but that rupture often leads to rapture.

SOUL CONTRACTS AND DIVINE ORDER

Ever since I read all of Edgar Cayce's work when I was about 12, I've resonated with the idea of reincarnation and soul contracts. (Edgar Cayce, known as the Sleeping Prophet, was a renowned healer who lived in the late 19th and early 20th century and assisted with the healings of thousands of individuals through tapping into the Universal Mind.) I believe that we make soul contracts with ourselves and other souls before incarnating into our human bodies. These contracts set up whom we're going to have primary relationships with, what types of things we intend to accomplish while we're here on Earth, and what unfinished business we're going to resolve. They are at work even when we don't realize it. And generally speaking, those with whom we have the most "unfinished business" end up being family members! So even when you study and work with the Law of Attraction, you will often find that your soul contracts supersede your ability to get what you want. Tosha Silver puts it this way:

> I once read a woman who took her "manifesting" very seriously. She had a vision board in every room, a personal coach, and a list of affirmations so long it took an hour a day to say them all. Yet for all her drive, most of her wishes never occurred. She was desperate, especially since her coach thought she was "blocking" the manifestation.
>
> "Well," I said to her, "actually, while our thoughts do attract reality, there's much more. Because in a given lifetime, we also have *prarabdha karma*, our soul's personal curriculum. The lessons we signed up to learn. So it's not just always visualize, get down, and jump on the party-train."
>
> With sufficient detachment, acceptance, and openness, things fall into place . . . effortlessly. They just line up. Here is a prayer to say when what you want isn't being manifested: "Change me, Divine Beloved, into One who wishes to genuinely let You take the lead. Let me know true surrender, openness, and acceptance. Take over my actions, so I know when to act, and when to pause."

One day, we look back and see a pattern and finally get what we were supposed to get all along. That's when we can move on to the next lesson. One reason I keep a journal is so I can look back and see how divinely guided I have been all along. Documenting my experiences in the journey and writing down my dreams are very practical and proactive ways to build trust in this divine guidance. If you think back to a painful time in your life that happened long ago, can you see how it served as a turning point to bring you to this moment when you are wise, joyful, and experienced in the art of triumphing over adversity? Now think back to a painful experience you had last week or last month or even this morning. Have you already made your way from grief, frustration, anger, or loss to joy? Would you have made that journey as quickly if that experience had happened 20 years ago? I bet not! You are stepping into your ageless years already. As Dr. Joe Dispenza says, wisdom is simply memory with the emotional charge removed. What a revelation—when we can look back on the painful parts of our journeys, appreciate the perfection in the unfolding of all of it, in retrospect, and no longer feel the pain. That is freedom, and it allows you to seize the days ahead with joy and delight.

ACTING IN ALIGNMENT

My daily intention is to give my life over to the Divine and then wait for the impulse to act. If I'm passionate about something, I always know that I'm meant to do it. Excitement about something always means that you're aligned with who you really are! Learning Argentine tango was like that. Sometimes, you just *know.* Sometimes, you get a sign. It could be a message on a truck or billboard, a dream, a snippet of a song lyric that you hear just when you need an answer—or you can seek a sign from oracle cards, or listen to your intuition if it is screaming "no!" or "yes!" A couple of days ago, I set the intention to experience magic, just for the fun of it. The next day, while driving to a friend's house, I saw a car in front of me with a license plate that read MAGIC. I laughed with delight. This kind of thing happens all the time once you begin to align with the Divine!

Acting in alignment doesn't mean you can't try to manifest something specific. I'm all for vision boards and focusing your intention. You can ask Spirit for whatever you want. But be flexible. Don't get exhausted trying to use your will instead of Divine Will. Be open to the fact that Spirit answers prayers three ways: "Yes!" and "Not now" and "No, because I love you too much." Think back to a time when the answer was "Not now." Does it make sense now? Do you see how the Divine had something better in mind? And what about a time when, in retrospect, you see that God wasn't saying, "No, because you don't deserve it," but "No, because I love you too much." You dodged a bullet on that one, correct?

The action you take to align with Divine Order needs to be both spiritual and practical. You have to let go of your expectations about what is supposed to happen in your life and be open to the divine plan. Recently, my youngest brother, who raises mule-horses, hybrid animals known for their gentleness, was bucked off as he was riding downhill and landed on his neck. As a physician, of course, I did what I could to get information from his doctors and help our family understand his condition and what could be done for it medically. That was the action part. But there was a spiritual part too. I knew that the accident could be something he was supposed to experience as part of his life story. I took spiritual action and said a prayer that he would recover completely. I also gathered with other family members to send Divine Love to him, and especially to his lungs, because I knew he would need strength in his lungs to survive the emergency surgery. But beyond doing what I could do, including praying and sending Divine Love, I had to let the Creator fill in the holes of my brother's story. To everyone's great relief, he made it through just fine. And by surrendering to Divine Order rather than trying to micromanage the situation as the designated know-it-all family member (every family seems to have one of those in a crisis), I saved myself and everyone around me a lot of suffering.

I can't guarantee that if you live joyously and agelessly, nothing bad is ever going to happen to you. Stuff happens on planet Earth. Even if your physical body ages, or suffers an accident, or develops a disease, living joyously and agelessly is going to maximize your healthspan and lifespan. And the source of all joy is Spirit. The ancient Sufi poet Rumi wrote, "There's a kiss we long for our whole lives: the kiss of the Beloved." Spirit or

Source is our true Beloved, who will always accept, forgive, and love us. It is the kiss of the Divine Beloved we're all looking for, and the Divine Beloved is willing to bestow it upon us. All we have to do is invite in the Beloved who has been patiently waiting. We don't have to wait until we've lost that last ten pounds, or cleaned out our junk drawer, or vacuumed the rug—we can have it right now!

THE BODY, THE SPIRIT, AND THE EARTH

I'm all for quieting the mind for 15 to 20 minutes or so to meditate, but we're here to live and enjoy our bodies, hearts, and minds, not escape them. Life is the real meditation. I know a meditation teacher who sits on a cushion ten hours a day, but his life off the cushion is a wreck. You can get addicted to the whole "woo woo" metaphysical thing as a distraction from the needs of your body and your daily life. You can go to India, trek to ancient Mayan sites, and sit at the base of the Great Pyramid and chant. But when you come back home, the relationships that drove you nuts when you left will still be there—and so will your laundry. You can't ignore your physicality and your connection to the earth.

The separation from our generative pelvic bowls and our sexual, sensual life force is mirrored by our sense of separation from Mother Earth. That painful disconnection began thousands of years ago when our reverence for the sacredness of the life-giving earth started to fade and a culture of domination, not collaboration, begin to take over. We developed the belief that we're supposed to dominate and exploit the planet. Intuitively, though, we know this isn't how we are supposed to relate to the natural world. Spirit and earth are completely connected. The Gaia hypothesis says that the earth is a living being and that we're not just living *on* the planet, we're *part of* the planet. After eons of separation, we're finally acknowledging that a relationship with Spirit, the earth, and each other based on domination instead of collaboration isn't healthy. And we're recognizing the sacredness of life on our home planet instead of thinking of God as existing far above us in the heavens, separate from us, our daily lives, and our experiences of our bodies.

Reconnecting with the earth—and sky—isn't just something you can do figuratively. The human body evolved to walk on the earth, drinking its water, breathing its air, and basking in its sunlight. You can actually improve your health by spending more time in nature and getting in touch with the earth and sky. When you do this, you experience the divinity of both the earth and your body.

A hundred or so years ago, the Victorians believed it was important to get fresh air and sunshine. They instinctively understood that public parks could help reduce crime and disorder and calm people who enjoyed them, which is why they built so many of them.[5] People would go off to a sanitarium in the mountains if they contracted tuberculosis. The cure often worked because the fresh air, relaxation, and relief from everyday stress helped the body heal. But then we started shipping people off to hospitals and clinics with electric lights and doctors who had prescription drugs and scalpels to treat us. Fortunately, we're starting to see research that backs what we all know: that spending time in the natural world revitalizes us and reduces our stress, which leads to better health.[6] Time in nature also lowers cortisol levels, boosting immunity.[7] Being outdoors in the sunshine increases vitamin D levels, reducing the risk of depression, cancer, heart disease, and other serious illnesses. One of the effects of nature deprivation is that we don't expose ourselves to natural light the way we did when we lived closer to the land, before artificial light came along. Think of natural light as a nutrient your body needs for good health and balanced mood. It is Mother Earth's gift to you.

If you live in the northern hemisphere, or have little exposure to sunlight because you're indoors all day under artificial lighting, you're probably low in vitamin D. You can improve your levels by getting enough light. Get outside more, especially on sunny days. I don't advocate baking in the sun for hours. But a 30-minute sunbath without sunscreen in the early morning or late afternoon can do a world of good for your mood and vitamin D levels. (Beyond that, use sunscreen.) Make sure you get plenty of natural light through windows. When that's not possible, use natural-spectrum lightbulbs. You can buy light boxes that will give you an extra burst of full-spectrum light that mimics outdoor lighting. To prevent eye strain, set them up so that you can see them in your peripheral vision. Let the light of the sky shine upon you and replenish you.

And speaking of eyes, being indoors most of the time is associated with nearsightedness, while being outdoors may prevent or halt its progression.[8] Be sure to spend some time outdoors—without sunglasses—like your ancestors did. Also, your retinas need natural light to produce serotonin, a "feel-good" neurotransmitter that boosts your mood and prevents depression. Seasonal affective disorder (SAD), a temporary condition that's most common in winter when there's less natural light, can be alleviated by exposure to sunshine or full-spectrum lighting. That said, respect and work with the natural cycles of your body and the sun's light. If you feel like sleeping in once in a while when it's dark and dreary, listen to your body. If you sleep a little more in winter, don't worry about it.

Another way that being in nature can improve your health is if you practice "earthing." Earthing means reconnecting with the earth's electromagnetic field (usually through walking barefoot on the ground) to stabilize your own electrical field. All the modern electrical devices surrounding us, such as cell phones, televisions, and other electronic equipment, affect our personal energy fields and the electromagnetic field we're constantly interacting with. I sleep with an earthing sheet that I plug into a grounded outlet, but I also spend as much time as I can with my bare feet touching the earth. The earth's negative ions counteract the positive ions that cause oxidative stress in your body, which is what causes damage to your tissues. In fact, studies have documented that standing on the earth herself decreases jet lag and also decreases cellular inflammation. Try this next time you have to fly somewhere so you can get back in touch with the natural rhythms of the earth and sun.

NATURAL CYCLES, COSMIC CYCLES

Part of aligning with Divine Order is aligning with the natural cycles of the earth and the cosmos. One of the natural cycles is the cycle of the sun, which creates two solstices each year: winter and summer, December 21 and June 21 in the northern hemisphere (the dates are reversed in the southern hemisphere). Winter solstice marks the return of the sun and a lengthening of days, and summer solstice marks the longest day of the year and the beginning of the nights becoming longer. Each one has a different significance. For those who lived closer to the earth, back when the Mother Goddess was at the center of spirituality and religion, summer solstice was a time for joyful celebration and dancing. Winter solstice was a time for reflection. As the light returned, it was a time for imagining what to create in the longer days to come. Since winter solstice falls near Christmas and New Year's Day, you might want to take either of those days, or the solstice itself, as a time to reflect on what you would like to bring into your life. Spending time resting and reflecting will nourish you, body and soul.

The moon has cycles, or phases, too. In ancient traditions, the sun was often seen as a male energy, but the moon was a goddess. After all, the moon rules the flow of fluids in the body, including our menstrual cycles. It also rules the flow of fluids on and in Mother Earth, including the tides in the ocean and the fertility cycles of many plants and animals. There are times of the month when the moon is full and abundant and times when it's invisible and has no light to shine on anyone. Those who work with plant medicine very often follow the cycles of the moon for planting and harvesting. It's also instructive to notice how the moon affects the cycles of your life. The waxing moon and full moon are times when things are birthed and come to fruition, while the waning moon is a releasing moon. When the moon is waning, it's a good time to release what is no longer needed—including old resentments and hurts. The new moon is the time to plant "seeds" of new intentions. Lunar eclipses and solar eclipses often cause agitation and upheaval in people, and there's research showing what we who have worked in obstetric wards have long noticed: that births occur more often when there's a full moon.[9] Pay attention to the phases of the moon and reflect on what you want to bring in and what you want to release because it's no longer serving you.

The planets have cycles of their own. While the astrology forecasts in newspapers and magazines are harmless fun, actual astrology, which uses detailed charts and looks at the positions of all the planets when you were born compared to their positions now, will help you see how your cycles fit in with larger cycles. If you choose not to believe in this form of divining based in nature, that's fine. But for many people, including me, astrology is a tool for becoming aware of life patterns and societal patterns. Astrological charts are blueprints of the soul's journey. I have a "solar return" chart done every year by a professional astrologer to see what major energies will be influencing my journey. Knowing my astrological forecast helps me be conscious and prepare for what I'll experience, including spiritual lessons. It's kind of like when you consult the weather forecast to see whether or not it would be a good idea to take an umbrella or light jacket. Being prepared keeps me from feeling victimized by circumstances. There are no "bad" charts, but sometimes the planets' positions show that you're going to be dealing with something challenging.

If you want to consult an astrologer, don't go to one who scares you with the information in your chart. Consult someone who uses astrology as a tool for consciousness. Doom-and-gloom astrologers are just as bad as doctors who always look for the worst instead of assisting you in truly flourishing.

Hippocrates, the father of Western medicine, whose oath all of us doctors take when we get our degrees, was an astrologer. But we have lost that sense of the connection between the earth, the cosmos, and our bodies that was present back in his day. If the moon rules the flow of fluids in our body, why wouldn't other planets besides the moon affect us? The subtle energies and how they move and interact in the energy field we all share are still mysterious to scientists, but they are transmitted to us through the electromagnetic grid, which we experience in our connective tissues. This is scientific fact. And it's very empowering to know that we have this tool!

As I was first writing this chapter in September 2013, the planet Saturn dove into what is called the north node of Fate. (The nodes mark the points where the orbit of the moon and the orbit of the sun intersect.) A slow-moving planet like Saturn joins those nodes rather infrequently. In this case, that node/Saturn conjunction had also occurred in June 2002, and before that in January 1991 and July 1979. I looked up those dates in my journals and saw that, in fact, each coincided with a major event involving one of my books. Many people shared with me that they, too, had experienced huge turning points in their lives during those periods. Knowing about astrological cycles like this and seeing how they have manifested in my life are ways to trust in Divine Order. I realized that it is no mere "coincidence" that I was writing another book at this time.

Pay attention to your body's natural cycles too. If you're a morning person, consciously choose to reserve your mornings for activities that are priorities for you. Don't give away your best time of day to just anyone or anything. If you find you're most reflective in the early evening, honor that by writing in your journal, pondering your dreams of last night, or meditating at that time. Respecting your natural cycles and those of the earth and sky will help you connect to Spirit and your own creativity and joy.

CONSCIOUS CONNECTIONS

Knowing the cycles of nature and the cosmos, you can consciously choose to align with them. When you do this, you're aligning with other people, and you're changing the relationship among humans as well as the relationship between humans and the earth.

In Chapter 4, I explained the phenomenon of aligned cardiac activity called coherence. The Global Coherence Initiative at www.glcoherence.org, launched by the Institute of Heart-Math, is a project that uses coherence to shift global consciousness toward balance and collaboration. It involves people using conscious intent, affirmation, prayer, and meditation to alter the electromagnetic field (EMF) of the earth that is affecting all of us. They've actually measured EMF activity and found correlations to global crises, such as 9/11, when our human hearts are all affected by something that big. On the other hand, they have also seen results when many concentrate their intention to raise the vibration of the EMF through joy. Our human energy fields affect the field of the earth herself! And yes, they're using scientific research methods to track their progress. They often send out a call for global prayer and meditation at a particular time, such as for ten minutes on a specific date. Robert Fritchie of the World Service Institute (www.worldserviceinstitute.org) and Lynne McTaggart (www.lynnemctaggart.com) both have large networks that coordinate these activities as well. And spiritual leaders are joining in the call—especially when a crisis is brewing. Everyone who participates in raising the vibration of the EMF is contributing to changing the EMF, and the effect is cumulative.[10]

Connecting with other people in prayer or meditation, whatever form it takes, is an excellent way to stay connected with Spirit. Churches or synagogues often help people feel a sense of safety and belonging, and they meet important social needs. Jesus said, "Whenever two or more are gathered in my name, there shall I be also." In other words, when at least two people choose to come together in vulnerability, with the intention of connecting to the Divine Beloved and their own spiritual selves, it is very powerful and nourishing for the soul. Research shows that regular church attendance is associated with better health and greater longevity. Twelve-step meetings of all kinds, too, work very nicely for bringing people together to remember that Spirit is the healer of addictions. Be forewarned, however: while a church, synagogue, sangha, prayer group, or 12-step group can give you emotional sustenance and help you feel your connection to the Divine Beloved and to the greater community, the group can also be weighted down in personal politics and psychological dysfunction. If you've had a bad experience with churches or spiritual communities, don't let that stop you from joining or creating one, or improving the one you're in so that it's more supportive of everyone's spiritual well-being. Look around in your own community. Talk to people you know who are tapped into various networks. You can also find a group through the Internet.

Or you can set the intention to connect with like-minded people who don't require a building or a schedule in order to tune in to their spirituality. We no longer need specific buildings called synagogues, mosques, churches, or temples in order to actively connect with Spirit. When I was growing up and attended church with my father, my mother always went out into the woods. She'd say to my father, "You go to your church. I'll go to mine." Now *that* was a profound childhood imprint about spirituality!

Where you hold your gatherings doesn't matter. All space is sacred space when you remember that God is within you. But you might find it's especially enriching to meet up in nature, in a beautiful public space, or in a place where people have prayed for centuries. Some of the old cathedrals in Europe sit atop sacred springs recognized by people who lived in those areas before Christianity came in. Sedona has always been considered a holy space by the indigenous people in that area, and it's become a magnet for people eager to experience and express their spiritual nature. When I first went there, my first thought was, *Wow. This place is holy. It's a sanctuary.*

You don't need the formal blessing of a religious leader to form a congregation or group of spiritual seekers or to explore your own spirituality. Reconnecting with the Divine Beloved means letting go of the old idea that you need someone to serve as a go-between whenever you want to feel connected to Spirit. What we're seeking is the Divine within, not something "out there." All of us are worthy of having a direct line to this nourishing force.

When we feel this connection, we know there *is* a divine plan. The plan also becomes easier to see as we get into our ageless years and have likely experienced the fact that the Divine does indeed work in mysterious, extraordinary, and exquisite ways.

GOOSE BUMPS AND INNER KNOWING

The Divine Beloved communicates with us in many ways, but we have to get out of our heads to receive the messages. That's controversial to say in a culture of domination that's dismissive of intuition and divining arts, but I'm saying it anyway! As women, we know deep down that intuition is powerful and that we can trust it. Intuitive, wise women have been shamed and marginalized for centuries. Saying, "I can't explain why, but I just know this situation isn't right for me"—listening to your inner knowing—can be difficult because we're told we need to logically justify what our hearts tell us. But as the feminine way of knowing becomes stronger and stronger, it's easier and easier to take this stance unapologetically.

You know yourself and your heart. If you feel resistance to something, explore your resistance. Once you sit with an idea for a while, or remain mindful in a situation, your true feelings and beliefs will become much clearer. Become still and listen to your inner knowing—and your goose bumps. I've always been fascinated by how our bodies can create this physical response in unfiltered form. If someone tells you about an uncanny coincidence, or you experience a perfect synchronicity, or you suddenly have a strong sense that you're being guided by a loving and protective force, you'll often get goose bumps. They're a sure sign that whatever you just heard has special significance. Here's the anatomy of a "goose bump": an electrical signal activates the tiny muscles in the skin that supply a hair follicle. The hair literally stands on end. That electrical signal itself is activated when a deep truth inside of us connects with the deep truth of something outside of us. We experience a resonance field between that outer truth and our own hearts that links them like points on a big grid. Goose bumps are the sign that our grids are in sync with a profound, intuitive truth that we may not be able to articulate fully.

If you find yourself feeling tired or sad for no reason and you've just been in a cemetery, bar, or hospital, it may be because you've picked up on energies there that are dark and heavy, or there are spirits lingering about. The late Peter Calhoun, a former Episcopal priest who became a shaman, told me that the native people he worked with often said, "You white people don't know how to let go of your dead. You're surrounded by dead people." Many of us were taught that if—and it was "if"—souls live after death, they go away to a place where we can't sense them and they can't communicate with us. But many souls don't get across the portal if their loved ones are still hanging on to unresolved feelings about them. I can't begin to tell you how many women have been helped by the knowledge that it's okay to release their mothers or other loved ones after death. One of my friends noticed that she felt her grandmother's presence more after she died than before. This grandmother had been mentally ill and, especially in later years, had been a major burden on the family. Sure enough, a healer friend of mine noted that her grandmother hadn't gone through the portal and was still hanging around, making life a bit heavier for everyone. When the healer helped the grandmother cross over, my friend said she could feel a weight lifting from around her ankles!

It's comforting to know that many people connect regularly with loved ones after their passing. This is beautifully depicted in the movie *What Dreams May Come,* which I highly recommend for those who may be having trouble letting go. Messages and communication from loved ones who have crossed over are common, but again, our intuition and experience of what can't be proven is shamed and dismissed in a dominator culture. Let's reclaim this experience. It's real and we know it. I like to think of life as similar to being at a big fairgrounds—you get disconnected from someone and you eventually hook up with them again.

COMMUNING WITH THE DIVINE

Each of us is a being of light with consciousness, a form of the Divine who has come back to Earth to remember and experience her sacred essence. The fact that we are beings of light—and that we, in fact, emit light—has been demonstrated by researcher Gary Schwartz, Ph.D., at his lab at the University of Arizona. (You can learn more at www.drgaryschwartz.com.) Your soul probably came here with the intention of doing some learning while you're in human form, but you aren't here to prove anything to anyone. You don't have to earn the love of your Creator. It's a given. Many religions say that God is love, and that's the truth. Divine love is bestowed on you regardless of what you do or think. It's up to you to accept it and connect to it. If you believe otherwise, it's a sign you need to reconnect to what you know deep down: that you are a divine, ageless, beloved goddess worthy of unconditional love. Own it!

Agelessness means engaging in the creative process of life itself, not being constricted by a preconceived notion of how you are "supposed" to act or to age or to commune with the Divine. The Divine just wants you to connect with it. It is not issuing orders about where to stand or sit or how to hold your hands or what words to say.

Though the Divine is always there for us, it's easy to feel disconnected in a culture that keeps God locked in a box labeled "religion" and tells us that we don't have access to God without specially trained go-betweens. Nevertheless, prayer is powerful because it invokes the Divine and helps you actually feel that connection. There are many different forms of prayer, so if one doesn't feel right to you, try a different one. Some people find that singing, speaking, or just silently reciting a prayer they know well allows Spirit to resonate in their bodies. The words evoke a feeling of being connected to everyone who ever said that particular prayer. Speaking words or prayers changes the vibration around you, too, so if your prayer is one you make up on the spot, it can still be very powerful. There's a Jewish tradition of prayer for everyday blessings. Why not make a habit of saying a prayer of gratitude for everything you can think of as you go about an everyday task? "Thank you for my good cookware and my knowledge about how to use it to prepare a delicious meal. Thank you for my full refrigerator, and for the zucchini being fresh and in season. Thank you for my knives being sharp." Try it sometime! Prayers of gratitude are powerful tools for wellness.

I absolutely love Tosha Silver's Divine Beloved prayers. I've already introduced several in the course of the book, and you'll find more in the 14-Day Ageless Goddess Program in the next chapter. Tosha says she invented this form of prayer after working with many spiritual teachers who instructed her to "just let go" and puzzling over how to do that. Eventually, she came up with her Change Me prayers as a way to engage the Self to help the self. The Change Me prayer is a very effective way to bypass the death grip of the ego that always wants to know "how, when, where, how high," and so forth. In effect, you are asking your

Higher Self to take the wheel and align you with Divine Order. When you pray, "Divine Beloved, please change me into someone who is open to this experience and all it has to offer me," you are also inviting Spirit to help you have faith in Divine Order. You are sending a message out over the crystalline structure of your body connected with your heart and waiting to receive guidance. Since your cytoskeleton is precisely designed to both send and receive, and is masterminded by your heartfelt desires, you can be sure that your prayers are being both sent out and received.

However, the vibration at which a request is made or a prayer is said is often quite different from the vibration of the answer. It might take several weeks or months or even years for your prayer to be answered. It may be that you won't get your response until you raise your vibration—and you do that by shedding old resentments, grief, or beliefs that are keeping you from experiencing your good. Sometimes, as I've said, Spirit's answer to a prayer is "No, not yet" because you have some work to do first. Remember, soul contracts are agreements to resolve what's been unresolved and to experience things we want to experience. You may need to do some growing and healing before you're ready to receive what your mind and heart are longing for.

I love invoking a wiser, stronger part of myself and asking it to change me into someone who is organized, who receives easily, who trusts, or whatever. The idea that you can ask for help, that it doesn't all have to come from you, is one that hasn't been as much a part of the New Age as it should have been. Women think it all has to come from them—we have to make it happen! But God is there to help us every time. When you ask for help from God, you acknowledge that being a perfectionist and trying to micromanage the world is too damn exhausting and that you are worthy of divine intervention! Here's a prayer you can say daily: "Divine Beloved, change me into someone who relishes my goddess nature and my connection to you and to the earth. Change me into someone who truly trusts in Divine Order. And while you're at it, please send me a few signs that remind me I'm always connected to you." When you say it, let yourself feel it.

Another form of prayer is affirmations. When you say them, you articulate what you wish for as if it were true right now, in the present moment. Thoughts have vibrations, evoke emotions, and change the electrical potential that gets sent out along your grid. If you want to change your emotions, you have to change your thoughts and be mindful of negative self-talk. Energy flows where awareness goes. And in the brain, neurons that fire together quite literally wire together. If you think about problems instead of solutions and opportunities, your problems expand. If you have a health challenge and that becomes your main focus—what you talk about, what you post about on social media to all your friends, family, and acquaintances—you give illness a lot of energy that could be directed toward joy and health. Think about what you want to affirm—that you're ill? Or that you're actively repairing your body's cells, organs, and tissues even as you're living a luscious, joyful life?

Say affirmations with your whole heart, as though what you're affirming were true right now, and your electromagnetic field and heart will send out messages that begin to attract to you the very things you are now vibrating. You probably affirm things all the time but don't realize it. Think about how many times you say, "I am" during a day. What are you affirming when you say that? Do you really want the universe reflecting "I am so overwhelmed" or "I am screwing this up"? No, you want the universe to reflect your affirmation that "I am flourishing! I am a joyful, ageless goddess!" The original name for Spirit is "I AM": Spirit is the power of intention to create something new.

Spirituality requires being present and mindful. Mindfulness practices support agelessness and health—and they are ways to commune with the Divine as well. Mindful meditation or breathing, and mindful partner dancing or other activities where you have to be fully present and aware of what is happening in the moment, are a few forms of mindfulness practice, but there are many. Mindfulness isn't something you have to take a course in. You just have to get out of your head and your anxiety and worries that you're not good enough. Forget that. If you're meditating and realize your mind has been wandering, laugh at it and pull your focus back to your breath or your mantra. Every time you replace judgment with a return to being present right now, you get better at keeping your mind from drifting away from your control. Don't worry that you weren't mindful when you can simply be mindful again.

Using Affirmations

Affirmations are strongest when they're in the present tense and completely positive. Here are a few you can use—but think about writing some of your own too, based on what you'd like to manifest in your life and what you're grateful for. Or check out Catherine Ponder's meditations, which I especially like to work with. (You can find some of them at www.absolute1.net/catherine-ponder.html.)

Say affirmations with meaning and passion. The emotion behind them, and repetition, are what change our biology over time.

I am health, strength, peace, happiness, and prosperity.

Divine Love, expressing through me, now draws to me all that is needed to make me happy and my life complete.

My life is unfolding perfectly in ways that are exciting and uplifting.

I love taking care of my body. My body responds beautifully to this loving care.

I am a magnet for wealth, health, and true love.

When I say yes to myself and my needs, my energy always increases and I feel wonderful.

I awaken each morning feeling the promise of a new day and a new beginning.

I love moving my body. I love getting stronger and more flexible every day.

I am a divine, ageless goddess and I am dearly loved!

Write down your favorites and say them out loud several times a day. Say them to yourself while exercising, while driving to work, when cleaning the sink, or whenever. I often say them out loud while on the elliptical trainer!

SYMBOLS AND RITUALS

Ritual and symbol are powerful because they bypass the intellect and give us a direct line to the Divine through our own goddess selves. I use ritual constantly. I often do new moon and full moon rituals with my friends, using free conference calls to connect if we can't be together. I light candles, and then I call in the four directions and Archangel Michael and his Legions of Light. I call on Power Animals that protect those four directions. I cut cords, say prayers, and invoke Divine Love. I smudge spaces with burning sage to cleanse the energy. I say Divine Beloved prayers, asking to be changed into someone who is already where I want to be. My rituals are alive and in the moment. I make them up as I go along. The late Peter Calhoun talked about being a priest who performed rituals that he came to realize had become rote, dry, and meaningless for him and the people participating in his church. But when he began to work with living energies of nature, and with the unseen, things began to change. Then he was really able to help people instead of just repeating tired old homilies passed down through the generations. (It's okay to use traditional words, but only if you infuse them with life!) We are programmed to respond to rituals that take place in natural areas or use natural objects. These rituals remind us of our connection to the great Mother Earth. Let the sun and the breeze bring energy in!

Rituals don't have to be perfect to be meaningful and powerful. The universe won't zap you with a lightning bolt if you don't say the words correctly or your smudge stick burns out and needs to be relit. I have a friend who liked doing rituals with a neopagan group, but they kept getting upset with her because her dyslexia inevitably made her turn "widdershins" (counterclockwise) instead of "sunward" (clockwise). Then she'd mumble, "Sorry!" as she stepped into the circle awkwardly to turn herself around, which broke the rules about keeping the container of sacred space intact. And then she'd start in the west instead of the east to call upon the four directions and stifle a fit of nervous giggling. In fact, there is nothing more Divine than laughing at yourself!

THE LAUGHING BUDDHA

In many religions, there's no symbol or story about humor and laughter as ways to raise your vibration and feel more connected to others and to God. In Buddhism, there's the Laughing

Buddha with his big, round belly and huge grin reminding us that God is laughter as well as love. Spirituality and irreverence aren't often seen as compatible, but truly spiritual people aren't self-conscious, grim, or judgmental. The Dalai Lama giggles all the time. However, many of us have been brought up to be far too serious when it comes to spirituality, religion, and God. More than that, we've been brought up to think that someone else has the answers for us and we don't. We're deadly serious about our gurus. And by the way, there's a marvelously funny documentary about the tendency to look outside of ourselves to someone else to guide us: *Kumaré: The True Story of a False Prophet*. This story of a man who was looking for a guru and decided to become one—and developed a devoted following almost by accident—is a great reminder that our connection with the Divine is always an inside job. And that the guru is you.

Stop waiting to be "worthy" of indulging your desire for joy, connection, and pleasure. You're already worthy, so get on with it. And cut out the harsh, ugly stimulation that brings you down. These days, you can be just about anywhere on the planet and take out a mobile device and access information. Do you need to know about every horror that is happening around the globe, in real time, 24/7? For some reason, we've become convinced that we're bad people if we don't pay attention to every gory detail of human and animal suffering. We now have the ability to be connected all day and all night with the entire planet, but we have to be very mindful about what we give our attention to—suffering or healing and flourishing. Over time, the images, thoughts, and emotions we experience are programming our biology.

Stop replaying that traumatic image, whether you're watching it on a screen or in your mind. Otherwise, you'll get stuck in a milder form of PTSD—post-traumatic stress disorder. This debilitating condition involves a nervous system that's become overreactive and causes a person to reexperience a trauma as if in real time, with the heart racing, the cortisol shooting through the bloodstream, and the eyes dilating as fear takes over the body. The body and nervous system don't know that the danger has passed—and the stress you experience while you're reliving the past wreaks havoc on your body. You can honor the past and its tragedies without putting your body and spirit through all of that trauma and stress again. We can be compassionate without reliving someone else's trauma as they replay the video over and over. Say this prayer when you realize you're falling back into the old habit of taking in too much negativity or reliving a trauma from the past: "Divine Beloved, please change me into one who knows how to focus on the positive. Change me into someone who easily shifts my focus from the negative to the positive. Show me how to do this."

The human body and its nervous system have not evolved to tolerate the onslaught of bad news and emotionally traumatizing information and images that are part and parcel of mainstream news. Focusing only on doom and gloom is neither an accurate depiction of reality nor a healthy practice. Remember that for every terribly depressing news story, there is an uplifting one. The good is just as real as murder, assault, kidnapping, or war.

And believe me, once you start looking for the good, you will see it everywhere. Shift your focus now. Limit the amount of negative news coming into your consciousness. Look for good news, uplifting ideas, and reminders that people are looking out for each other and the earth and her creatures. As a daily spiritual practice, laugh often and look for the magic of everyday life. Understand that the more joyful you feel, the more you will uplift the entire world. Joy and laughter replenish you at a cellular level, so go for the comedy in life, not the tragedy.

As you deepen your connection to the Divine, you will find you see life differently. The little things won't bother you so much, and your anxiety and perfectionism will start to fade as you relax into trusting in Divine Order. Here's a cultural norm to replace: living your life as an emergency. I was trained as a doctor to be "on call" at all times, vigilant about every disaster that might befall a patient. This was not in keeping with the prayer "Thy kingdom come, thy will be done, on earth as it is in heaven," which I learned as a child. Life on earth ought to be heavenly. Heaven shouldn't be experienced only after death, and then, only if you're a good girl. You are a divine goddess. Bring heaven to earth now, through your heart, your hips, and your sheer joy. Get rid of the old ideas about your relationship with Spirit and step into an embrace with the Divine Beloved, whose kiss awaits you.

CHAPTER TWELVE

THE 14-DAY AGELESS GODDESS PROGRAM

*Old age is the only disease you can
catch by imitating its symptoms.*

— MARIO E. MARTINEZ, PSY.D.

When I was in medical school, a professor showed us a slide of the dendrites that branched off from individual neurons in the brain. Each neuron had dozens of dendritic connections for communication between different brain cells. To make the connections visible, a golden orange-yellow stain was used on the brain tissue. Against the background, the dendrites appeared black. As I sat in the dark lecture hall, I was taken aback by the sheer beauty of the image on the projector screen. It resembled a tree late in autumn, branching outward to connect with other branches on other trees. Like trees, our minds and bodies are always growing and expanding, forming new connections between thoughts, ideas, activities, and experiences. Our minds, bodies, and organs are formed and constantly remodeled every day. The quality of these connections—which we can change at any age—has everything to do with what we believe and how we behave.

To maintain and even enhance your physical well-being, your attitude, and your experience of life—all of which are core to agelessness—you have to be connected to your life force. Creativity, joy, prosperity, pleasure, lushness, love, and faith are all part of being ageless. Each is both an emotional state and a biochemical reality that results in the free flow of life energy throughout the body. Dr. Joe Dispenza's work has documented how thinking thoughts with enough amplitude (as measured by EEGs) literally changes the neural connections in our brains. Modern brain-scanning techniques have documented beyond a shadow of a doubt how powerful our minds are to, quite literally, change and heal our bodies—and our lives. What we refer to as "faith" translates into the amount of time and intention it takes for new nerve cell connections to form from new habits of thought. That intention and that desire are what you must tap within yourself to become an ageless goddess. (These astonishing neural pattern changes are beautifully documented in Dispenza's TEDx talk—which is well worth watching.)

So now that you've learned about the power of your mind, heart, and spirit to transform your body and transcend outdated cultural portals about age, the question is, how are you going to incorporate into your life practices that contribute to agelessness? What do you need to do to allow your true goddess self to emerge and flourish? In other words, what will it take for you to become happy, healthy, energized, and ageless? How are you going to apply the ideas in this book to your life right now?

Remember that to find answers, you start by looking within. What do *you* know about what you have to do to be ageless? Physicians, healers, diagnostic tests, and checklists are all valuable tools, but becoming an ageless goddess means letting go of the fear that you aren't smart enough, educated enough, or intuitive enough to make the right decisions for yourself. If you're reading this, you have what it takes to be in charge of your health and work effectively with the tools and resources available to you.

What do you most need to do to begin living agelessly instead of in fear of aging?

I've provided many ideas in this book to help you answer that question for yourself, but I've also created a 14-day program or checklist to keep it simple and make it easy for you to begin living agelessly. The program is tied in to the chapters in this book and incorporates two days that are to be devoted to affirming new thoughts. There's plenty of room for personalization in this program. You have to tailor these formulas to your own life and listen to your body's wisdom about what's right for you. Pay attention to your instincts and your body's signals as you work the program for two weeks. When you get to Day 3 or Day 4, you'll find that your energy, mood, and well-being are better than they were before. After you've completed the program, notice how revitalized you feel.

As you start the Ageless Goddess Program, you may find yourself releasing physical and emotional toxins from deep within your tissues, fascia, and cells. Because toxins of all types leave the body the same way they went in, you're likely to feel a little more achy, tired, or irritable than usual, so be prepared. Change can be difficult. If it were easy to live joyfully and agelessly, everyone would be doing it! In part, it's difficult to change because we often get more support from our family or friends for being stuck than for doing what it takes to truly flourish. Notice whether that has been true for you.

The activities for each day of the program won't take more than a few minutes—after all, you can look into your eyes in your bathroom mirror and say, "I love you. I really love you!" out loud, and create a genuine feeling of love, in about 15 seconds. If you can't do all the suggested activities in one day, do as many as you can. And if on a given day you decide you can do no more than affirm that you love yourself, that affirmation is powerful, because you've rejected perfectionism, self-criticism, and self-neglect and replaced them with nourishing love for yourself. Tomorrow is another day, so don't stress yourself out when you can reconnect with Divine Love and replenish yourself.

As part of the program, keep an Ageless Goddess journal in which you chronicle your activities and thoughts. This will help enormously in the future, because you'll be able to joyfully look back and see how far you've come. Before going to sleep at night, reflect back on your day and savor all the delicious moments that were part of it. Notice what part of the program really spoke to you, what nourished you and filled you up, and what stressed you out. Can you do an activity differently so that instead of being a chore that drains you, it's something you don't mind, or something you actually look forward to?

As you reflect on the activities you did and the thoughts associated with them, you'll learn what deeply nourishes you and what doesn't. As you look at the activities you skipped, reflect on why you didn't do them. Why didn't you make the time for self-nourishment? We're always changing around our calendars and agendas to fit in everyone else's needs, but we feel guilty blocking out time for our own pleasure and well-being. But making yourself a priority is absolutely vital for ageless living! And if you skipped an activity because you were afraid it would make you feel uncomfortable, consider the payoff of holding on to old emotions and avoiding discomfort compared to the payoff of ageless living. If you were reluctant to do the grieving and raging exercises, remember that your feelings don't have to overwhelm you. Prepare for the exercises with a Divine Beloved prayer affirming that you are always connected to Divine Love and support, and set the intention to do something pleasurable after you've done the hard work of opening up to your grief and rage so they can be released.

Because it's easier to tack a new habit onto an old one than to completely change the way you operate, plan to do the activities in the Ageless Goddess Program at times of the day when you're most likely to remember to do them and be uninterrupted. If you're not a morning person and you're usually rushing to get out of the house after you wake up, don't add more items to your already overstuffed morning routine and create more stress for yourself because of some old belief about early birds catching the worms. If you are most productive later in the day, when things are calmer, take a look at your afternoon or evening habits. Maybe that's when you can add on journaling, or getting in touch with your body's need for pleasure—whatever habit you'd like to add to your life so that you can be an ageless goddess.

If you usually collapse onto the couch with a glass of wine and a remote control or your phone after work, try doing a couple of affirmations before you pour that wine. Or simply close your eyes and just remain fully present with yourself, being aware of the sensations in your body and what emotions come up for you, for five minutes. You might find you don't really want or need the alcohol after all! And you'll soon realize that you really aren't replenished by calling your old friend who always has a sob story or a cynical attitude that change is impossible. Soon, you'll find yourself eager to replace the old after-work routine with some stretches that revitalize you, plus a Divine Beloved prayer or two.

THE 14-DAY AGELESS GODDESS PROGRAM

Every day:

Follow a low-glycemic diet that keeps blood sugar stable. Many volumes have been written on this topic, but it's still new information for some. As I've said, it takes a long time to replace old ideas with new ones. Low-fat diets are outdated and obsolete; remember, we almost always make up for the lack of fat by eating more sugar when we should be eating plenty of *healthy* fats to keep our brains, skin, and organs healthy. Be sure to enjoy cheese, eggs, avocados, butter, healthy oils, grass-fed meats, and fish. If you're a vegan, make sure you're not eating too many high-glycemic carbs. As I explained in detail in Chapter 8, it's not fat or cholesterol that's the culprit. It's sugar in all its many forms, including alcohol.

But don't overthink this or stress out about what you should and shouldn't eat. Healthy centenarians sure don't. Remember that eating should be a pleasurable ritual, not some kind of fundamentalist activity. Eat lots of greens, healthy fats, and protein. Cut out or at least cut down on sugars and grains. Avoid processed foods. Get in those cruciferous vegetables! And enjoy eating with others.

Take supplements that support health and wellness. The most important ones, and recommended dosages, are in the list that follows. The list can be used as a guideline. With any supplement, look on the label for "GMP," which stands for "good manufacturing practice," and the term "guaranteed potency" to ensure it's a high-quality supplement. You won't be able to get everything you need in just one tablet, but start with a good multivitamin, check the amounts of various vitamins and minerals in it, and use the chart below to fill in with nutrients that will support agelessness.

Table 1
Recommended Daily Supplementation

Vitamins	
Multivitamin	(See note above)
Vitamin C	1,000 to 5,000 mg
Vitamin D3	2,000 to 5,000 IU
Vitamin A (as beta-carotene)	25,000 IU
Vitamin E (as mixed tocopherols)	200 to 800 IU
Alpha-lipoic acid	10 to 100 mg
Coenzyme Q10 (ubiquinone)	10 to 100 mg*

* Use 70 to 100 mg coenzyme Q10 if you're at high risk for breast cancer. If you take a statin drug to lower your cholesterol, be sure to get your coenzyme Q10, because statin drugs reduce the levels of this important nutrient that's rare in our diets anyway (unless we eat a lot of organ meats).

Omega-3 fats	
DHA	200 to 2,500 mg
EPA	50 to 2,500 mg
B-complex vitamins	
Thiamine (B1)	8 to 100 mg
Riboflavin (B2)	9 to 50 mg
Niacin (B3)	20 to 100 mg
Pantothenic acid (B5)	15 to 400 mg
Pyridoxine (B6)	10 to 100 mcg
Cobalamin (B12)	20 to 250 mcg
Folic acid	1,000 mcg
Biotin	40 to 500 mcg
Inositol	10 to 500 mg
Choline	425 mg

Minerals (use chelated versions for optimal absorption)	
Calcium	500 to 1,200 mg
Magnesium	400 to 1,000 mg
Potassium	200 to 500 mg
Zinc	6 to 50 mg
Manganese	1 to 15 mg
Boron	2 to 9 mg
Copper	1 to 2 mg
Iron	15 to 30 mg
Chromium	100 to 400 mcg
Selenium	50 to 200 mcg
Molybdenum	45 mcg
Vanadium	50 to 100 mcg
Iodine	3 to 12.5 mg/day (from kelp or organic eggs, or from supplements)

Trace minerals from marine sources

For hormonal support in perimenopause or menopause to alleviate symptoms such as hot flashes and vaginal dryness, you can take *Pueraria mirifica* 80 to 100 mg twice per day. Make sure that the source is reputable and that the active ingredient, Puresterol, is on the label. (See my website, www.a-ma-ta.com, for *Pueraria mirifica* products.) Alternately, you can use maca, black cohosh, or ground flaxseed. If you have vaginal dryness, you can use any number of lubricants on the market, including those that contain *Pueraria mirifica,* which has been found to have a very beneficial effect on vaginal tissue. You can also ask your health care provider for a prescription for estriol vaginal cream, which is available through formulary pharmacies. Vaginal dryness is very, very easy to reverse.

Connect with the Divine. Say Divine Beloved prayers, do affirmations, or simply surrender your life to the Divine. I've provided examples throughout the book, and I'll suggest some specific ones for each day, but you can make up your own. It's important to allow emotions to come up naturally when you say prayers or affirmations. If you find yourself resisting them, know that beneath your resistance is the actual treasure—insight! Maybe you have to alter the wording you use, or substitute a prayer for an affirmation or vice versa. So if you're uncomfortable saying, "I am a beautiful, sexy goddess," word it differently to get past your mind's tendency toward negativity or doubt. Try this: "Divine Beloved, please change me into someone who feels and enjoys her divine beauty, sensuality, and sexual attractiveness. Help me experience my own lushness."

If affirmations or Divine Beloved prayers make you feel uncomfortable, it's probably because, generally speaking, our minds don't have a clue how to do any of this stuff. No one teaches us to say, "I'm wonderful!" And you may have bad memories about prayer. Honor that experience—I'm not asking you to deny its power. But recognize the power inherent in asking for the help of a loving, Divine force in feeling your worth. It's infinitely helpful to simply pray for assistance in changing your beliefs, but you have to ask! As the Bible says, "Ask and it is given. Knock and the door shall be opened unto you." It's true. Believe me, a Divine Beloved Change Me prayer can work wonders in your life. Don't let any initial discomfort or old baggage about God, religion, or prayer keep you from empowering, replenishing, and revitalizing yourself with these remarkable tools. You deserve to feel deeply beloved.

ACTIVITIES FOR DAYS 1 THROUGH 14

Day 1: Close cultural portals!

Affirmation: *"I am eternally youthful and vibrant."*

Prayer: *"Please change me into someone who is completely free of the cage of age!"*

The focus of Day 1 is closing cultural portals and replacing old perceptions that prevent you from being ageless. Take some time on Day 1 of the program to think about these ideas and make some decisions and commitments that will nourish agelessness.

Don't act your age! In fact, don't even think about it. Do something that might be considered "too young" for someone of "your age." You could dress or style your hair differently, or go to a party or event where everyone's younger than you are. The idea is to stop assigning meaning to numbers and thinking that a certain age is "old" or that you should or shouldn't do something when you are in your 50s, your 70s, or your 90s because it's "inappropriate."

Be aware of your self-talk and make sure it supports ageless-ness. Delete the sentence "I'm having a senior moment" from your vocabulary for good. Remove the phrase "at my age" as a preface for anything you're about to say. If you forget something, it's probably because you're overtaxing your brain by multitask-ing, or you're skipping sleep or eating poorly. Over time, yes, your brain will pay the price for chronically ignoring your body's needs and stressing yourself out, but if you forgot where you put your phone, don't reinforce the idea that you're aging and becom-ing senile. Stop, breathe, and ask yourself, "What do I need to do for myself right now?" Maybe misplacing your phone is the universe's way of telling you to stop checking in with your boss or clients to make sure they're not disappointed in you.

Choose how you will respond to questions about your age. You might say, "I'm in my ageless years," or "I was born in the twentieth century." Here's my personal favorite: "My biological age is thirty-five and my mental/emotional age is three hundred."

Reject the senior discount. Cultural beliefs about age are far more potent than your genes. Taking the "senior discount" lands you in the category we culturally associate with deterioration and decline. Now, if you're taking the discount mindfully so you can get a break on seeing the midnight sci-fi movie with the crowd of teenagers, or attending a concert featuring a hot new band, that's another story. Trust your gut on this one.

Find a couple of role models who are your age or above and let yourself be inspired. If you have no role models for agelessness, find some. You might want to print out a photograph and quote of theirs and place it somewhere in your home so you see it daily. Spend a few minutes reading an interview with these ageless role models or watching a video of them.

Day 2: Experience the power of pleasure.

Affirmation: *"I allow myself to experience pleasure, and my body, mind, and spirit rejoice."*

Prayer: *"Divine Beloved, please change me into someone who revels in the joy of life and in allowing others the supreme pleasure of delighting me."*

Day 2 is a day for pure pleasure and fun. Rediscover what gives you pleasure and indulge in it, fully aware that by letting yourself be a joyful goddess, you're boosting your immunity and helping your body repair cellular damage.

Make today a special occasion. What have you been putting off for a special occasion? Using your good china and silverware? Dressing up? Saying no to chores or work? Declare today a special occasion. As humorist and stress-management consultant Loretta LaRoche says, "Life is short, so wear your party pants." Experience pleasure that you would typically put off for a holiday or special occasion.

Practice exalted emotions by experiencing pleasure and joy. If you're not feeling enthusiastic about the day, try the inner smile exercise: Close your eyes. Smile. And then use the power of your mind to smile into your liver, your kidneys, your lungs, your heart, your genitals, your brain, your eyes, your ears, your nose—your entire body. This exercise instantly takes you into a better mood and builds immunity. Then find something that will give you pure pleasure—and do it.

Watch funny videos for ten minutes. The ones of cats never fail to make me laugh, but you get to choose whichever ones appeal to you. Laughter releases nitric oxide and beta-endorphins into your bloodstream, boosting immunity.

Day 3: Empower your inner healer.

Affirmation: *"My body is powered by Divine Radiant Substance and Divine Love. I am flourishing now!"*

Prayer: *"Divine Beloved, please change me into someone who totally trusts my body and all the messages it gives me about how it wants to be treated."*

On Day 3, the focus is on the mind/body connection. Find a balance between action and rest, and change your mind-set to support better physical and emotional health. There are many actions that can help your body heal itself, one of which is to tune in to your inner awareness of what you need to flourish. Honor that, regardless of what advice you encounter about how you "should" do this or "should" do that. Be mindful of what you eat today and make sure your food is nourishing. If you know you're not moving very much throughout the day, move more. If you're not sure you feel up to exercising, then just put on your workout gear and vow to be active for ten minutes. Often, those ten minutes will expand very pleasurably when you get past the initial inertia.

Counteract stress by beginning to establish a habit of rest and restoration. A habit of relaxation is a must if you want to live agelessly. It doesn't matter what you do—yoga, mindful breathing, listening to the reverberations of a brass singing bowl (used in meditation practice), bathing by candlelight, breathing in the smell of nature as you walk by a beach or in a park, or simply standing barefoot on the ground for 15 minutes. Even if you can only fit in 15 or 20 minutes, take that time for yourself. And think about how you can actually schedule in relaxation time. Where will it fit into your life? Make a commitment to resting and relaxing.

Turn off the bad news. Don't unnecessarily expose yourself to stressful situations and information that trigger an emotional response of anxiety, depression, or anger. Being a good mother, or daughter, or friend doesn't mean you have to be the dumping ground for every negative thought or feeling your daughter, mother, or friend wants to express. Being informed doesn't mean you have to expose yourself to a barrage of depressing information. Turn off CNN—the initials seem to stand for constantly negative news! Read good news or at least benign news that helps you have a better understanding of the world but gives you a sense of hope and helps you see what you can do to make a difference. Hang up, disconnect, and turn off your sources of stress today.

Ask your body what it needs for you to flourish. Your body has wisdom. Take a few moments to let your intuitive vision of what you need for good health come to you. You might get an image of lemon juice, symbolizing the need to detoxify your body. You might realize you really need a nap. If nothing comes to you when you ask yourself the question "What does my body need to heal and flourish?" ask it before you go to sleep and set the intention to get an answer in a dream.

Make a God Box. Worry is by far the most common drainer of joy and enthusiasm that I know of. Make a God Box—it can be any box you designate for this purpose. Any time you have a worry, just write it down and put it in the box. Then, when the same worry arises, tell yourself, "It's in the box." It's no longer on *your* To Do list—God is taking care of it. This practice can work wonders for alleviating worry and stress.

Day 4: Understand and implement the causes of health.

Affirmation: *"Divine Love is now magnified throughout my body, mind, and spirit. I release all my problems to the Creator. I am alive with energy and radiant with glowing health."*

Prayer: *"May I be healed with Divine Love according to the Creator's Will."*

On Day 4, begin to reset any old habits of going on a "search and destroy" mission to seek out problems in your body and fix them. Commit to getting to know your body, expressing love to it, and listening to it. Agelessness is having faith in your body and in the future.

Send love to your body. Affirm the health of your heart, breasts, and erotic anatomy. Envision sending love and appreciation to these parts of your body as you caress them. You might try the Body Love exercise from Chapter 4 and admire your body by candlelight. Pay attention to all that's working about your body and affirm it. Close your eyes and feel how good it feels to have feet on the ground, a spine that holds you up, and so on. Take your time with this so you truly feel grateful and amazed by your beautiful, strong body. Do the same for any part of your body you would like to improve in some way, or any part of your body you're concerned about. Create the expectation that your body is becoming healthier and even better at serving you. For instance, you might draw your focus to your eyes, express gratitude for your eyesight, and affirm that it's improving.

Get enough sleep, and be sure you eat well. Sleep in if your body tells you to rest. Take a little time to consider your sleep habits and how you might improve them. Make the best possible choices about what to eat. If you can't eat the best food at every meal or snack today, send Divine Love into your food before you eat it, knowing that the Divine has changed it into something that will nourish you. Let go of any guilt. Think about and even journal about what's stopping you from giving your body the rest, sleep, and nourishment it needs.

Flex and tone your pelvic floor muscles. Use a Squatty Potty stool or at least lean forward when you use the toilet to put your pelvic floor muscles into a natural position for eliminating waste, and don't rush to relieve yourself. Let it come naturally. Identify the feeling of tightening your pelvic floor muscles and squeeze them today for at least a couple of minutes. In this way, you help build the muscles that will keep you from developing incontinence (and if you have it to any degree, building up your pelvic floor muscles will help).

Day 5: Grieve, rage, and move on.

Affirmation: *"It is safe for me to feel my emotions fully and to release them. The crying will stop when it needs to stop. I have the strength to tolerate my strong emotions."*

Prayer: *"With my spirit, I focus Divine Love throughout my system. I ask my spirit to identify all the causes of and symptoms of my discomfort, resentment, grief, and anger and release them to the Creator according to the Creator's Will.*

Releasing old, toxic emotions is one of the most important things you can do for your health, but most people were never taught how to do it. On Day 5, begin letting go of anger, hurt, resentment, and the grief you're holding on to because of something that happened in the past. Realize that the reason resentments are so difficult to release is that we have unwittingly given our sense of worthiness and self-love to those who have hurt us. Create a ritual for release that will contain your emotions so you don't become overwhelmed by them. Set a timer or decide what you want to do to complete the ritual once you've experienced the feeling of letting go of the difficult feelings that come up for you. You might say an affirmation or do something that makes you laugh so that you can clear the air of the old emotions. This part of a ritual is often called grounding because it brings you back to ordinary consciousness. Having something to eat is another way to ground after a releasing ritual. You might also ask someone to hug you, or you might say a prayer of gratitude as you cuddle your pet. You could simply say aloud, "That's enough of that. Onward!"

Consciously choose to forgive someone. Write a letter to someone who has hurt you. Say everything you always wanted to say. Don't stop writing until you feel as though the resentment and hurt are drained onto the paper. This exercise is for you and you alone. Expressing what you experienced—acknowledging it consciously—is a step you must take before you can truly release yourself from this other person. Now burn the letter and take a soothing Epsom salts bath. When you pull the plug, imagine all that negativity going down the drain. Repeat if necessary. Remember that forgiveness is something that you do for you, not for the other person. Forgiveness frees you.

If you don't want to write a letter, you can say today's prayer or affirm that you're consciously choosing to let go of negative thoughts and emotions about a past experience and forgive the other person. You might say, "Divine Beloved, change me into someone who is free from my past and the beliefs I held when I was a child. Change me into someone who is no longer angry at my parents." Then do the Epsom salts bath to detox and release old toxins down the drain.

The choice to forgive and express your truth is an important first step in actually forgiving someone, *but it is only a first step.* You have to release old emotions of anger, fear, and grief too, and you can start that work today. The body tends to hold on to old emotions deep in its tissues, so be sure to follow this first step with at least one if not several exercises for releasing the emotions.

Release buried emotions in a contained way. This will return you to a state of natural happiness. Old emotions get buried in your personal energy field and your body. Over time, they penetrate your tissues very deeply and even result in thickened and scarred connective tissue. Massage therapists and yoga teachers often notice that their clients begin to cry when these fascial areas are released during bodywork. Releasing these patterns regularly is part of being an ageless goddess. Think of it as being like flossing your teeth.

You can use the Snapping Out of Grief and Rage exercise, where you face a chair and express your emotions (see page 133), or the Cutting Energetic Cords exercise, where you cut the cords of grief, anger, hurt, and sadness that bind you to people who have hurt you (see page 221). You can also meditate with the intention of having a good cry, or watch a movie that will get your tears flowing, or play a recording of a song that gets you in touch with your anger, and dance fiercely. Remember: we heal through movement, sound, and tears.

Be mindful that you're not avoiding your difficult emotions, skimming their surface because it's hard for you to tolerate them. If there's no emotion associated with your forgiving someone, chances are that no permanent forgiveness is happening. I get callers to my radio show who begin to do an imprint removal with me, and I can tell that they're consciously choosing to forgive but they're resisting the release of the old emotions. They'll say something like, "Mom, I forgive you for neglecting me and criticizing me whenever you did pay attention to me—" and then they'll quickly add "—but I understand you were going through a lot of stress and your own mother wasn't nurturing . . ." They start making excuses for the other person and stuffing their feelings again. You *must* let the feelings out if you ever expect to truly move on. This is not an intellectual exercise. It's a release process in the emotional body!

Forgiving and blessing those who have hurt you is the only way to get them or their toxic patterns out of your life permanently. It liberates you from self-entrapment. Remember that forgiveness is not about the other person, nor does it mean you're condoning what they did. Grief and rage are very sticky: they will keep attracting their energetic equivalents to you if you don't release them. For more help with emotional release, try the "21 Days of Forgiveness" program by Iyanla Vanzant, from her book *Forgiveness: 21 Days to Forgive Everyone for Everything* (SmileyBooks, 2013). *You Can Heal Your Life* by Louise Hay and *A Course in Miracles* also have lots of forgiveness suggestions.

It can take more than one session to release strong emotions you're holding on to, so you may need to come back to do more emotional releasing later on. And remember what you learned earlier—neurons that fire together, wire together—so if you create a habit of releasing emotions, your brain will actually rewire itself for optimism and forgiveness. You want to release the emotion and move on—not wallow in it forever—so that you can establish habits for ageless living.

Day 6: Be sexy and sensual.

Affirmation: *"I am Aphrodite—I am a goddess of divine pleasure, beauty, and passion. And I am irresistible."*

Prayer: *"Divine Beloved, please change me into someone who owns and enjoys her own beauty and sensuality."*

Sexuality and sensuality are connected with the pelvic bowl, and we need to get out of our heads and back into our hips. Doing so also helps the brain! We also need time, space, and freedom to experience pleasure in our bodies, and to honor ourselves and our desire for sensual pleasures. That means carving out time for ourselves—uninterrupted. That's the delight waiting for you on Day 6.

Reconnect with your pelvic bowl. There's much to be gained from reconnecting with your pelvic bowl through movement, touch, and focus. Swing your hips or belly dance to music. Self-pleasure, or explore your erotic anatomy with your hands (not a vibrator) and maybe a mirror too—and learn the feeling of slowly and sensually contracting your pelvic floor muscles, as described on pages 110–111.

Create a sensual playlist. Music goes right to the emotional centers of the brain. To further enhance your ability to connect with your sensual self, I suggest a "self-cultivation" playlist of music that you listen to while doing hip circles or self-pleasuring.

Creating this list and updating it is sheer pleasure! Here are some of my favorites:

- ~ "Feelin' Love" (Paula Cole)
- ~ "Sacred Love" (Sting)
- ~ "Glory Box" (Portishead)
- ~ "Porcelain" (Moby)
- ~ "Cream" (Prince)
- ~ "Lick" (Joi)
- ~ "Beautiful" (Meshell Ndegeocello)
- ~ "Chocolate" (Kylie Minogue)
- ~ "I'm Kissing You" (Des'ree)
- ~ "Buttons" (Pussycat Dolls)
- ~ "I Touch Myself" (Divinyls)
- ~ "Slow Down" (Morcheeba)

Use aromatherapy. Like music, smell has a powerful effect on the emotions. Use perfume, scented candles, essential oils, or aromatherapy to bring more pleasure to whatever activity you enjoy. You can look up aromatherapy oils and see which are typically the most relaxing, or you can just use whichever make you feel calm. See Resources for some of my favorites.

Enjoy luscious lubrication. Many women experience vaginal dryness. Again, this is very easy to remedy, allowing you to enjoy penetration. There are many effective lubricants available. You can even use organic coconut oil.

Own the power of your "Lady Garden." Ob/gyn Dr. Sara Gottfried calls the female genitals the "Lady Garden"—a term that I love! This area of the body has great power once it is awakened. Do the following: Sometime today when you are getting a cup of coffee or standing in a checkout line, bring your attention to your Lady Garden. Feel the tingling that happens with attention. Then smile at someone or give someone a compliment.

Notice what happens—especially with men. Just the thought of this makes you smile, doesn't it?

Day 7: Love without losing yourself.

Affirmation: *"I am a unique embodiment of Divine Love. My life is powered by my connection with Source. I feel whole, complete, and lacking in nothing."*

Prayer: *"Divine Beloved, please let me feel the truth about myself. Let me truly feel whole, complete, and lacking in nothing."*

Relationships are meant to connect us to our hearts and replenish us, not drain us. Today, take pleasure in your relationships, starting with your relationship with yourself. Make it a love affair—imagine you are the love of your life. How would you treat yourself? If you have a partner, imagine that the person you're with relishes the fact that, ultimately, it's *you* who are the love of your life.

Taking pleasure in your relationships also means saying no when someone else's needs become a burden for you. This can be a challenge because many of us have spent years putting the needs of others before our own. Saying no is very likely to fill you with doubt and guilt at first. With practice, you'll find out how freeing this is. There's a reason why my favorite chapter in Cheryl Richardson's book *The Art of Extreme Self-Care* (Hay House, 2009) is the one titled "Let Me Disappoint You." You will *never* be able to become ageless if you're always donating your energy to others at your own expense!

Have fun with your tribe. Have a girls' night, invite friends over, or call a friend to go out and have fun. If you're married or partnered, go out just for the fun of it and don't put pressure on yourself to make it a "perfect" date night. Let go of any agenda other than having fun bonding with each other.

Set a healthy boundary. As you wake up in the morning, set the intention to clarify or set a boundary with someone. It could be a friend or family member, or it could be someone you work with—or even an acquaintance or stranger. Remember that when you honor your own needs, you're inspiring others to honor theirs too, so when asked to do something you don't want to do, don't be afraid to say, "No, I can't. I simply can't." In fact, memorize this phrase! Be assertive by smiling and repeating the same simple statement as often as needed: "No. I just don't feel comfortable with that." "No, thank you." "I understand. Again, I simply can't." Saying no can be very invigorating! And if you feel someone is looking to you to rescue him or her, you can say something like, "I'm sorry you're going through this, but I know you're going to find the solution." Or "I'm so sorry. I wish I had the solution for you, but I have faith that it will come to you." We often feel compelled to rescue others in order to soothe our own worry and sense of powerlessness. Remember, people often go through difficulties because they need to reconnect with their own Divine Source. You are actually causing them harm when you bail them out. Don't stand in their way just to alleviate your own worry that they won't be okay. Be loving and supportive, and assist someone if it feels right to do so and won't deplete you. But if your heart (or body) tells you that the best course of action is to express compassion and not take on their troubles and try to fix them, listen to it!

Reflect on your relationship with a man in your life. All of us have men in our lives. Spend some time thinking about how a man or boy you care about is feeling pressured to be a certain way regardless of how he feels. Whether it's a son who feels he has to be good at sports or a brother who feels he can't show his vulnerability and fear when it comes to dealing with your aging parents, there's a man in your life who can benefit when you connect with your ageless goddess self and let go of old ideas about how we are "supposed" to act and feel to fit into a culture that diminishes all that's feminine or womanly.

Express gratitude for what you learned from your mother or daughter, and work to heal that relationship. There's nothing like the mother-daughter bond to cause you extreme joy or extreme pain. Whatever your mother-daughter relationships are, however troubled they might be, there is something your soul can learn from that. Honor and cherish that today. Then, for your own sake, make a move toward healing the mother-daughter bond you have with your mother or daughter. It can be something small, like simply telling her, "I haven't said this in a while, but I love you." It can be setting a boundary that's healthy for both of you (for example, not picking up the phone when your mother calls if you know that she's just going to complain). Even if you don't have daughters or if your mother has passed, think about your girlfriends or female family members who occasionally drain you. Learn to express your love to yourself by doing a cord-cutting exercise to ensure that you're not maintaining any draining energetic cords to your late mother or anyone else.

Day 8: Eat like a goddess.

Affirmation: *"I eat slowly and sensually, with great pleasure, savoring every bite."*

Prayer: *"Divine Beloved, change me into someone who enjoys my body and the healthy food I choose to eat. Help me make the best possible choices for nourishing myself."*

For many of us, food has become a chore, a threat, a necessity—anything but a pleasure. For today, banish the food police and your internal guilt and judgment about what you eat, and put fresh and delicious foods on the menu. Nourish your body while truly enjoying your food. Eat sensually, like a divine goddess infusing her body with the luscious fruits of the earth.

Savor the foods you eat, whatever they are. Arrange food on your plate beautifully, and then eat slowly and sensually as though you were slow dancing in the moonlight. You might also make a point of eating with people whose company gives you pleasure. As you eat, pay attention to how good it feels and what a delicious experience eating is. Try to eat as healthfully as possible, and if you end up indulging in a treat, relish every bite of it. Chew slowly! Inhale the aroma of your food or drink before you bring it to your lips. Then enjoy every mouthful or sip. Think about how it feels to have a pleasurable relationship with food that's good for you—and how it feels to enjoy a treat without feeling guilty or ashamed. Eat as though you are making love with your food.

Try a new, healthy food or recipe—especially if it involves vegetables. Let's face it—underneath all the advice about diet, and beyond all our individual differences, every one of us could eat more vegetables. Sometimes it's just easier to reach for something else to put on our plates. Make a point today of trying a new vegetable or preparing a new vegetable dish. You can find recipes on the Internet very easily and even search by vegetable, which is helpful when a particular vegetable is in season, plentiful, and at the height of its taste and nutritional quality.

Do tapping, using EFT (the Emotional Freedom Techniques) before each meal or snack. The technique, which you can see demonstrated in videos at www.TheTappingSolution.com, will help you to release any shame or guilt you have about what you've eaten in the past, your weight, and your relationship with food. Try it for a day, using it before you begin to eat a meal or snack. Pay attention to how you feel during the exercise and afterward.

Day 9: Move joyously and sensually—like a cat!

Affirmation: *"My body was designed to move and stretch and feel strong, flexible, and alive. I love the feeling."*

Prayer: *"Divine Beloved, change me into someone who enjoys moving in my body. Help me find ways to move my body throughout the day, in ways that build my strength and vitality."*

Don't worry about "exercise." Today's the day to get back in touch with your body by moving it in ways that give you pleasure, stretch your muscles, and get your energy flowing so that you feel alive.

Dance or have fun trying a new type of movement. Whether you dance or do interval training, whether you go to an exercise class or simply do some yoga poses in your living room, move your body and enjoy doing it. If you dance or hike for exercise, do it a little differently today. Walk in a place where you've never walked before, or try a new dance class. And pay attention to what feels good and what doesn't when you stretch or move. Does a little discomfort make you feel good while you're doing it? Does it feel good afterward? Be honest with yourself about how the movement feels, and don't do it simply because it's on your list or because you associate exercise with weight loss. Switch to a more joyful form of movement for today and see how that feels for you. You might make a playlist and dance around the house dusting or decluttering, or get together with friends and go for a walk outside.

If you sit most of the day, set a timer and stand up every 15 minutes. Do a little stretching or yoga, even if just for a minute. Do some hip circles and some stretches. Notice how much more energized you feel at the end of the day.

Practice balancing. Stand on one foot (when you're not wearing heels). Close your eyes. Balance for as long as you can. Repeat on the other foot. Do this throughout the day.

Pretend you are a cat. Stretch like a cat. Yawn like a cat or dog. And really feel how great it feels to tense your muscles as you stretch. Do a catlike stretch a few times throughout the day.

Day 10: Be gorgeous.

Affirmations: *"I am a beautiful, divine, gorgeous creature."* Try saying this while looking deeply into your eyes in a mirror in the morning and again at bedtime: *"I love you, gorgeous woman. I really love you."*

Prayer: *"Divine Beloved, please change me into someone who sees how very beautiful I am."*

Day 10 is for connecting with your inner Venus, the energy of beauty that lies within you, and venerating it simply because you deserve to feel and see yourself as gorgeous. Today is a day for redefining what it means to be beautiful and for discovering ageless beauty. Be conscious of cultural portals about beauty today and reject them. Don't dress for your age!

Do a beauty ritual or have a beauty treatment. Whether you do it at home or at a salon, do something to enhance your beauty or adorn yourself—and take pleasure in doing it. What's important isn't how much time or money you spend attending to what you look like, but enjoying the ritual of adorning and enhancing your body so that you feel beautiful. If you're not comfortable getting a facial or manicure, go to a boutique and get some personalized service in trying on and choosing clothes, do a hair treatment at home, or go to a makeup counter for a free makeover. Here's a simple home beauty ritual: pour a tablespoon of sugar or salt into your palm with some olive oil, mix it, and rub it into your hands to soften them. Then wash them with gentle soap. Luxuriate in the feel of your soft hands.

Close a cultural portal about beauty. Wear something that you once might have thought was "too young" or "too daring" for you to wear. Or style your hair or nails differently, in a way that suits you, regardless of whether someone might say that it looks too youthful on you. If there's something in your closet that you bought but never wore because it seemed too "out there" compared to what you usually wear, put it on today. Be sure to affirm your beauty and sense of style—and remember that taking chances with how you adorn yourself is part of an ageless attitude.

Make an entrance. Hold your head up as though you are suspended by a string from the ceiling. Relax your shoulders. Walk as though you are the Queen of the Universe entering a room, slowly and beautifully. Notice what feelings arise when you consciously do this.

Day 11: Know yourself as divine.

Affirmation: "I am the Divine Source, I am, I am, I am. God comes through me as me."

Prayer: "Divine Beloved, change me into someone who feels your presence in my life, who sees the Divinity within me."

You've no doubt heard this before, but it bears repeating here. You are a spiritual being currently inhabiting a human body. Day 11 is for remembering and reconnecting with who you really are: your spiritual essence.

Pick up your journal. One way to reconnect with who you are as a spiritual being—with the essence of you—is to write in your journal, or read past entries, or both. If you don't journal, start one today. There aren't any rules about how much you have to write, or whether you have to write every day or most days. You might even want to draw in your journal—drawing is a wonderful way to express yourself and your feelings. When you take quiet time alone with your journal, you can reconnect to your spirit and to Spirit.

Remind yourself of your spirit. Often, we feel pressured to act inauthentically, out of sync with our spirit. Today's a day to reconnect with your spirit and remind yourself why it's important to be who you really are instead of who others want you to be. Today you might look at old photos of yourself from a time when you were expressing your spirit fully. You might go outside and walk barefoot on the earth or spend time among the trees, reconnecting to your sense of yourself as a spiritual being integrated with nature. Get an astrological chart done and spend some time pondering whether what it reveals rings true for you. Or simply ponder some of the cycles you've been through and the challenges you've overcome.

Practice mindfulness. Pray and say affirmations if you like, but make a point today of drawing your attention to what you're doing or feeling in the moment, without judgment. See what feelings and sensations come up and sit with them. You might find yourself feeling pride at having made it through the chaos of last week, or the stress of a challenging time at work, or you might realize you're tired—or angry. Honor your spirit by practicing mindfulness so that you can notice what you're experiencing.

Find a way to connect with others in spirit and community. The power of the experience of spiritual reconnection can be magnified in a group, so consider joining one, whether it's a 12-step program, a meditation group, or a prayer group. I also know countless women who gather at full moons or on solstices and equinoxes to connect with the Divine Beloved and the divine within each of them. I do this myself and have found it invaluable. If you feel more comfortable being a part of a community effort, take pleasure in that today while remaining aware of how it feels to be integrated into a community of people sharing an experience together.

Say a prayer or an affirmation. If you have been avoiding saying prayers or affirmations, today's the day to try it. Maybe it will feel strange to you, but maybe you'll realize you get something out of the experience that you hadn't anticipated. Say some of the prayers or affirmations in this book, silently or aloud. Feel free to change the wording to make it more comfortable for you—and to make your prayer or affirmation a better tool for reconnecting to your spirit and to Spirit.

Day 12. Create a personal paradise worthy of Aphrodite.

Affirmation: *"I am worthy of my own personal paradise—a place for renewal and rejuvenation."*

Prayer: *"Divine Beloved, change me into someone who honors herself by surrounding herself with space that reflects my inner beauty and divinity."*

Day 12 is about altering your space, because too often we deny how important it is to be in physical space that rejuvenates us. We too often settle for ugly rooms, or being in dark, artificially lit spaces, and forget how great it feels to be out in nature, our natural home.

So on Day 12, create a personal paradise that's a physical manifestation of beauty and peace. Keep this simple and doable.

Take 15 minutes to rearrange your space to be more supportive of your ageless goddess mind-set. Set a timer for 15 minutes and do one of the following:

- ~ Make a small, beautiful altar—with candles, flowers, a favorite photo, or a beautiful piece of fabric.

- ~ Clean a drawer, clear off a bathroom counter, or clean off a cluttered dresser top. Notice how good this "white space" feels whenever you enter the room.

It's important to take that minute or two to get in touch with how you feel after arranging the space. That's what will reinforce the idea that what your space looks and feels like matters. Today is the day to begin establishing the habit of creating beautiful spaces in your home, even if you can only do it 15 minutes at a time.

Create a boudoir or powder room worthy of a goddess by making simple changes to the space. You'll want to use high-quality essential oils and music that energizes and relaxes you when you're in this space. Today, you might simply order some new recordings to listen to when you're bathing or use candles, flowers, and luscious scents to enhance these rooms. Then spend some time enjoying the sensual space you've just sculpted for yourself. Think of it as your personal paradise.

Find the perfect place in nature to replenish yourself. Get out into nature, choosing a special spot where you feel comfortable. Spend at least 20 minutes there, being mindful of how it feels to have the sun on your face, the wind in your hair, and the earth underneath your feet. This is your natural home, so visit it often!

Day 13: Affirm your goddess nature.

Affirmation: *"I deserve pleasure and joy. I am ageless, strong, and powerful. I relish great health. I am an ageless goddess, an expression of the creative, divine life force."*

Prayer: *"Divine Beloved, please change me into someone who feels ageless. Allow me to feel the eternal Source within me."*

On Day 13, choose one of the activities you have done in the past 12 days and repeat it—and be sure to do something pleasurable, not just something that's good for you. Remember, living as an ageless goddess means bringing more and more pleasure into your life and leaving worry and fear behind. Be joyful and affirm your right to pleasure, using affirmations or Divine Beloved prayers. Becoming and then living as an ageless goddess is a way of life, not a destination. It means living from the inside out and knowing that the soul enters your body through your hips, not your intellect. You can't think your way into being happy (although a positive attitude helps quite a lot). You also have to experience pleasure in your body and especially in your pelvis.

Day 14. Align with Divine Order.

Affirmation: *"Divine Order is in charge of my life. I now turn my life over to Divine Order, knowing that the perfect solution to every situation in my life has already been chosen."*

Prayer: *"Divine Beloved, please change me into someone who trusts that what's meant for me will always come, in exactly the right way and at exactly the right time for my highest good."*

Living agelessly takes courage and discipline. Nothing is easier than complaining and acting old, which some people do when they're only 30! To be ageless, you have to align with Divine Order and let yourself be shown what to do. Agelessness requires living in the moment, in alignment with the rhythms of nature. It's simple, but it's not easy because we're under a lot of pressure to think ahead and plan out everything. And we habitually worry that we did the wrong thing, and we beat ourselves up for not being perfect. The path of imperfection is the only one that is sustainable. Here's a Divine Beloved prayer to say if you have trouble staying in the moment: "Divine Beloved, please change me into someone who knows exactly how to live as an ageless goddess." Aligning with Divine Order requires surrendering to the divine part of yourself that knows more than your intellect (your ego). The divine part of you is your soul. It means having faith that what's meant for you will always come—and if it's not meant for you, you won't want it anyway.

AGELESS LIVING

Once you have completed the 14-Day Ageless Goddess Program, your mission is to create an ageless goddess life and make sure you're surrounded by others who support you in living this way. Find at least one friend to walk this path with you. Connect with other ageless goddesses in person and on the Internet (which is especially important if it's difficult for you to get out to be with people every day—or with people who support ageless living). Each day, journal about your experiences so you can get a sense of which activities you want to do more of. Use calendars, reminder apps, and appointments with yourself to make sure you're honoring the ageless goddess you are.

From now on, remember this: you have the power to be an ageless goddess and to be a living, breathing embodiment of joyful, ageless living—*no matter what has gone before*. As the saying goes, "What you are seeking is also seeking you." So who do you really want to be? Who would you be if your age weren't a factor? Ask yourself these questions every morning and then live them throughout your day. Make that ageless goddess within you feel at home. Bless her, please her, welcome her. Little by little she will show up more and more until one day soon, you will look in the mirror and see a whole new woman smiling back at you. This is your new chapter, your new life. The best is yet to come. I promise.

RESOURCES

Chapter 1

Learn more about Dr. Mario E. Martinez's work on cultural portals at the website of the Biocognitive Science Institute, www.biocognitive.com, and follow him on Facebook at www.facebook.com/TheMindBodyCode. His posts are wonderful. He also has a whole series of YouTube videos. And do check out his book *The MindBody Code* (Boulder, CO: Sounds True, 2014).

I highly recommend Tosha Silver's books *Outrageous Openness: Letting the Divine Take the Lead* (New York: Atria Books, 2014) and *Make Me Your Own: Poems to the Divine Beloved* (Alameda, CA: Urban Kali Productions, 2013). Her website is www.toshasilver.com, and you can follow her on Twitter at www.twitter.com/toshasil as well as on Facebook at www.facebook .com/ToshaSilver13.

Chapter 2

Jill Bolte Taylor, Ph.D., told her story of being awoken to the abilities of her right, intuitive brain in her book *My Stroke of Insight: A Brain Scientist's Personal Journey* (New York: Viking, 2008) and her TED talk of the same name, March 2008, at: http://new.ted.com/talks/jill_bolte_taylor_s_powerful _stroke_of_insight.

Anita Moorjani's story of returning from a near-death experience after a serious illness is very inspiring and enlightening. Her book is *Dying to Be Me: My Journey from Cancer, to Near Death, to True Healing* (Carlsbad, CA: Hay House, 2012).

You can learn more about pleasure in your ageless years, and the role of nitric oxide, in my book *The Secret Pleasures of Menopause* (Carlsbad, CA: Hay House, 2008).

Colette Baron-Reid's *Weight Loss for People Who Feel Too Much: A 4-Step, 8-Week Plan to Finally Lose the Weight, Manage Emotional Eating, and Find Your Fabulous Self* (New York: Harmony, 2013), is about overcoming the habit of using pleasurable food to compensate for having porous emotional boundaries.

"Mama Gena" (Regena Thomashauer) has a school for reclaiming your sexuality and sensuality. You can learn about her ideas in her book *Mama Gena's School of Womanly Arts: Using the Power of Pleasure to Have Your Way with the World* (New York: Simon & Schuster, 2002). To learn about her classes, visit her website, www.mamagenas.com. Her online community can be found at www.sistergoddess.com.

Chapters 3 and 4

There are many herbs that have been successfully used to quell menopausal symptoms. These include chasteberry, dong quai, maca, and the Thai herb *Pueraria mirifica,* which contains a unique and effective phytoestrogen called miroestrol. I have been so impressed with *Pueraria mirifica* that I started a new company to bring the most effective form of this supplement to women everywhere: www.a-ma-ta.com.

For more information on postmenopausal breast health and breast cancer, see www.breasthealthcancerprevention.com/What_is_breast_cancer.htm.

Serial urine testing, which tests for not only estrogen, progesterone, and testosterone, but also your patterns of stress hormone release, can be done through www.precisionhormones.com.

You can buy bath gel, oil, or bath crystals from Health and Wisdom at www.health-and-wisdom.com.

A biofeedback device such as the emWave from the Institute of HeartMath can help you learn how to get into the state called "cardiac coherence," in which HRV (heart rate variability) is optimized. See www.heartmath.org.

An NMR lipid profile for cholesterol can only be obtained through LabCorp, www.labcorp.com, or LipoScience, www.liposcience.com.

You can learn more about home versions of the 25(OH)D test for vitamin D yourself at http://www.vitamindcouncil.org/about-vitamin-d/testing-for -vitamin-d. You can order a home test through ZRT Labs or New Century Diagnostic's Home Health Testing website or City Assays in the United Kingdom.

Learn more about ancient Taoist exercises such as the Female Deer Exercise in Stephen T. Chang's book *The Tao of Sexology: The Book of Infinite Wisdom* (San Francisco, CA: Tao Publishing, 1986).

You can buy pomegranate breast oil (for sending love to your breasts as you massage them) at www.pomegranatebreastoil.com.

If you want to find a practitioner who performs and interprets thermograms so that you can monitor your breasts regularly as part of your plan for loving self-care, visit www.breastthermography.com, www.breastthermography.org, or the websites of the International Academy of Clinical Thermology (www.iact-org.org) or the American College of Clinical Thermology (www.thermologyonline.org).

The Squatty Potty toilet stool for supporting a healthy pelvic floor can be found at www.squattypotty.com. You can learn more about toning the pelvic muscle group in a book by Kathryn Kassai, P.T., C.E.S., and Kim Perelli, *The Bathroom Key: Put an End to Incontinence* (New York: Demos Health, 2012, www.demoshealth.com).

I highly recommend USANA pharmaceutical-grade supplements and have been using them and recommending them for many years. I am also a distributor. For more information, go to www.usana.com.

Chapter 5

You can learn about Unity minister Jill Rogers's Seven Sacred Steps workshops at www.thesevensacredsteps.com.

Eve Ensler, author of *The Vagina Monologues,* organized a global movement called One Billion Rising, www.onebillionrising.org, and creates events for celebrating the survivors of sexual abuse.

Information on the findings of the ACE study of adverse childhood experiences can be found at www.acestudy.org.

Declutter your life with the help of Marla Cilley, The Fly Lady (www.flylady .net), a woman who teaches millions how to overcome CHAOS ("can't have anyone over syndrome").

Chapter 6

I recommend the following books on women's sexuality:

Jenny Wade, *Transcendent Sex: When Lovemaking Opens the Veil* (New York: Gallery Books, 2004).

Tami Lynn Kent, *Wild Feminine: Finding Power, Spirit & Joy in the Female Body* (New York: Atria Books/Beyond Words, 2011).

Sheri Winston, *Women's Anatomy of Arousal: Secret Maps to Buried Pleasure* (Kingston, NY: Mango Garden Press, 2009).

Barbara Hand Clow, *Liquid Light of Sex: Kundalini, Astrology, and the Key Life Transitions* (Rochester, VT: Bear and Company, 2001).

Steve and Vera Bodansky, *Extended Massive Orgasm: How You Can Give and Receive Intense Sexual Pleasure,* 2nd edition (Alameda, CA. Hunter House, 2013).

David Deida, *Finding God Through Sex: Awakening the One of Spirit Through the Two of Flesh*, 2nd edition (Boulder, CO: Sounds True, 2005).

Mantak Chia and Rachel Carlton-Abrams, M.D., *The Multi-Orgasmic Woman: Sexual Secrets Every Woman Should Know* (New York: HarperOne, 2009).

I highly recommend a DVD called *A Guide to Your Orgasm*, produced by the Welcomed Consensus (www.welcomed.com).

Mama Gena's School of Womanly Arts in New York City, run by Regena Thomashauer (www.mamagenas.com), is an incredible source for learning how to reconnect with your pelvic bowl and your sexuality. Check out her books *Mama Gena's School of Womanly Arts: Using the Power of Pleasure to Have Your Way with the World* (New York: Simon & Schuster, 2002) and *Mama Gena's Owner's and Operator's Guide to Men* (New York: Simon & Schuster, 2004).

Gina Ogden, Ph.D., a pioneering researcher whose ISIS study revealed new information about women's sexuality, has written several books on the topic, including *Women Who Love Sex: Ordinary Women Describe Their Paths to Pleasure, Intimacy, and Ecstasy* (Boston, MA: Trumpeter Books, 2007). Her website is www.expandingsextherapy.com.

Betty Dodson, a pioneer in encouraging women's self-pleasuring who is now in her 80s, has a marvelous website devoted to this topic at www.dodson andross.com.

Student of tantric sex Layla Martin offers an effective and fun online course in femininity and sexuality on her website at www.layla-martin.com.

Women's health physical therapist Tami Lynn Kent (www.wildfeminine .com) as well as Larry and Belinda Wurn (www.clearpassage.com), who developed the Wurn Technique and have trained many other physical thera-pists, report some incredible results with using manual therapy on women who find sex painful due to fascial scarring and lesions. Jennifer Mercier, M.D. (www.drjennifermercier.com), is also an expert in this area and has trained other practitioners in manual therapy for pelvic scarring. You can also find more information about women's health physical therapists at www.thebathroomkey.com or www.obgyn-physicaltherapy.com.

My favorite essential oils that can be used for aromatherapy are Uttati oils from www.gabrielleyoung.com and Young Living Essential Oils from www .youngliving.com.

Chapter 7

Peter Calhoun and Astrid Ganz's book *Last Hope on Earth* (Knoxville, TN: World Service Institute, 2013) offers energetic healing techniques including imprint removals.

Miriam E. Nelson, Ph.D., a nutritionist at Tufts University, and Jennifer Ackerman wrote *The Social Network Diet: Change Yourself, Change the World* (Campbell, CA: FastPencil, 2011), about how social networks affect our eating and exercising behaviors and what you can do to give and receive support for healthy lifestyle choices. Available from http://premiere.fastpencil.com /social-network-diet. Miriam Nelson's website is www.strongwomen.com.

For more on energetic connections, read Robin Kelly, M.D.'s *The Human Antenna: Reading the Language of the Universe in the Songs of Our Cells* (Fulton, CA: Elite Books/Energy Psychology Press, 2007). www.human antenna.com.

Chapter 8

The most up-to-date way to test your cholesterol is the NMR lipid profile, which you can obtain through LabCorp, www.labcorp.com, or LipoScience, www.liposcience.com.

You can order many of your own lab tests through SaveOnLabs at www .saveonlabs.com. You can learn more about home versions of the 25(OH)D test for vitamin D yourself at http://www.vitamindcouncil.org/about-vitamin-d /testing-for-vitamin-d. You can order a home test through ZRT Labs or New Century Diagnostic's Home Health Testing website or City Assays in the United Kingdom.

A good source for Paleo diet recipes is www.fastpaleo.com.

The best thyroid site I've found is Mary Shomon's http://thyroid.about.com.

Everyone with a thyroid problem needs to know about iodine. Please read *Iodine: Why You Need It, Why You Can't Live Without It*, 5th edition, by David Brownstein, M.D. (West Bloomfield, MI: Medical Alternatives Press, 2014).

To overcome old blocks about food and weight, I recommend Jessica Ortner's *The Tapping Solution for Weight Loss & Body Confidence: A Woman's Guide to Stressing Less, Weighing Less, and Loving More* (Carlsbad, CA: Hay House, 2014). See her website too, at www.TheTappingSolution.com.

I also recommend *Women, Food, and Desire: Embrace Your Cravings, Make Peace with Food, Reclaim Your Body* by Alexandra Jamieson (New York: Gallery Books, 2015) and *Pleasurable Weight Loss: The Secrets to Feeling Great, Losing Weight and Loving Your Life Today* by Jena la Flamme (Boulder, CO: Sounds True, 2015). Or visit Jena la Flamme's website, www .PleasurableWeightLoss.com.

Chapter 9

Bob Cooley's Resistance Flexibility program is outlined in his book *The Genius of Flexibility: The Smart Way to Stretch and Strengthen Your Body* (New

York: Touchstone, 2005). You can also go to his website to learn more: www.thegeniusofflexibility.com.

Information on John Barnes's work can be found at www.myofascial release.com.

Information on myofascial release techniques such as those used by Larry and Belinda Wurn can be found at www.clearpassage.com.

You can learn more about Sprint 8 and its benefits at http://fitness .mercola.com.

Chapter 10

Llorraine Neithardt, an intuitive with a radio show called *Venus Unplugged*, designs shoes as an offering to Aphrodite. You can see some of her designs at www.shoefineart.com.

Chapter 11

Bob Fritchie, who wrote the marvelous book *Being at One with the Divine: Self-Healing with Divine Love* (Knoxville, TN: World Service Institute, 2013), teaches the power of Divine Love to people all around the world and has spent decades documenting the healing power of this energy. You can learn more and buy his book at his website: www.worldserviceinstitute.org. I encourage you to participate in at least one of his webinars—they can be life-changing.

Lynne McTaggart (www.lynnemctaggart.com), like Bob Fritchie, has a large network that coordinates mass events for raising the vibration of the planet. She has written several books about energy connections, including *The Bond: How to Fix Your Falling-Down World* (New York: Atria Books, 2011).

The fact that we are beings of light—and that we, in fact, emit light—has been demonstrated by researcher Gary Schwartz, Ph.D., at his lab at the University of Arizona. (You can learn more at www.drgaryschwartz.com.)

Sera Beak's *Red Hot and Holy: A Heretic's Love Story* (Boulder, CO: Sounds True, 2013) and Meggan Watterson's *Reveal: A Sacred Manual for Getting Spiritually Naked* (Carlsbad, CA: Hay House, 2013) are rich explorations of the relationship between spirituality, pleasure, and the divine feminine.

You can find affirmations by Catherine Ponder at www.absolute1.net /catherine-ponder.html.

ENDNOTES

Introduction

1. "Centenarians Are the Fastest-Growing Age Segment: Number of 100-Year-Olds to Hit 6 Million by 2050," *New York Daily News,* July 21, 2009.

2. Sue Campbell, "What's Your Plan If You Live to 100?" *Next Avenue,* May 27, 2014. http://www.ncxtavenue.org/blog/whats-your-plan-if-you-live-100.

3. Mario E. Martinez, Hay House radio interview with Christiane Northrup, "Your Culture Is Stronger Than Your Genes," *Flourish!,* November 6, 2013.

Chapter 1

1. I heard this Abraham quote, "happy, healthy, dead," in an Esther Hicks lecture many years ago, and it has stayed with me!

2. HeLa cells used in scientific experiments are derived from one woman, Henrietta Lacks, who unknowingly made an incredible contribution to science in 1951 when a scientist took cells from a cancerous tumor that ultimately killed her. It was found that these cells could serve as stem cells from which new cells could be grown again and again without the original cells dying. Something was different about the cells in Ms. Lacks's tumor that made them, in a sense, immortal—yet the "immortal" cells also killed her with cancer. Other research has connected telomerase, the enzyme that seems to repair telomeres, with cancer as well. There's much research to be done in extending telomeres without causing cancer. One study shows that it's possible to increase telomere length in mice, which leads to a reversal in the aging process. M. Jaskelioff et al, "Telomerase Reactivation Reverses Tissue Degeneration in Aged Telomerase-Deficient Mice."

Nature 469 (January 6, 2011): 102–6. http://www.nature.com /nature/journal/v469/n7328/full/nature09603.html.

3. E. Epel et al, "Can Meditation Slow Rate of Cellular Aging? Cognitive Stress, Mindfulness, and Telomeres," *Annals of the New York Academy of Sciences* 1172 (August 2009): 34–53.

4. R. Davidson et al, "Alterations in Brain and Immune Function Produced by Mindfulness Meditation," *Psychosomatic Medicine* 65, no. 4 (July/August 2003): 564–70. http://www.ncbi.nlm.nih.gov/pubmed/12883106.

5. Mindfulness Matters: http://www.mindfulness-matters.org/.

6. Mark Hamer et al, "Taking Up Physical Activity in Later Life and Healthy Ageing: The English Longitudinal Study of Ageing," *British Journal of Sports Medicine* 48 (2014): 239–43. DOI:10.1136/bjsports-2013-092993. http://bjsm.bmj.com/content/48/3/239.abstract.

7. Michael F. Roizen, *RealAge: Are You as Young as You Can Be?* (New York: HarperCollins, 2001).

8. Becca R. Levy et al, "Longevity Increased by Positive Self-perceptions of Aging," *Journal of Personality and Social Psychology* 83, no. 2 (August 2002): 261–70.

9. J. M. Hausdorff et al, "The Power of Ageism on Physical Function of Older Persons: Reversibility of Age-Related Gait Changes," *Journal of the American Geriatric Society* 47, no. 11 (November 1999): 1346–49.

10. Kathryn P. Riley et al, "Early Life Linguistic Ability, Late Life Cognitive Function, and Neuropathology: Findings from the Nun Study," *Neurobiology of Aging* 26, no. 3 (2005): 341–47.

11. Martinez, "Your Culture Is Stronger Than Your Genes."

12. Susan Kuchinskas, "The Alpha Goddess: Open to Anything, Including Technology," *Adweek,* February 27, 2012. http://www.adweek.com /news/advertising-branding/alpha-goddess-138528.

13. Robert Love, "The Smart Money Is on the 50+ Crowd," *AARP: The Magazine,* June/July 2014. http://www.aarp.org/entertainment/style -trends/info-2014/baby-boomer-economic-power.html.

14. Tosha Silver's Twitter post about absolute and unconditional self-acceptance can be found at http://twitter.com/toshasil.

15. *When God Was a Woman* by Merlin Stone (Orlando, FL: Harvest Books, 1978) and *The Chalice and the Blade: Our History, Our Future* by Riane Eisler (New York: HarperCollins, 1987) are two of the first books that explored the history of the goddess religion.

Chapter 2

1. Audre Lorde, *A Burst of Light: Essays* (Firebrand Books, 1988), 131.

2. Herbert Benson and William Proctor, *The Breakout Principle: How to Activate the Natural Trigger That Maximizes Creativity, Athletic Performance, Productivity and Personal Well-Being* (New York: Scribner, 2003), 56.

3. Rick Strassman, *DMT: The Spirit Molecule: A Doctor's Revolutionary Research into the Biology of Near-Death and Mystical Experiences* (Rochester Press, VT: Park Street Press, 2000), 73. DMT, derived from the ayahuasca plant, is used by South American shamans to induce what Strassman calls a "psychedelic" state.

Chapter 3

1. Christiane Northrup, *Women's Bodies, Women's Wisdom: Creating Physical and Emotional Health and Healing*, rev. ed. (New York: Bantam, 2010), 99.

2. Marshall Kirkpatrick, "Google CEO Schmidt: 'People Aren't Ready for the Technology Revolution,'" *ReadWrite*, August 4, 2010. http://readwrite .com/2010/08/04/google_ceo_schmidt_people_arent_ready_for_the _tech#awesm=~or9ZvGJTDdkf01.

3. H. Gilbert Welch, M.D., M.P.H., *Should I Be Tested for Cancer? Maybe Not and Here's Why* (Berkeley, CA: University of California Press, 2006).

4. Per-Henrik Zahl et al., "The Natural History of Invasive Breast Cancers Detected by Screening Mammography," *Archives of Internal Medicine* 168, no. 21 (2008): 2311–16.

5. Archie Bleyer and H. Gilbert Welch, "Effect of Three Decades of Screening Mammography on Breast-Cancer Incidence," *New England Journal of Medicine* 367 (November 22, 2012): 1998–2005. DOI: 10.1056 /NEJMoa1206809.

6. Maryland Coalition on Mental Health and Aging, "Effects of Medications." http://www.mhamd.org/aging/agingconsiderations /effectsofmeds.htm.

7. Kazi Stastna, "'Junk DNA' Has a Purpose, New Map of Human Genome Reveals," CBC News, September 5, 2012. http://www.cbc.ca/news /technology/junk-dna-has-a-purpose-new-map-of-human-genome -reveals-1.1238937.

8. James Gallagher, "'Memories' Pass Between Generations," BBC News, December 1, 2013. http://www.bbc.co.uk/news/health-25156510.

9. Earle Holland, "Stress Hormones May Play New Role in Speeding Up Cancer Growth," *Ohio State University Research News* (November 2006). http://researchnews.osu.edu/archive/epinorepi.htm.

10. L. S. Massad et al, "2012 Updated Consensus Guidelines for the Management of Abnormal Cervical Cancer Screening Tests and Cancer Precursors," *Journal of Lower Genital Tract Disease* 17, no. 3 (July 2013): S1–S27. http://www.omniaeducation.com/images/hpv_resource2.pdf.

Chapter 4

1. Stephani Sutherland, "Bright Screens Could Delay Bedtime," *Scientific American*, December 19, 2012. http://www.scientificamerican.com /article/bright-screens-could-delay-bedtime/.

2. J. Manonai et al, "Effect of Pueraria Mirifica on Vaginal Health," *Menopause* 14, no. 5 (September/October 2007): 919–24. http://www.ncbi .nlm.nih.gov/m/pubmed/17415017/.

3. Sukanya Jaroenporn et al, "Improvements of Vaginal Atrophy Without Systemic Side Effects after Topical Application of *Pueraria mirifica,* a Phytoestrogen-rich Herb, in Postmenopausal Cynomolgus Macaques," *Journal of Reproduction and Development* 60, no. 3 (April 21, 2014): 238–45.

4. The Bogalusa heart study, conducted through Tulane University, has generated research articles in several journals and can be found at http://tulane .edu/som/cardiohealth/.

5. K. Miyagawa et al, "Medroxyprogesterone Interferes with Ovarian Steroid Protection Against Coronary Vasospasm," *Nature Medicine* 3, no. 3 (1997): 324–27.

6. For more specifics on the research into statin drugs, see pages 586 to 590 in *The Wisdom of Menopause;* and Jonny Bowden and Stephen Sinatra, *The Great Cholesterol Myth: Why Lowering Your Cholesterol Won't Prevent Heart Disease—and the Statin-free Plan That Will* (Beverly, MA: Fair Winds Press, 2012).

7. The American Society for Aesthetic Plastic Surgery (ASAPS) statistics are from its website, http://www.surgery.org/media/statistics.

8. Lynne McTaggart, "What Doctors Didn't Tell Angelina Jolie," on her blog, May 21, 2013, citing D. de Jong et al, "Anaplastic Large-Cell Lymphoma in Women with Breast Implants," *Journal of the American Medical Association* 300, no. 17 (November 2008): 2030–5. DOI: 10.1001 /jama.2008.585. McTaggart writes, "Breast implants have been linked to a rare type of breast cancer known as 'anaplastic large-cell lymphoma' (ALCL), a form of non-Hodgkin lymphoma, increasing risk of contracting the disease by 18 times." http://www.lynnemctaggart.com/blog /226-what-doctors-didnt-tell-angelina-jolie.

9. Stephen T. Chang, *The Tao of Sexology: The Book of Infinite Wisdom* (San Francisco, CA: Tao Publishing, 1986).

10. Inger Thune et al, "Physical Activity and the Risk of Breast Cancer," *New England Journal of Medicine* 336 (May 1, 1997): 1269–75.

11. C. F. Garland et al, "Vitamin D for Cancer Prevention: Global Perspective," *Annals of Epidemiology* 19, no. 7 (July 2009): 468–83. Also, C. F. Garland et al, "Vitamin D and Prevention of Breast Cancer: Pooled Analysis," *Journal of Steroid Biochemistry and Molecular Biology* 103 (March 2007): 708–11.

12. The complete U.S. Preventive Services Task Force mammogram guidelines can be found at http://www.uspreventiveservicestaskforce.org/uspstf09 /breastcancer/brcanrs.htm.

13. Bleyer and Welch, "Effect of Three Decades of Screening," 1998–2005.

14. Sarah C. Darby et al, "Risk of Ischemic Heart Disease in Women After Radiotherapy for Breast Cancer," *New England Journal of Medicine* 368 (March 14, 2013): 987–98 http://www.nejm.org/doi/full/10.1056 /NEJMoa1209825.

15. As researcher Laura Esserman states, "The word *cancer* often invokes the specter of an inexorably lethal process; however, cancers are heterogeneous and can follow multiple paths, not all of which progress to metastases and death, and include indolent disease that causes no harm during the patient's lifetime." Laura J. Esserman et al, "Overdiagnosis and Overtreatment in Cancer: An Opportunity for Improvement," *Journal of the American Medical Association* 310, no. 8 (August 28, 2013), 797–98. http://jama.jamanetwork.com/article.aspx?articleid=1722196.

16. Nikola Biller-Adorno, M.D., Ph.D., and Peter Jüni, M.D., "Abolishing Mammography Screening Programs? A View from the Swiss Medical Board," *New England Journal of Medicine* 370 (May 22, 2014): 1965–67.

17. Ibid.

18. Genetics Home Reference, National Institutes of Health, "Breast Cancer," August 2007. http://ghr.nlm.nih.gov/condition/breast-cancer.

19. American College of Obstetricians and Gynecologists, Committee on Genetics (October 1996), *Breast-Ovarian Cancer Screening* (Committee Opinion no. 176), Washington, DC. Cited in Christiane Northrup, *The Wisdom of Menopause,* rev. ed. (New York: Bantam Books, 2012), 544.

20. National Human Genome Research Institute, National Institutes of Health, May 1997, reviewed September 2006, "Three Breast Cancer Gene Alterations in Jewish Community Carry Increased Cancer Risk, but Lower Than in Previous Studies." http://www.genome.gov/10000939.

21. McTaggart, "What Doctors Didn't Tell Angelina Jolie." As McTaggart points out, "New evidence shows that even a faulty BRCA1 gene, as Jolie has, may require epigenetic modification, or 'silencing,' before cancer progresses (V. Birgisdottir et al, 'Epigenetic silencing and deletion of the BRCA1 gene in sporadic breast cancer,' *Breast Cancer Res,* 2006; 8: R38). And

diets during critical times in a daughter's life (as a fetus and then during puberty) have a big influence on the expression of genes like BRCA1 (S. de Assis and L. Hilakivi-Clarke, 'Timing of dietary estrogenic exposures and breast cancer risk,' *Ann NY Acad Sci,* 2006; 1089: 14–35)." Also, see Karolyn Gazella, "Angelina Jolie Missed an Important Opportunity," *The Healing Factor, Psychology Today,* May 16, 2013. Retrieved February 19, 2014. http://www.psychologytoday.com/blog/the-healing-factor /201305/angelina-jolie-missed-important-opportunity. "Specific to BRCA1 and BRCA2, a 2009 study featured in the journal *Breast Cancer Research and Treatment* demonstrated that women with the inherited mutation who ate more fruits and vegetables significantly reduced their risk of developing cancer compared to the women with the mutation who ate fewer fruits and vegetables. In a 2006 study also featured in *Breast Cancer Research and Treatment,* women who carried the mutation and had normal weight and prevented weight gain as they aged also had much lower risk of developing cancer than women with the mutation who were overweight."

22. Shoshana M. Rosenberg, Sc.D., M.P.H., et al., "Perceptions, Knowledge, and Satisfaction with Contralateral Prophylactic Mastectomy among Young Women with Breast Cancer: A Cross-Sectional Survey," *Annals of Internal Medicine* 159, no. 6 (September 17, 2013): 373–81. DOI: 10.7326/0003-4819-159-6-201309170-00003.

23. Kathryn Kassai, P.T., C.E.S., and Kim Perelli, *The Bathroom Key: Put an End to Incontinence* (New York: Demos Health, 2012).

Chapter 5

1. Brené Brown, *Daring Greatly: How the Courage to Be Vulnerable Transforms the Way We Live, Love, Parent, and Lead* (New York: Gotham Books, 2012), 68.

2. Joe Dispenza, Hay House radio interview with Christiane Northrup, "You Are the Placebo," *Flourish!,* August 13, 2014.

3. Gay Hendricks, *The Big Leap: Conquer Your Hidden Fear and Take Life to the Next Level* (New York: HarperOne, 2010).

4. Mario Martinez, *The MindBody Code* (Boulder, CO: Sounds True, 2014).

5. Stephen Levine, *Healing into Life and Death* (New York: Anchor Books, 1987).

6. Llorraine Neithardt, personal correspondence, June 13, 2013.

7. Tina Rosenberg, "For Veterans, a Surge of New Treatments for Trauma," *The Opinionator, New York Times,* September 26, 2012. http:// opinionator.blogs.nytimes.com/2012/09/26/for-veterans-a-surge-of -new-treatments-for-trauma/.

8. Erin Largo-Wight et al, "Healthy Workplaces: The Effects of Nature Contact

at Work on Employee Stress and Health," Public Health Report 126, supplement 1 (2011): 124–30. http://www.ncbi.nlm.nih.gov/pmc/articles /PMC3072911/.

Chapter 6

1. J. Shifren et al, "Sexual Problems and Distress in United States Women: Prevalence and Correlates," *Obstetrics and Gynecology* 112, no. 5 (November 2008): 970–78.

2. Regena Thomashauer, Hay House radio interview with Christiane Northrup, "Pleasure and Health: The Vital Connection," *Flourish!*, November 24, 2010.

3. Gina Ogden, *The Return of Desire: A Guide to Rediscovering Your Sexual Passion* (Boston: Trumpeter, 2008).

4. ———. *The Heart and Soul of Sex: Making the ISIS Connection* (Boston: Trumpeter, 2006).

5. Andrew Newberg, Eugene D'Aquili, Vince Rause, *Why God Won't Go Away: Brain Science and the Biology of Belief* (New York: Ballantine Books, 2001), 9.

6. Judy Harrow, *Gnosis.* http://goddessofsacredsex.com/the-goddesses/.

7. Laura Bushnell, *Life Magic: The Renowned Psychic Healer Shares the 7 Keys to Finding Your Power and Living Your Purpose* (New York: Miramax Books, 2005).

8. John Harvey Kellogg, *Plain Facts for Old and Young* (Burlington, IA: Segner and Condit, 1881, available from the Gutenberg Project). http://www .gutenberg.org/files/19924/19924-h/19924-h.htm#chapi100.

9. Brené Brown, "Listening to Shame" TED video. http://www.ted.com /talks/brene_brown_listening_to_shame.

10. Dave Itzkoff, "Melissa McCarthy Goes Over the Top," *New York Times,* June 13, 2013. http://www.nytimes.com/2013/06/16/movies /melissa-mccarthy-goes-over-the-top.html?pagewanted=all&_r=0.

11. Jeanne-Philippe Gouin et al, "Marital Behavior, Oxytocin, Vasopressin, and Wound Healing," *Psychoneuroendocrinology* 35, no. 7 (August 2010): 1082–90. DOI: 10.1016/j.psyneuen.2010.01.009.

Chapter 7

1. Anita Moorjani, *Dying to Be Me: My Journey from Cancer, to Near Death, to True Healing* (Carlsbad, CA: Hay House, 2012), 172, 140.

2. Diane Fassel, *Working Ourselves to Death: The High Cost of Workaholism and the Rewards of Recovery* (San Francisco: HarperSanFrancisco, 1990), 58.

3. Gail Sheehy, *Passages in Caregiving: Turning Chaos into Confidence* (New York: William Morrow, 2010), 12.

4. Ira Byock, Hay House Radio interview with Christiane Northrup, "A Good Death," *Flourish!*, March 14, 2012.

5. J. S. House et al., "Social Relationships and Health," *Science* 241, no. 4865 (July 29, 1988): 540–545.

Chapter 8

1. Mark Hyman, *The Blood Sugar Solution 10-Day Detox Diet* (Boston: Little, Brown, 2014), 80.

2. Joseph Mercola, "To Achieve Optimal Health, Eat 50–70% of This Frequently Demonized Food," Mercola.com, December 28, 2011. Retrieved November 4, 2013. http://articles.mercola.com/sites/articles/archive /2011/12/28/what-you-dont-know-about-fats.aspx.

3. Patty W. Siri-Tarino et al, "Meta-analysis of Prospective Cohort Studies Evaluating the Association of Saturated Fat with Cardiovascular Disease," *American Journal of Clinical Nutrition* 91, no. 3 (March 2010): 535–46. http://ajcn.nutrition.org/content/91/3/535.abstract.

4. Fernando Gómez-Pinilla, "Brain Foods: The Effects of Nutrients on Brain Function," *Nature Reviews Neuroscience* 9, no. 7 (July 2008): 568–78. http://www.ncbi.nlm.nih.gov/pmc/articles/PMC2805706/.

5. Joseph Mercola's site has some excellent articles on the nuanced differences between types of fats, sugars, and carbohydrates. See, for example, "Heart Specialist Calls for Major Repositioning on Saturated Fat, as It's NOT the Cause of Heart Disease," November 04, 2013. http://articles .mercola.com/sites/articles/archive/2013/11/04/saturated-fat-intake.aspx.

6. Sanjay Basu et al, "The Relationship of Sugar to Population-Level Diabetes Prevalence: An Econometric Analysis of Repeated Cross-Sectional Analysis," *PLOS ONE* 8, no. 2 (February 27, 2013): e57873. http://www .plosone.org/article/info:doi/10.1371/journal.pone.0057873.

7. Nicolas Cherbuin et al, "Higher Normal Fasting Glucose Is Associated with Hippocampal Atrophy: The PATH Study," *Neurology* 79, no. 10 (September 4, 2012): 1019–26. http://www.neurology.org/content/79/10 /1019.short.

8. A great source of information on aspartame is my friend Joseph Mercola's website: http://aspartame.mercola.com.

9. R. Molteni et al, "A High-Fat, Refined Sugar Diet Reduces Hippocampal Brain-Derived Neurotrophic Factor, Neuronal Plasticity, and Learning,"

Neuroscience 112, no. 4 (2002): 803–14. http://www.ncbi.nlm.nih.gov /pubmed/12088740.

10. Theodore T. Zava and David T. Zava, "Assessment of Japanese Iodine Intake Based on Seaweed Consumption in Japan: A Literature-Based Analysis," *Thyroid Research* 4 (2011): 14. http://www.thyroidresearch journal.com/content/4/1/14.

11. Lyle MacWilliam, M.Sc., F.P., *NutriSearch Comparative Guide to Nutritional Supplements,* 5th edition (Summerland, BC: Northern Dimensions Publishing, 2014).

12. Lawrence A. David et al., "Diet Rapidly and Reproducibly Alters the Human Gut Microbiome," *Nature* 505 (December 11, 2013): 559–63. DOI:10.1038/nature12820. http://www.nature.com/nature/journal/vaop /ncurrent/full/nature12820.html.

Chapter 9

1. Kellie Bisset, press release, "Stand Up: Your Life Could Depend on It," EurekAlert, March 26, 2012. http://www.eurekalert.org/pub_releases /2012-03/si-suy032612.php.

2. Kelly McGonigal, Ph.D., *The Willpower Instinct: How Self-Control Works, Why It Matters, and What You Can Do to Get More of It* (New York: Avery, 2011).

3. Joe Verghese et al, "Leisure Activities and the Risk of Dementia in the Elderly," *New England Journal of Medicine* 348 (June 19, 2003): 2508–16. http://www.nejm.org/doi/full/10.1056/NEJMoa022252.DOI: 10.1056 /NEJMoa022252.

4. Richard Powers, "Use It or Lose It: Dancing Makes You Smarter," Social Dance at Stanford website, July 30, 2010. Retrieved February 27, 2014. http://socialdance.stanford.edu/syllabi/smarter.htm.

5. Tiiu Poldma et al, "The Use of Argentine Tango Dancing in an Interior Environment to Enhance Mobility and Social Activity in Seniors: A Multidisciplinary Research Study," IDEC 2012 Annual Conference, posted January 11, 2012. Retrieved August 19, 2014. http://conf.idec.org/2012 /the-use-of-argentine-tango-dancing-in-an-inte/.

6. Kathleen Facklemann, "Doing the Tango Keeps the Brain in Step, Too," *USA Today,* November 15, 2005. http://usatoday30.usatoday.com/tech /science/2005-11-15-tango_x.htm.

7. Leon Speroff, "Is Long-Term Alendronate Treatment a Problem?" *Ob/Gyn Clinical Alert* 22, no. 2 (June 1, 2005): 9–10.

8. S. L. Ruggiero et al, "Osteonecrosis of the Jaws Associated with the Use of Bisphosphonates: A Review of 63 Cases," *Journal of Oral and Maxillofacial Surgery* 62, no. 5 (May 2004): 527–34.

9. Rick Nauert, Ph.D., "The Role of Exercise in Bolstering Memory," Psych-Central, July 30, 2013. http://psychcentral.com/news/2013/07/31/the-role-of-exercise-in-bolstering-memory/57812.html.

10. K. Erickson et al, "Exercise Training Increases Size of Hippocampus and Improves Memory." *Proceedings of the National Academy of Sciences* 108, no. 7 (February 15, 2011): 3017–22.

11. L. S. Nagamatsu et al, "Physical Activity Improves Verbal and Spatial Memory in Older Adults with Probable Mild Cognitive Impairment: A 6-Month Randomized Controlled Trial," *Journal of Aging Research* (2013): 861893, DOI: 1155/2013/861893. Epub 2013 Feb 24. Retrieved February 27, 2014. http://www.ncbi.nlm.nih.gov/pubmed/23509628.

Chapter 11

1. Robin Kelly, M.D., *The Human Antenna: Reading the Language of the Universe in the Songs of Our Cells* (Fulton, CA: Elite Books/Energy Psychology Press, 2007), 65–66. http://www.humanantenna.com.

2. Marion Dejosez et al, "Safeguards for Cell Cooperation in Mouse Embryogenesis Shown by Genome-Wide Cheater Screen," *Science* 341, no. 6153 (September 27, 2013): 1511–14. DOI: 10.1126/science.1241628.

3. Lynne McTaggart, "Cancer Is a Selfish Gene," September 17, 2013, retrieved February 25, 2014. http://www.lynnemctaggart.com/blog /237-cancer-is-a-selfish-gene.

4. Rob Kirby, "Wild Elephants Gather Inexplicably, Mourn Death of 'Elephant Whisperer,'" The Delight Makers, retrieved February 25, 2014. http://delightmakers.com/news/wild-elephants-gather-inexplicably -mourn-death-of-elephant-whisperer/.

5. David M. Scobey wrote, "New York's city builders . . . believed . . . public parks would educate the masses from riotousness to refinement." David M. Scobey, *Empire City: The Making and Meaning of the New York City Landscape* (Philadelphia: Temple University Press, 2003), 10–11.

6. The University of Rochester, "Spending Time in Nature Makes People Feel More Alive, Study Shows," June 3, 2010. http://www.rochester.edu/news /show.php?id=3639.

7. Anahad O'Connor, "The Claim: Exposure to Plants and Parks Can Boost Immunity," *New York Times,* July 5, 2010. http://www.nytimes.com /2010/07/06/health/06real.html?_r=1&.

8. American Academy of Ophthalmology, "Outdoor Recess Time Can Reduce the Risk of Nearsightedness in Children," *Science Daily,* May 1, 2013. http://www.sciencedaily.com/releases/2013/05/130501101258.htm.

9. P. Guillon et al, "Births, Fertility, Rhythms, and Lunar Cycle: A Statistical Study of 5,927,978 Births," *Journal of Gynecology, Obstetrics, and*

Biological Reproduction (Paris) 15, no. 3 (1986): 265–71. http://www
.ncbi.nlm.nih.gov/pubmed/3734339.

10. Lynne McTaggart, "When You Wish upon a Star: Results of the Heal
America Intention Experiments," July 12, 2013. Retrieved February 26,
2014. http://www.lynnemctaggart.com/blog/233-when-you-wish-upon-a
-star-results-of-the-heal-america-intention-experiments.

INDEX

ACKNOWLEDGMENTS

The first thing I'd like to acknowledge here is my own trajectory around writing a book. The first edition of *Women's Bodies, Women's Wisdom* was a kind of forced march—a "do or die" mission to change the language and practice of women's health. I felt as though I were hiking up a mountain overgrown with brush and strewn with treacherous rocks. And there were no trails. But I was compelled. And I succeeded. Karmic debt paid.

And though that first book was a most painful process, I have always believed that creation doesn't need to be that way. After all, I know that some women give birth to their babies with orgasmic pleasure. Why not create a book the same way? And I finally did just that! The writing and editing of *Goddesses Never Age* has been a most pleasurable process. Part of that has been simple evolution. We now have the tools and the science that have documented the profound connection between the mind, the emotions, and the body, so my work isn't being questioned at every turn, requiring me to "prove" what I know repeatedly. And the other part is, of course, my own personal evolution. I am now able to recognize and receive the kind of support and assistance I have always dreamed of—much of which has been there all along! I just needed to let it in. And so with that, I joyfully acknowledge the following individuals.

Nancy Peske, editorial assistant and researcher extraordinaire, whose Midwestern practicality and work ethic have been right up my alley. You have been a Godsend and were instrumental in making this book so much fun to create.

Anne Barthel, my editor at Hay House—you "got it" from the beginning, and all of your suggestions have made a much better book. You made the editorial process pure pleasure.

Patty Gift—for bringing such bracing editorial East Coast rigor to your work, as well as the joys of tango, Paris, and all things pleasurable.

Reid Tracy, Margaret Nielsen, Christy Salinas—and the whole staff at Hay House. I pinch myself that I get to work with such a simpatico and fun group.

Hope Matthews—Intuitive Movement healer extraordinaire. You have borne witness to and catalyzed my personal transformation for many years through your knowledge of both classical Pilates and the impact of emotions on the body. I am profoundly grateful.

Julie Hofheimer—my massage therapist and intuitive healer who has kept my muscles and my spirit supple and tuned for many years and has borne witness to and documented the rebirth of my body.

Bob Cooley and the elite trainers at The Genius of Flexibility Center in Boston. Bob—what a gift you and your work have been in my life. Your generosity, your genius, and your knowledge continue to amaze, delight, and transform me and my body.

Paulina Carr—my girl Friday, who does whatever it takes to keep my company and my life afloat and does it with good humor and willingness.

Janet Lambert—my trusty bookkeeper, who keeps all the finances on the straight and narrow, when she is not skydiving or waterskiing and demonstrating the physical prowess of an ageless goddess!

Judie Harvey—for your editing skills and sense of humor with the e-letter, website, and social media.

Fern Tsao and her daughter Maureen Manetti—I have been so blessed to have you both as the most skilled practitioners of TCM right in my backyard. You practice the medicine of the future—here and now.

Tosha Silver—you arrived in my life at precisely the right moment to remind me of Divine Order and how to use it. The healing of my life and heart have been profound.

Mario Martinez—your work has given me the scientific foundation upon which the message of this book is built. I can't thank you enough for having the courage to reframe health the way you have and for articulating an entirely new language of actual health and flourishing. You are a gift in my life.

Bob Fritchie—thank you, thank you, thank you for your dedication to Divine Love and for creating a practical method for bringing this to everyone in the world, and for personally being available to me and my family. Thank you also for being such a good friend.

Doris E. Cohen—for coming up with the phrase that became the title for this book. You have been a spiritual midwife and skilled guide through my deepest sorrows and the dark night of the soul. You have fanned the flames of my deepest desires and given me the courage to keep on going. I can't thank you enough.

Melanie Ericksen —my magical mermaid medicine woman. From the first session I ever had with you, I knew that I had found the real deal. You are a goddess of healing, joy, beauty, high magic, and skill. And I am thrilled to have you and your consort Thor in my life.

Deborah Kern—for your friendship, your mirroring, your Divine presence, your moon in Pisces, all of it.

Regena Thomashauer (aka Mama Gena)—thank you, dear sister, for the courage and cheekiness required to bring the discipline of pleasure and joy into the hearts, minds, and bodies of women throughout the world. May our dance of joy continue forever.

To all the skilled and loyal members of my "assisted living" program here at home. Stephen Meehan, whose skill with flowers and plants is otherworldly. You have created a personal paradise for me that never ceases to amaze me. Mike Meehan for the plowing and shoveling and tree work, cheerfully accomplished at 5 A.M. Mike Brewer for being a most reliable and cheerful handyman for many years. Carlo Dorio for being the most amazing plumber on planet Earth. To Vern and Mike Cassidy, my father-son electrical geniuses, for maintaining all the things that keep it "lit up" around here. Charlie Grover for the weekly trips to the recycling center—and also for making sure Diane gets fed and watered. And for that twinkle in your eye that we can always count on. And Barbara McGivaren for housekeeping skill and charm—and for loving Mr. Moon.

For my brothers and my incredible sisters-in-law—John and Annie, Bill and Lori. Your love and support mean the world to me. To my sister, Penny, and her husband, Phil (who calls us his sister-wives). What a pleasure it has been to share so many adventures with you during the writing of this book.

Mom—your physical prowess and adventuresome spirit have blazed this trail from the very beginning. Without you, I would never have developed the backbone to carry me through until now.

Annie and Katie, my beautiful daughters. Watching you both flourish in your adult lives has been such a gift, and so has spending so much time together. Thank you for hanging in there with me despite my eccentricities and occasional fierceness. Plus there is all the falling-down-laughter part. And to Mike Watts, my new son-in-law, a man who is "all in," handsome, *and* handy. Seriously, how did I get so lucky?

And finally, to Diane Grover—my CEO of Everything, my business partner, my close friend. My sister-in-arms. From the beginning, for decades, you have been there for me and this work—in ways too numerous to list. You are truly the pearl of great price, and I have no idea how I would have done any of this without you. I bow at your feet.

ABOUT
THE AUTHOR

Christiane Northrup, M.D., board-certified ob/gyn, former assistant clinical professor of ob/gyn at the University of Vermont College of Medicine, *New York Times* best-selling author, is a visionary pioneer in women's health. After decades on the front lines of her profession as a practicing physician in obstetrics and gynecology, she is now dedicating her life to helping women truly flourish by learning how to enhance all that can go right with their bodies. Dr. Northrup is a leading proponent of medicine that acknowledges the unity of mind, body, emotions, and spirit. Internationally known for her empowering approach to women's health and wellness, she teaches women how to thrive at every stage of life and encourages them to create health on all levels by tuning in to their inner wisdom.

As a business owner, physician, former surgeon, mother, writer, and speaker, Dr. Northrup acknowledges our individual and collective capacity for growth, freedom, joy, and balance. She is also thrilled with her company Amata, whose name is derived from Thai words meaning "ageless" and "eternal." This company is devoted to creating and distributing products to support ageless goddesses everywhere.

When she's not traveling, Dr. Northrup loves devoting her leisure time to dancing Argentine tango, going to the movies, getting together with friends and family, boating, and reading.

Dr. Northrup stays in touch with her worldwide community through her Internet radio show *Flourish!*, Facebook, Twitter, her monthly e-letter, and her website, www.drnorthrup.com.

Hay House Titles of Related Interest

YOU CAN HEAL YOUR LIFE, the movie,
starring Louise Hay & Friends
(available as a 1-DVD program and an expanded 2-DVD set)
Watch the trailer at: www.LouiseHayMovie.com

THE SHIFT, the movie,
starring Dr. Wayne W. Dyer
(available as a 1-DVD program and an expanded 2-DVD set)
Watch the trailer at: www.DyerMovie.com

❦ ❦ ❦

THE ART OF EXTREME SELF-CARE:
Transform Your Life One Month at a Time, by Cheryl Richardson

CALM: A Proven Four-Step Process Designed Specifically
for Women Who Worry, by Denise Marek

THE SECRET FEMALE HORMONE:
How Testosterone Replacement Can Change Your Life,
by Kathy C. Maupin, M.D.

THE TAPPING SOLUTION FOR WEIGHT LOSS & BODY
CONFIDENCE: A Woman's Guide to Stressing Less, Weighing Less,
and Loving More, by Jessica Ortner

All of the above are available at your local bookstore,
or may be ordered by contacting Hay House (see next page).

❦ ❦ ❦

We hope you enjoyed this Hay House book. If you'd like to receive our online catalog featuring additional information on Hay House books and products, or if you'd like to find out more about the Hay Foundation, please contact:

Hay House, Inc., P.O. Box 5100, Carlsbad, CA 92018-5100
(760) 431-7695 or (800) 654-5126
(760) 431-6948 (fax) or (800) 650-5115 (fax)
www.hayhouse.com® • www.hayfoundation.org

Published and distributed in Australia by:
Hay House Australia Pty. Ltd., 18/36 Ralph St., Alexandria NSW 2015
Phone: 612-9669-4299 • *Fax:* 612-9669-4144 • www.hayhouse.com.au

Published and distributed in the United Kingdom by:
Hay House UK, Ltd., Astley House, 33 Notting Hill Gate, London W11 3JQ
Phone: 44-20-3675-2450 • *Fax:* 44-20-3675-2451 • www.hayhouse.co.uk

Published and distributed in the Republic of South Africa by:
Hay House SA (Pty), Ltd., P.O. Box 990, Witkoppen 2068
Phone/Fax: 27-11-467-8904 • www.hayhouse.co.za

Published in India by: Hay House Publishers India, Muskaan Complex,
Plot No. 3, B-2, Vasant Kunj, New Delhi 110 070 • *Phone:* 91-11-4176-1620
Fax: 91-11-4176-1630 • www.hayhouse.co.in

Distributed in Canada by:
Raincoast Books, 2440 Viking Way, Richmond, B.C. V6V 1N2
Phone: 1-800-663-5714 • *Fax:* 1-800-565-3770 • www.raincoast.com

Take Your Soul on a Vacation

Visit www.HealYourLife.com® to regroup, recharge, and reconnect with your own magnificence. Featuring blogs, mind-body-spirit news, and life-changing wisdom from Louise Hay and friends.

Visit www.HealYourLife.com today!

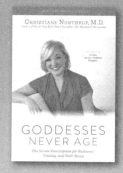
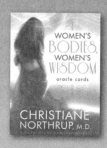
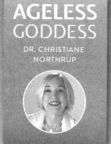

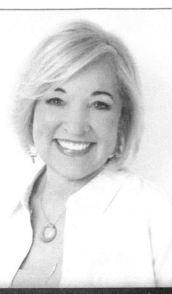
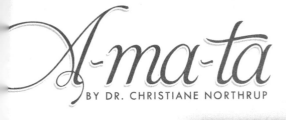
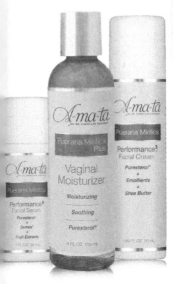
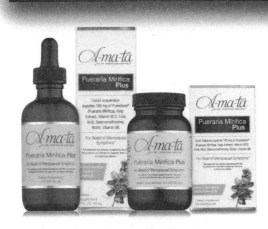